PROBLEM-BASED PSYCHIATRY
Second Editi

Problem-based Psychiatry

SECOND EDITION

BEN GREEN

Consultant Psychiatrist in Psychiatric Intensive Care
Cheadle Royal Hospital

Radcliffe Publishing
Oxford • New York

Radcliffe Publishing Ltd
18 Marcham Road
Abingdon
Oxon OX14 1AA
United Kingdom

www.radcliffe-oxford.com
Electronic catalogue and worldwide online ordering facility.

British Library Cataloguing in Publication Data

A catalogue record for this book is available from the British Library.

ISBN-13: 978 184619 042 1

The paper used for the text pages of this book is FSC certified. FSC (The Forest Stewardship Council) is an international network to promote responsible management of the world's forests.

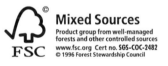

Mixed Sources
Product group from well-managed forests and other controlled sources
www.fsc.org Cert no. SGS-COC-2482
© 1996 Forest Stewardship Council

Typeset by Pindar NZ, Auckland, New Zealand
Printed and bound by TJI Digital, Padstow, Cornwall, UK

Contents

Preface to the second edition

This second edition is upgraded, expanded and updated. It includes details of the best modern web-based resources. Its problem-based approach to teaching is at the forefront of the delivery of modern medical school curricula. This edition has additional new case scenarios and includes current opinion about mental disorders and their treatment, using both drug therapy and psychotherapy according to the latest research. It includes the latest Mental Health Act (2007) and recent changes in mental health provision, and has been fine-tuned after more than 10 years' teaching experience on one of the UK's leading problem-based medical courses. It has been written for student doctors, mental health nurses, social workers, occupational therapists, mental health advocates and mental health therapists.

Ben Green
May 2009

About the author

Professor Ben Green is a Consultant Psychiatrist in Psychiatric Intensive Care at Cheadle Royal Hospital, Visiting Professor at the University of Chester and an Honorary Senior Lecturer at the University of Liverpool. He has designed and taught on undergraduate and postgraduate courses in Psychiatry, and has researched post-traumatic stress disorder and depression. He is an undergraduate examiner for the University of Liverpool and a postgraduate examiner for the Royal College of Psychiatrists. He is a medico-legal expert and has published 10 books. He has edited *Psychiatry On-Line* since 1994.

For Toby Green, my son

CHAPTER 1

The fundamentals of psychiatry

Psychiatry is a rich and diverse medical specialty concerned with abnormalities of the mind, namely abnormal emotions and thoughts, which may result in abnormal behaviour. Psychiatric illness may have social, psychological and biological causes. The symptoms and signs of mental disorder are known as psychopathology. Doctors analyse a patient's psychopathology using the psychiatric history and the mental state examination.

CONTENTS

INTRODUCTION

Psychiatrists use four methods of assessment: the **psychiatric history**, the **mental state examination,** a **physical examination** and relevant medical, social and psychological **investigations**. Information from these assessment methods is built into a differential diagnosis from which a management plan is formulated. The assessment is a holistic one in that it incorporates physical, social and psychological components. Similarly, treatments for mental illness may involve physical, social and psychological treatments.

- ➤ Physical treatments may include drugs such as antidepressants and antipsychotics, electroconvulsive therapy (ECT) and, very rarely, psychosurgery.
- ➤ Social treatments may involve rehousing in special rehabilitation settings, attendance at day hospital or day centres, some family interventions such as giving information and counselling to relatives and socio-legal advice.
- ➤ Psychological treatments may include one-to-one psychotherapy, group psychotherapy and family therapy. One-to-one psychotherapy is sometimes called interpersonal therapy. There are many different forms, such as psychoanalysis and cognitive behavioural therapy (CBT).

However, such treatment plans can only be put into place once a diagnosis is made. Before a doctor can make a diagnosis, he or she must first recognise the symptoms and signs of mental illness. Such symptoms and signs are referred to as psychopathology.

THE PSYCHIATRIC ASSESSMENT

The four cases here demonstrate that mental illness can occur at any age and that it can have a rich variety of presentations. Making a full assessment helps make sense of these different presentations and helps psychiatrists avoid dangerous diagnostic errors such as missing treatable organic disease (like hypothyroidism)

CASE HISTORY 1

A 24-year-old man is brought to accident and emergency by the police after picking a fight with a taxi driver. He paces up and down restlessly and talks non-stop about an alien space craft from Betelgeuse which is transmitting thoughts into his head. His speech is difficult to understand. From his appearance it looks as if he has not changed his clothes or washed for several weeks.

CASE HISTORY 2

A 72-year-old woman is seen by her family doctor. She complains of not being able to sleep because of 'the people upstairs'. They keep her awake all night with their conversations about her. Sometimes they sing rude limericks about her virginity. The family doctor protests that she lives on the top floor of a block of flats and so there is nobody living above her. However, the old lady is adamant: 'They must be living in the roof space then. I hear them all day long.'

CASE HISTORY 3

A 20-year-old man goes to see his primary care doctor with feelings of panic and anxiety that have come on since the death of his mother four weeks before. He is finding it difficult to concentrate on his work and is crying most days. Sometimes he walks round the house expecting to see her. Sometime he thinks he catches glimpses of her out of the corner of his eye.

CASE HISTORY 4

A 70-year-old man is reluctantly brought to the surgery by his wife. He denies that there is anything wrong, but when alone with the doctor his wife says that his memory is rapidly failing him and recently he has been doing 'odd things' like putting his shoes in the fridge and wearing his vest outside his shirt.

and preventing suicide (by assessing whether the patient has suicidal thoughts or plans).

Traditionally, the psychiatrist then draws the information from this assessment together into a *formulation* which includes a summary, a *differential diagnosis* and a *management plan.*

The differential diagnosis depends upon the psychiatrist being aware of how different psychiatric illnesses are classified. The most important or likely diagnoses are considered first and are usually followed by a brief summary of evidence for and against each diagnosis. The differential diagnosis should cover any possible organic causes of symptoms together with the contribution that the patient's personality makes.

In order to ensure that all possibilities are covered, the psychiatrist may use a diagnostic hierarchy. Later chapters will explain the differences between the categories in the hierarchy. The first group considered in the hierarchy approach are organic disorder candidates, then possible psychotic disorders, then affective disorders, then neurotic disorders and finally personality disorders.

A glossary is placed at the end of this chapter, but before we go any further, we need to explore some of the range of symptoms and signs that occur in everyday psychiatry in more depth.

PSYCHOPATHOLOGY
ABNORMAL MOOD

Affect is our emotional state at any particular time. *Mood* is our prevailing emotional state over a longer period of time. Generally, people's mood does vary according to events (that is to say it is *reactive*). Welcome events, like passing exams or getting promotion, make us feel happy. Untoward events, like sudden bereavement or failure, make us feel sad. On the whole, our mood is fairly constant, equable and *euthymic. Dysthymia* suggests an abnormality of mood. Abnormal mood is usually very different from normal in severity and persistence and may be low (*depression*) or high (*mania* or *hypomania,* a lesser form of mania).

Depression is associated with pervasive feelings of sadness, which are persistent. Bouts of crying or feeling like crying may be frequent. A depressed person's thoughts are usually gloomy. Depressed people think the worst of themselves, the world around them and the future. Usually enjoyable activities are no longer of interest or enjoyment (this is a symptom known as *anhedonia*). Concentration on tasks, such as reading, is difficult for the depressed individual, leading to poor function at work or home. Thoughts themselves may seem slowed down and the depressed person may even move less (*psychomotor retardation*), to such an extent that they may become stuporose. Important symptoms associated with depression are the so-called *biological features of depression* which usually include:

➤ insomnia (particularly intermittent waking through the night and waking earlier in the morning and being unable to return to sleep)
➤ anorexia (a loss of appetite and subsequently reduced food intake)
➤ weight loss
➤ diurnal mood variation – variation in mood through the day, e.g. feel low and slowed down in the morning and brightening towards the evening)
➤ reduced sex drive (reduced sexual appetite/libido)
➤ constipation.

Feelings that life is not worth living or thoughts about ending one's life are very common among depressed people and must be asked about in clinical encounters. Asking about these thoughts does not provoke suicidal thoughts or acts, but may allow the patient to express some difficult ideas, feel better understood and ultimately may help prevent suicide. Indeed, failure to ask would be negligent.

Mania (or its lesser form hypomania) is usually associated with an elated mood in marked contrast to the depressive's gloom. The manic patient's thoughts and feelings correspond with elation and are expansive and generally exceedingly positive. Instead of being psycho-motor retarded as in depression, the manic patient's thoughts seem to race along; their activity may be greater than normal, even frantic. The rapid pace of thoughts may lead to very rapid speech (*pressure of speech*) and a rapid flow of connected ideas (*flight of ideas*), usually of a grandiose kind. The manic patient often exhibits poor judgement and might have grandiose plans based on an overvaluation of their own potential or abilities. They may feel that they are inordinately wealthy. This lack of judgement may lead to *overspending* or other errors at work or business. Sexual disinhibition may lead to risky sexual encounters. The elated mood exhibited by such patients can be temporarily enjoyable for those around them, but the elation may also be associated with irritability. When confronted the disinhibited manic patient may become violent. Mood swings are possible and the previously elevated mood may easily switch into a depressed one. Suicidal feelings may occur.

Insomnia is nearly always present and patient may give a history of intense activity at times when they would normally be asleep, e.g. spring cleaning the entire house at 3 a.m.

ABNORMAL THOUGHTS

Through the course of a normal day a variety of thoughts and fantasies pass through the average person's mind. Sometimes people are *preoccupied* with certain thoughts and these may be relevant and understandable, e.g. often thinking about a driving test in the days beforehand. Occasionally, some thoughts may enter a person's mind unbidden and, though the person knows that these thoughts of theirs are irrational or nonsensical, the thoughts keep on recurring no matter how hard they try to resist them. Such thoughts are *obsessions*. An example might be a vicar who has a repeated *intrusive thought* that someone has urinated in the holy water in the church font. Sometimes a person may dwell on an unusual topic to a

morbid degree, e.g. a sweet shop owner who campaigns outside Parliament every day to say that chocolate should be recommended by doctors for its mood-enhancing properties. Such a thought could be described as an *overvalued idea*. It is sometimes difficult to fault the detail of an overvalued idea. After all, as in the example, chocolate is reputed to have some mood-enhancing properties, but is the idea worth campaigning about to the exclusion of other pursuits?

Where a person holds a belief that is manifestly untrue, is not culturally accepted, and holds it with an intensity that cannot be argued against, then this is a *delusion*. A delusion is an example of a severe or *psychotic* symptom. The presence of a delusion suggests a major psychiatric illness or *psychotic* disorder.

There are different types of delusion. In severe depressive illness patients may have delusions of poverty (for instance, that they have no money when they are in fact very comfortably off). A patient with severely depressed mood can also have *hypochondriacal delusions* (for instance that they have terminal cancer when there is no evidence for this at all). Other depressive delusions may include *infestation* (perhaps that they are infested with insects after an illicit sexual liaison), or sometimes so-called *nihilistic* delusions, such that they may say, 'I have no head' or 'I have no heart'. Delusions of guilt may accompany psychotic depression where someone might incorrectly believe that they have murdered someone or caused a war.

The content of delusions in some patients is *mood congruent*. In mania, delusions may follow the underlying mood and be expansive or *grandiose*, e.g. 'I am related to the King and he will send me a million pounds next week.'

Sometimes delusions, as in schizophrenia, may be bizarre, e.g. 'I was born from a Vulcan father and an Andromedan mother who gave birth to me in a McDonald's restaurant last week.'

In paranoid, or persecutory, schizophrenia there may be *delusions of reference* in which the patient is certain that a variety of cues in the environment are particularly and specifically related to them, e.g. a patient called Brian Murray Walker who is convinced that all BMW advertisements relate to him or another patient who believes that the television news reader is giving him coded messages when he blinks on screen.

ABNORMAL EXPERIENCES

Some experiences may be infrequent or unusual; others may be so very unusual as to immediately suggest a major or psychotic illness. *Depersonalisation* is an example of an experience that is not everyday, but may occasionally be experienced in 'normal' people. It is the sense that something has changed in the perception of the self, a feeling of unreality, which may be quite unpleasant. Depersonalisation may occur in those who are tired or unwell. *Derealisation* is a related phenomenon where one feels that the world around one (rather than the self) has become unreal. A variant of this is a change in the experience of time – the feeling of *déjà vu* where the person feels that they have experienced an exactly similar event previously. *Jamais vu* occurs when the person feels that they have never experienced a familiar event before, such as feeling they have never been in their own sitting room before. Such experiences may occur in anyone given the setting of tiredness or physical ill health but may also occur in any psychiatric illness. These experiences may also be suggestive of temporal lobe epilepsy.

We experience the world through our senses. An experience is often the same thing as a perception. In other words, our perception of reality usually accords with reality, i.e. we see what is actually there. We perceive real stimuli or real objects. When we misperceive real stimuli this may be an example of an *illusion*. In an illusion our brain misinterprets a real object. The misinterpretation may be because of an extreme affect, e.g. fear, or some problem in processing the information, e.g. tiredness or disorientation due, say, to an infectious illness.

An example of an illusion secondary to fear is the scene in Disney's *Snow White* where the princess runs through the dark forest seconds after nearly being killed by the huntsman. In her fright the princess misperceives the hollows in the trees around her as gaping eyes and mouths and the trees' branches as claw-like hands: this, then, is a visual illusion. Illusions may occur in other sensory systems too. For illusions, though, remember that there must be an object.

Hallucinations are sensory perceptions where there is no stimulus, i.e. no object. Hallucinations can occur in any sensory system. An example of an auditory hallucination might be hearing a voice talking to you when there is nobody or nothing around to produce that voice. If you look at Case History 2 again you may agree that the patient here might be hallucinating.

Hallucinations when they are experienced are very real in quality – just as real as any voice or any real-life image. They are also experienced in *external space*, that is to say they are not experienced as being inside the patient's head.

Hallucinations can occasionally occur in people when they are just tired or physically unwell. *Hypnagogic* hallucinations are hallucinations occurring on the edge of falling asleep, such as hearing one's name called when there is nobody there. Hallucinations on waking are called *hypnopompic* hallucinations. Occasionally, people who have been bereaved may transiently hear or see the lost one (*see* Case History 3). These experiences are known as *pseudohallucinations of mourning*. However, persistent hallucinations outside these rare circumstances are deemed psychotic symptoms and suggestive of psychotic illness.

Severe depressive illness may be associated with derogatory auditory hallucinations such as voices telling the patient they smell, are guilty or are doomed. These hallucinations are mood congruent. In mania, auditory hallucinations may correspond to the expansive mood and praise the patient. Visual hallucinations are less common than auditory ones and suggest the possibility of organic factors such as brain lesions or drug side-effects. Olfactory hallucinations are rare and may suggest a frontal lobe tumour. Somatic hallucinations occasionally occur with some drugs of abuse and in delirium tremens, but may occur in schizophrenia. Auditory hallucinations may be of a voice or voices talking to the patient (*second person auditory hallucinations*). Voices telling the patient to do something are known as *command hallucinations*. Voices talking about the patient, say in a discussion among themselves are known as *third person auditory hallucinations*. Third person hallucinations are suggestive of schizophrenia.

Still more unusual experiences involve the nature of thought itself. In *thought interference* the patient may feel that their thoughts are being tampered with. Normally, we experience owning our 'own' thoughts. In some psychotic illnesses people may feel as if their thoughts are not their own. They may feel that thoughts have been put into their head (*thought insertion* as in Case History 1), or taken out of their head (*thought withdrawal*) or feel that their thoughts are simultaneously known by others (*thought broadcasting*).

Thought interference is an example of a *passivity phenomenon* where the patient feels that the ownership of thoughts, feelings or actions is in doubt. Other passivity phenomena may include *made feelings*, e.g. 'This isn't my happiness, it's someone else's' or *made actions*, e.g. 'My leg can move, but it isn't me moving it'. Passivity phenomena are suggestive of schizophrenia.

ABNORMAL FORMS OF THOUGHT

You can describe thought in terms of its *content*, i.e. what it is about, or in terms of its *form*, i.e. how it is shaped. In mania there may be a flood of thoughts, rapidly spilling out of the mind and expressed in a pressure of speech. The form of these thoughts may be so-called *flight of ideas* in which there are a large number of ideas but where each idea is linked one to another by subject matter, by puns or sounds:

> 'I see you're wearing sandals, Third World shoes, sandy shoes, Road to Damascus shoes, conversion shoes, brilliant light shoes, on your knees in front of the Spirit, the Spirit inside the bottle, the genial genie genius of my soul.'

Although such speech may seem unintelligible at first, when analysed later each item can be linked to another. In the above example the speaker is reminded of St Paul's conversion on the road to Damascus by the sandals that someone else is wearing.

When the associations between the items of speech are lost (*loosening of associations*), this may represent *thought disorder*, which is seen in schizophrenia and other states. Here it is much less easy to spot an association between thoughts:

> 'On the albigisty of Kama Sutra I swear that the lazy dog leapt twice and danced on the afternoon sun, buthga, buthga, buthagee, where in fact the News at Ten is never at two. Have you a cigarette he asks, she asks. Never.'

The above example contains some examples of *neologisms* or new words, such as 'albigisty'. Such neologisms may occur in schizophrenic speech. Similarly, more familiar words may be used inappropriately.

ABNORMAL MOVEMENTS

Since psychological symptoms and treatments often involve the central nervous system, abnormal movements may be associated with a mental disorder. They may be idiopathic, symptomatic of the illness, a side-effect of drug treatment or signify a neurological disease such as neurosyphilis or Huntington's chorea.

Tics, occasional rhythmic involuntary movements such as eye blinking or occasionally vocalisations, may be common in childhood and of little prognostic significance. They tend to diminish of their own accord, but often worsen if attention is drawn to them or the patient is made to feel anxious. Rarely, tics may be progressive and disabling as in *Gilles de la Tourette's syndrome*, which is sometimes associated with obscene vocal tics (*coprolalia*).

Mannerisms are repeated voluntary movements that are idiosyncratic to the point of oddness, e.g. saluting twice before entering a room. *Posturing* may be prolonged and stereotyped or manneristic. Posturing is sometimes seen in schizophrenic illnesses. *Catatonia* in its most severe form involves the patient becoming mute, stuporose and prone to abnormal preservation of postures. In this catatonic state patients' limbs may be moved by observers and the resulting posture preserved for hours.

Akathisia, tardive dyskinesia and *Parkinsonism* are often seen in patients taking psychiatric medications (*see* Chapter 13, 'Physical treatments'). Akathisia is a drug-induced restlessness which may be described by the patient or observed as agitated fidgeting in a chair or restless pacing about the room. Tardive dyskinesia is a basal ganglia movement disorder manifesting as a combination of involuntary rhythmic movements of any of the following: lips, tongue, face, arms, hands, legs, feet or trunk. Sometimes it may be observed as choreoathetoid movements. Tardive dyskinesia is thought to be a late side-effect of some antipsychotic drugs. Parkinsonism may be an early side-effect of such drugs (extra-pyramidal side-effects) and may manifest with classical Parkinsonian features such as mask-like features, pill-rolling tremor and bradykinesia.

INTERVIEW SKILLS

The psychiatric history is lengthier and more detailed than in other fields of medicine. It covers aspects of personality, psychiatric illness and personal biography as well as a detailed medical history. To get this information the psychiatrist must interview the patient and an informant such as a relative or friend or other close acquaintance (with the patient's consent).

Since the history seeks to include sensitive information about past events and feelings past and present, the style is different from a conventional medical history. When you start taking full psychiatric histories, the interview may extend to 90 minutes.

With practice you will be able to gather the most relevant information more quickly, but it is important to remember that patients need time and to feel that their doctor is genuinely interested if they are to disclose personal details. Accordingly, psychiatric interviews sometimes appear less controlled by the doctor, who uses more open questions and empathic statements. Open questions are often used at the beginning of a section of questions on, say, family history, and will allow the patient to talk about important aspects as they see them, e.g. 'Can you begin by telling me about your family?' To regain control of the interview or gather specific information closed questions need to be used, e.g. 'What age was your father when he died?' or 'Which drugs helped you in the past?' or 'Do you ever feel like harming yourself?'

Statements, if used carefully, show that you understand what the patient is talking about from their point of view. Psychotic experiences are distressing ones, often associated with fear. Acknowledging this in some way would make a patient think that their doctor knew something about the symptoms and also understood how they really felt. Being understood is a positive experience for anyone and is reassuring.

THE PSYCHIATRIC HISTORY

Think how you might begin a long interview with someone. What would you do? How would you greet the person? How would you introduce yourself? Would you say how long the interview was going to take? Perhaps you might explain why you want to talk at all. Would you reassure the person about confidentiality?

> ### CASE HISTORY 5
> Alan was talking to the doctor. Tears of anxiety and fear came to his eyes when he was describing the voices that afflicted him. A strong male voice threatened him night and day, telling him he was about to be killed. 'That must be very frightening,' said his doctor. Alan looked up and nodded vigorously.

Verbal and non-verbal cues can also show interest. Nodding your head or making occasional noises such as 'uh-huh' can be encouraging if they are not overdone. Remaining silent for a short time or pausing before making further statements or questions may allow the patient space to disclose something else. Sometimes inexperienced doctors feel that silence is a bad or uncomfortable thing and that it must be filled with some statement. However, the statements may be ill-thought out, e.g. false reassurance such as 'I'm sure everything will be all right' can appear inappropriate or just plain wrong. In such cases the doctor is often trying to reassure him- or herself rather than the patient.

How will you cope with any expressions of emotion that the patient makes? What if they cry? What if they are irritable, angry or shout? What if they will not sit still long enough? A useful technique is to *reflect* the emotion back – acknowledge that you have noticed their distress or their anger, perhaps even ask about it. Sometimes people cry just before they say something really important, so do not shut them up: support them and let them speak. Anger may precede violence, especially if the patient is afraid. Whatever you do, try to stay calm. Saying that you have noticed how angry they are and asking them to talk about it may defuse the anger. Try not to appear threatening yourself. If an attack seems likely call for help or leave the room. Before you interview potentially dangerous patients always make sure that you have checked with staff who know the patient and that you interview the patient in a known safe place, with ready back-up in case of trouble. Having said this, violence is uncommon, and most patients you interview will probably be very cooperative.

People are sensitive to the moods of those they are speaking to. Just as the doctor can pick up on cues as to the patient's mood, the patient can pick up on whether their doctor is anxious, tired and ill-disposed towards them. It is important, therefore, to think about how you appear to the patient and to concentrate on the patient you are with in the here and now. Plenty of agencies will try to distort the doctor–patient relationship for their own ends. It is important not to be distracted from this central relationship by time considerations or matters of politics such as budgetary and rationing decisions. Every communication with the patient is special.

DEMOGRAPHIC DETAILS
You can begin the history proper by taking demographic details – age, marital status, employment status and, if in hospital, whether they are there voluntarily or are detained compulsorily. The patient's age, marital and employment status all have a bearing on diagnosis and management. Different mental illnesses have different ages of onset. Schizophrenia has its main onset in the third decade, dementia in the seventh and subsequent decades. The unemployed are more likely to suffer from depression and suicides are more common in the unmarried, widowed and divorced.

PRESENTING COMPLAINT
The presenting complaint is usually a brief list of the major problems as explained by the patient, e.g. 'hearing voices all the time' or 'drinking too much'.

HISTORY OF PRESENTING COMPLAINT
The history of presenting complaint (HPC) records further details. In terms of details it is sometimes useful to compare psychological pain (such as depression) with physical pain. Surgeons will enquire as to the severity of the

pain, its character, its onset, whether it is persistent or not and whether it is getting better or is aggravated by any particular thing. Similarly, in a case of depression, psychiatrists are interested in how it started: did it start suddenly or gradually? Did anything happen to bring on the depression such as a bereavement or a loss of job, or was the onset insidious and gradual? Is the mood getting worse or better? Can it be made better by visitors or entertainment or is it persistent? Psychiatrists would ask at this time about the so-called biological features of depression as described above.

The HPC would also focus on how severe the patient felt the depression was – is the patient crying every day or only once a week? It is sometimes appropriate to ask at this point whether the patient feels that life is not worth living and, if not, then has the depressed patient thought about harming themselves and do they have any definite plans?

Students are often unsure about how to ask about suicidal feelings. Usually, psychiatrists ask a hierarchy of questions to elicit these feelings; for an example, *see* Case History 6.

If a patient complained of hearing voices, an attempt would be made to discern exactly what these voices were like – were they hallucinations or illusions, for instance. If the doctor suspected schizophrenia, it would be appropriate in the HPC to ask for other features of schizophrenia, just as in a case of suspected appendicitis the surgeon would ask about fever and features of urinary tract infection to aid in making his or her differential diagnosis.

PAST PSYCHIATRIC HISTORY

A useful probe at the beginning of this section might be 'Have you ever felt like this before?' or 'Have you ever seen a psychiatrist before?' In the past psychiatric history the doctor is trying to build up a picture of how the illness has affected the patient in the past. The psychiatrist wishes to learn when the illness began and how many episodes there have been, who treated these illnesses and how

> ### CASE HISTORY 6
> Adam seemed very low to the interviewing doctor. He had biological features of depression such as early morning wakening, diurnal mood variation and poor appetite. He said that he was crying most days but was almost ashamed to tell the doctor. 'Makes me feel like a baby,' he said. He had felt this way for two months ever since he had lost his job and his girlfriend.
>
> 'It sounds as if things feel really bad,' said the doctor. Adam grunted, but avoided the doctor's gaze. 'Have you ever felt that life wasn't worth living at all?' Adam nodded slowly. 'That you'd rather it was all over?' Another nod. 'Have you thought about doing anything about that?'
>
> 'I keep thinking about it. Not all the time, I just see this picture suddenly, for a few seconds, of me running my car into a motorway bridge.
>
> 'Would you do anything like that? Or anything else to harm yourself?'
>
> 'No,' said Adam. 'I push the thought out of my head. If I did anything like that it would be too hurtful for my friends and my mum.'

successful treatment was – in particular which treatments were most useful. Bear in mind, though, that not all psychiatric illness presents to psychiatrists or even to doctors at all, so that the true onset of an illness may be a long time before the psychiatrist is called in. Try to get a picture of how many episodes of illness there have been. How long did each episode last? And between episodes, how well was the patient? Were they able to resume their work or care for their family as usual? Some illnesses impair function even between acute episodes. For any hospital admission you need to know which hospital it was (useful for getting past notes), which consultant, how long the admission was for and whether they were detained formally or informally (voluntarily). Record any use of antipsychotics, antidepressants, benzodiazepines and electroconvulsive therapy (ECT).

People often find it difficult to accurately recall past episodes of illness and a corroborative history may be necessary, as might be consulting past medical records.

PAST MEDICAL HISTORY

The past medical history is particularly relevant because various physical illnesses may mimic mental illness: hypothyroidism may present with depression, serum B12 deficiency may present with dementia and hyperthyroidism may present with persecutory ideas. Drugs that are used to treat physical illnesses may cause psychiatric presentations: digoxin may cause confusion and some drugs such as methotrexate and statins may cause depression. The psychiatrist is, therefore, interested in current and past physical problems including major operations, e.g. orchidectomy and hysterectomy may be complicated by depression and low esteem, and past head trauma may provoke epileptic phenomena.

FAMILY HISTORY

The family history should include details of parents, siblings and sometimes children. You should probe for occurrences of mental illness and suicide in any other relatives. It sometimes helps to record the family history in a family tree diagram with notes about each family member on the tree (*see* Figure 1.1). You should not be purely interested in the psychiatric history of other family members, although it is very relevant because certain psychiatric illnesses cluster in families. This is an opportunity to discuss the patient's feelings about parents, brothers and sisters (siblings). It is of great value to know, for instance, that a patient has never felt able to burden their mother with their anxieties because the mother had suffered with depression as well, or that the father was an argumentative man with an alcohol problem who used to beat his wife (the patient's mother). The family has been found to be important in the aetiology of personality difficulties, anorexia nervosa, bulimia nervosa and the prognosis of schizophrenia. Patients with schizophrenia are more likely

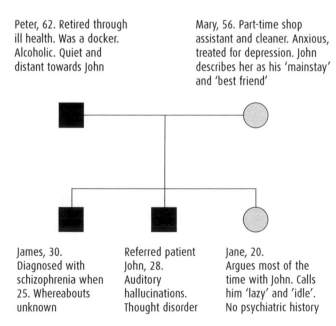

Peter, 62. Retired through ill health. Was a docker. Alcoholic. Quiet and distant towards John

Mary, 56. Part-time shop assistant and cleaner. Anxious, treated for depression. John describes her as his 'mainstay' and 'best friend'

James, 30. Diagnosed with schizophrenia when 25. Whereabouts unknown

Referred patient John, 28. Auditory hallucinations. Thought disorder

Jane, 20. Argues most of the time with John. Calls him 'lazy' and 'idle'. No psychiatric history

Figure 1.1 John's family tree with family history notes

to relapse in families where there is a high level of expressed emotion (hostility, over-involvement by other members and high levels of face-to-face contact).

PERSONAL HISTORY

In order to understand someone better it is often important to know what has happened to them in the past. The personal history seeks to build up a biography from birth to the present day. Early events in a person's life can fundamentally change the course their life takes. Early separation can colour just how secure people are in all their subsequent relationships. Early perinatal brain damage can affect IQ or lead to disabling epilepsy. There are hypotheses linking perinatal damage, febrile convulsions and adult psychotic illnesses. It is, therefore, important to know details as far back as possible. Gather information about the individual's birth – was it a normal full-term vaginal delivery or an induced or instrumental birth? Was there any event, such as time spent in a special care baby unit, which might have affected the maternal-infant relationship (perhaps making it a distant one or even over-close)? Is there any evidence for delay in reaching milestones such as the first steps or the first words? Can the person remember any details of what life was like when they were small? Were they hospitalised for any reason? Were their memories happy or not? Did they get on with their siblings?

Can they remember what it was like when they first went to school? Did they mix easily and find happiness with plenty of friends or were they lonely individuals, constantly being bullied? How did their parents get along? Were there numerous rows or was their home filled with mutual affection? If there were rows, did the child feel responsible for them in any way? Sometimes children feel that they cause marital breakdowns, especially if these occur at the 'age of magical thinking', i.e. when everything that happens in the outside world can be seen as a consequence of personal action. Examples of magical thinking include 'If I don't step on the lines in the pavement Mum and Dad will stay together'.

How did the person find the work at school: was it easy or was it very difficult for them? Were there any difficulties with reading delay or illiteracy? Were there any 'neurotic *traits*' such as prolonged bedwetting not due to organic causes, nail biting, hair pulling, head-banging or encopresis?

When the time came to move from primary to secondary education, how was that transition? Was it a smooth and easy one or was it fraught with anxiety? Was any time taken off school for exaggerated illness (*school* refusal) or was there any truancy (with others or alone)? Did the person make new friends after the move? What were their favourite subjects at school? Any hobbies?

What qualifications or examinations did the person gain by the time they left school? This may give an indication of their intelligence level. What did they do after they left school? Put together a work history of where people worked, what they did and for how long. If they left a job, why did they leave? Was it because they were made redundant, got bored or found a better post? Were they fired because they were difficult personalities or because they were becoming mentally ill? In the early phases of illness people often underperform at work, especially in depression and schizophrenia. Because of their low self-esteem in depression, the depressed individual may think that their sacking is entirely justified and make no protest when in fact they are ill.

There are aspects of a person's life which they tend to keep to themselves unless they are prompted to talk about them. This may be because they are embarrassing aspects of their life or are aspects which will damage the way they are seen by others.

A person may not discuss their impotence because they feel embarrassed by this. Another person may choose not to disclose his conviction for fraud because it will colour what you think of them. One of the barriers to disclosure is if the patient feels that their doctor is easily embarrassed or does not wish to discuss sensitive aspects of their lives. Unfortunately, such sensitive aspects of people's lives are often the ones that cause them the most anxiety. Such patients suffer in silence. The doctor who shows a willingness to discuss such matters openly helps his or her patients disclose. Such aspects are often crucial to diagnosis and management and must not be ignored. At first you may feel embarrassed in such discussions but your discomfort will ease with experience. Two such areas that you will need to cover in the personal history are the patient's psychosexual history and their forensic history (or criminal record).

PSYCHOSEXUAL HISTORY

What relevance is a patient's sexual history? It is important to realise that sexuality is inherent in all people regardless of their age, physical well-being or mental condition and is a major factor in their lives. Psychosexual functioning seems to have some bearing on prognosis. Good function often correlates with a better prognosis. Sexual orientation is a problem for some people and this may provide a focus for psychotherapeutic interventions. Psychosexual function is also of value in making judgements about dangerousness in some sexual offenders. Psychiatrists are, therefore, interested in what kind of relationships the person builds up. Schizoid personalities tend to avoid contact with other people, especially sexual relationships, so their psychosexual history may be characterised by a complete absence or avoidance of sexuality. Their sexuality may, however, be expressed in isolation, by fantasy or masturbation. Borderline personalities sometimes have many intense but fleeting sexual relationships. The relationships may be affected by discord or violence. In depressive illness and post-traumatic stress disorder there is often a reduced or absent sexual drive and this may cause difficulties for the patient with their partner. Similarly, mania may lead to a heightened sex drive and a lack of judgement which may put patients at risk because they have unprotected sex with people they might not normally consider as sexual partners.

What is included in the psychosexual history? We wish to know generally about the patient's current and past loving relationships. Are they a source of general pleasure and satisfaction or are they characterised by rows or unhappiness? Specifically we need to know when the person began building relationships – at what age? What was their source of sexual education? What were their feelings about sex? How long did their first relationships last? Were they happy experiences or were there problems? How did they manage those problems? When was the first experience of sexual intercourse? Are the relationships heterosexual or homosexual? You need to know whether sex is pleasurable, merely satisfactory or if there are any specific sexual dysfunctions like impotence, vaginismus and premature ejaculation.

A history of childhood sexual abuse may affect an individual's capacity to enjoy subsequent sexual relationships and may also have relevance to abnormal personality development, alcoholism, eating disorders and depression. Some psychiatrists include a screening question for sexual abuse in all their initial interviews. It could take this form: 'These days more people seem able to talk about difficult things which have happened in their childhood. Some people are able to talk about how they were beaten as a child or how sometimes older people took advantage of them sexually. Has anything like that ever happened to you?' Other psychiatrists prefer to allow their patients to disclose at their own pace, although they create an atmosphere of trust and safety where the person can disclose what they wish when they wish. For some people disclosing past abuse is relatively easy, for others the disclosure and the fear of subsequent rejection by the doctor may make disclosure very threatening. Disclosures of ongoing abuse or violence, or where there is disclosure that a minor is at risk, may necessitate action to protect the individual or a third party.

FORENSIC HISTORY

The forensic history concerns the overlap between criminal behaviour and psychiatry and might be started by a question such as 'Have you ever been in trouble with the police?' You will need to record all charges and convictions, together with whether these tie in with periods of mental illness.

SOCIAL HISTORY

The social history needs to record information such as where the patient is living and who they are living with. How do they get on with these people? A hostile environment may predispose to relapse in certain psychiatric illnesses. Are there any financial problems? Finally, unless previously recorded, how much does the patient smoke and drink? Smoking is a long-term risk factor for depression. In relapse or in times of stress or anxiety, a smoker's tobacco consumption increases. Similarly, alcohol consumption may rise. People with alcohol problems are notoriously evasive about exactly how much they drink. You will need to press the point. Sometimes alcoholics are reluctant themselves to face up to how much they consume. How much do they drink a day? What time of day do they start drinking? When they wake do they have a tremor that goes away with the first drink of the morning? Have they ever had the DTs (delirium tremens), blackouts or fits? Withdrawal fits occur in up to 10% of alcoholics. Have they any memory problems? Failure to remember the events of the night before is sometimes referred to as a *palimpsest*, especially when the individual then begins to make up what they think happened the night before. These false memories are often likely things that might have happened. For example, an individual may tell you a long story about doing the washing that morning and hanging it out to dry in the back garden when in fact they have been on the ward all morning. The story is 'invented' to fill the gap in their memory which occurs because alcohol-induced brain damage has affected their ability to lay down new memories. The whole process of telling

these false memories, which may appear valid to the individual, is known as confabulation. Ask also about street drugs use – what types, how often and how recently. Street drugs are linked to the development of short- and long-term psychoses. Besides street drugs you will need to take details of all currently prescribed drugs, with dosages and side-effects.

PRE-MORBID PERSONALITY

The penultimate history item is the pre-morbid personality. This is an idea of the patient's personality before the first signs of any mental illness. You can ask people to describe themselves as individuals. You may need to prompt them with adjectives such as shy, easy-going, nervous or extrovert. You might wish to probe for hobbies or interests, favourite books or films to build up a picture of the person opposite you.

CORROBORATIVE HISTORY

An individual's view of him or herself is necessarily subjective, so psychiatrists often ask for permission to speak to a relative or friend. This corroborative history might shed greater light on the patient's pre-morbid personality and how the illness has affected them. It will allow you to check details of alcohol and drug consumption. An important point to bear in mind is that in most cases you are taking information after gaining consent from the patient. You should not spontaneously offer inappropriate information to the relative or friend regarding other aspects of the history or diagnosis. There is a matter of confidentiality here. However, should the patient agree and want you to, such things may be discussed, but this probably should not arise during the history taking because your assessment and diagnosis is as yet incomplete.

When the history is complete there are still other components of your assessment to be done, but this is a useful time to pause and take stock of things with the patient. A useful thing to do is to summarise the history back to the patient. This has two benefits: it enables the patient to correct any mistakes you have made and, therefore, clarify your view of things and it also allows the patient to feel understood by another person, sometimes for the first time in their lives. This exploration of how things have been can turn up new information and may offer some insight to the patient that they never had before. Some studies have found that patients do benefit from one-off interviews of this type.

THE MENTAL STATE EXAMINATION

The mental state examination involves:
➤ eliciting psychiatric symptoms and signs
➤ recording these symptoms and signs in an objective and systematic way.

This allows you to distinguish organic brain syndromes from other illnesses and to put evidence together to make a differential diagnosis.

The mental state examination is used in every assessment but, particularly when a patient is too ill to give a history, the mental state examination can be useful in making a diagnosis. The examination has a logical sequence to it so that the first item (appearance) can give evidence which affects the conduct of the rest of the examination; for instance, if the patient appears to be unconscious or is very drowsy, assessment of mood or abstract thought is rendered unreliable or even worthless.

COMPONENTS

The components of the mental state examination are:
➤ appearance
➤ behaviour
➤ manner
➤ speech
➤ mood
➤ thought
➤ cognition
➤ insight.

Appearance

Briefly describe the patient's appearance, such as, 'A thin 80-year-old man, smartly dressed in a three-piece suit, carrying a leather-bound bible'. The description should not be a pejorative judgement of the person. You should be prepared to justify everything you ever write about a patient. Having said that, it is of great value to record exactly what you do see because this will influence your diagnosis and management. So that if you see a 'frail, elderly Caucasian man, with grimy clothing and smelling of urine', then all these points may have some relevance – this appearance might suggest self-neglect, which can be a feature of general ill-health, depression or dementia. Other more bizarre features of appearance will need documentation, e.g. 'A 24-year-old man, wearing few clothes and with his head in a skull-cap of tin foil, allegedly "to keep out the cosmic rays"', or 'A large 40-year-old lady, dressed only in a thin nightdress, standing in casualty, with her make-up over-liberally applied, and waving a bag of pig's trotters'. The former bizarre description accurately described a young man suffering from schizophrenia who had survived alone in a derelict flat for months eating raw meat and vegetables and the latter neatly fitted a lady with mania who had just been shopping in the local market. She had not felt the need to dress that morning and having grown tired of carefully applying her make-up, slapped it on.

Behaviour

The patient's behaviour may be altogether appropriate to the interview situation; he or she may sit quietly, answering each question carefully enough. Other patients may pace the room in an agitated way while the doctor tries to persuade them to stay in the room to answer more questions. Patients might leap out of their chair suddenly at the behest of unseen voices or they may be too preoccupied with visual hallucinations to concentrate on the doctor's questions. Some patients may appear unduly still, with their eyes unmoving and their limbs held tensely – these may be catatonic patients whose limbs if moved by the doctor may be put into unusual postures and have increased tone (waxy flexibility or *cereas flexibilitas*). The postures may then be held for minutes or hours (*preservation of posture*). Alternatively, the patient may be mute and still because they have psychomotor retardation, as in depression (this lacks the features of increased tone and abnormal posturing). It may be appropriate to include other movement disorders under behaviour and manner – psychotropic drugs sometimes cause restlessness (akathisia) or acute dystonic reactions (torticollis, oculogyric crises, etc.) or late-onset rhythmic involuntary lip-smacking, abnormal tongue movements, limb athetosis and truncal movements (tardive dyskinesia). Patients who mimic your every move are showing echopraxia.

Manner

Patients are usually cooperative in manner, but some may be suspicious, guarded or hostile to your questions. Record this. Also try to record how well you got on with the patient in terms of rapport.

Could you establish rapport with the patient? Could you both maintain eye contact or did the patient look down at the floor throughout the interview and answer questions reluctantly or not at all? Patients may also be over-friendly in manner (disinhibited as in mania) or over-hostile. Hostility may arise because patients are irritated with you or afraid of you – manic patients can be frustrated if you do not follow their fast thinking and paranoid patients may be suspicious of your motives and feel you are part of 'the plot'.

Speech

The speech of the patient may be totally spontaneous or may occur only when you ask questions. The answers to questions are usually relevant, but may be wildly off the point. Sometimes all the patient's speech is spontaneous and irrelevant and any intervention by the doctor is unheeded. When answers to questions begin relevantly but drift from the point this may be termed circumstantial speech, e.g. in answer to a question about their mother's age at death: 'Well, she died young, not to say tragically, through an accident. I think there are too many accidents now. They're becoming more and more common. It's a violent world. Look at the gang wars about drugs . . .' There is a conversational logic to this kind of speech, but it is difficult to focus in history taking as the actual information that the patient's mother died at 45 is never given.

Alternatively, answers to questions may be given in the minutest detail: 'My normal working day? I get up at 7.36, and wash in the bathroom while listening to Radio 4. I shave with a razor. I like it better than an electric shaver. Then I get dressed in the clothes my wife has put out for me the night before. I like a newly ironed shirt every morning. Then I go downstairs and have two pieces of toast and a mug of freshly brewed coffee . . .' This kind of speech is over-inclusive – there is just too much information.

Other speech types include tangential speech which veers markedly away from the topic under discussion and may be a feature of thought disordered speech. In mania speech may be pressured – the speech is rapid and crammed with ideas that tumble over one another to be expressed. In schizophrenia and some organic disorders there may be perseverative features such as the rhythmic repetition of the last words you said, known as echolalia, or the last syllable, palilalia.

Speech may be slowed down (as in psychomotor retardation). Speech disorders also include the results of brain damage (e.g. due to cerebrovascular ischaemia), which may produce dysarthrias, expressive and receptive dysphasias and word-finding difficulties.

Mood

The evidence derived from observations of appearance, behaviour, manner and speech can be used to form an idea of the patient's affect or mood. The patient's affect during the interview may have been one of sadness or elation. The affect may have remained the same throughout the interview or it may have varied in response to your questions (it is normal for people to be sad when recalling past traumas and happy when sharing a joke). When people's affect changes suddenly and repeatedly without due cause this is known as lability of affect, which is sometimes a feature of organic brain damage. A patient's affect seems incongruous if it does not match the topic being discussed, e.g. laughter when discussing their mother's death. In patients with severe depression it may be difficult to see their affect because they are psychomotor retarded. The severely depressed person's face may lack emotional expression, sometimes called flattened affect. In schizophrenia the patient may complain that they never feel highs or lows in their mood (blunted affect).

Using what you have found during the preceding assessment you can now build up an 'objective' view of the patient's mood, with the evidence to back this up. Ask the patient for their subjective view of their mood and record this. A suitable question might be: 'Can you tell me how you've been feeling, in your mood or in your spirits, over the past few days or weeks?' You might like to give prompts such as 'High or low? Sad or happy?' If they give a reply of sad or happy try to gauge whether this has been excessive: e.g. 'How sad?' 'The saddest you've ever been?' And in all patients probe for any suicidal ideation, 'Have you ever felt life was not worth living? Have you felt like this recently?' And if the answers are 'yes', then ask, 'Have you thought of doing anything about that?' or 'Have you got any plans to harm yourself? How would you kill yourself? When would you do it? What might stop you doing that?'

Also record again any biological features of mood disturbance: sleep abnormalities (initial insomnia, waking and early morning wakening), poor appetite, weight loss (exactly how much?), diurnal mood variation, altered sexual drive and constipation.

Thought

In the section on thought we are concerned with two main headings: form and content. The form of thought may be reflected by speech. Thus if speech is thought disordered it may be reasonable to assume that thought (which occurs before speech) is similarly disordered. Thoughts may also be pressured, which may lead to pressure of speech; they may be dominated by intrusive thoughts (as in obsessive compulsive disorder); they may exhibit flights of ideas (as in mania) or sudden unpleasant gaps (as in thought blocking in schizophrenia). To assess the content of thought you might ask for the main thoughts that dominate a person's recent thinking life: 'What kind of things do you think about most?', 'What kind of things do you worry about nowadays?' Record any worries, preoccupations, intrusive thoughts, overvalued ideas or delusions. Under thought content you may also record any abnormal experiences such as hallucinatory experiences or thought interference (withdrawal, insertion or broadcasting).

Cognition

Cognitive testing seeks to elicit signs that may point to an organic psychiatric disease. For instance, in a hallucinated patient if consciousness is diminished or 'clouded', this may mean that the hallucinations are the product of a delirious state (acute organic brain syndrome) perhaps due to infection or hypoxia. If there are memory problems on cognitive testing, it may be that there is a dementing process at work.

A basic scheme for cognitive testing might be:

➣ **Orientation:** Normally, in daytime people are aware of the time, the place they are in and the people they are with. In organic brain syndromes this orientation to time, place and person is often lost. It is possible to be disorientated just in time or disorientated in all three aspects. Ask for the current date (day, date, month, year) and the time of day. Ask for the place – 'Where are we now?' – find out if the patient knows which ward, hospital or clinic they are in. Finally, do they know who you are or do they imagine you to be a priest or a social worker (assuming that you have introduced yourself properly at some time during the interview)?

➤ **Attention and concentration:** An inability to focus attention may be seen in agitated depression, anxiety, mania or organic syndromes. Tests which can be used include: 'Please say the months of the year for me in reverse order, that is working backwards from December through to January . . .' or 'Please say the days of the week in reverse order, staring with Sunday and working back to Monday', or 'Please take 7 away from 100, now carry on taking 7 away from that, and again . . . (known as 'serial 7s') or 'Please take 3 away from 21 and keep on taking 3 away until there is nothing left'. Other tests may include digit spans – seeing how many numbers an individual can repeat back to you in sequence or reverse sequence, e.g. 364 . . . 463, 7924 . . . 4297. These tests help you assess attention, but do involve other skills too, so that if these other skills are lost, it may appear that attention is poor when it is not. If some one is poor at maths or has a specific brain defect which causes dyscalculia (a parietal lobe deficit), serial 7s or serial 3s will not produce useful results.

➤ **Memory:** Some people define short-term memory as everything remembered up to three minutes ago and everything retained beyond three minutes or so as medium- or long-term memory. Definitions of short- and long-term memory are contentious and you will observe that different psychiatrists and psychologists have different ideas about this. In a basic cognitive screening

we are interested in fairly crude tests of memory function – short-term testing may involve asking someone to remember a new name and address for a few minutes. 'I would like you to listen to and remember a new name and address I am going to say to you. I will repeat it until you are happy you have got it in mind.' The name and address may have, say, seven components. See initially how many times you have to repeat the name and address before the individual can repeat it back word perfect (i.e. how many times does it take before they register the address). Then ask them to recall the address at fixed intervals, for example 30 seconds, one minute, three minutes and five minutes and then record how many components they can give back to you (see table below).

This gives you an 'objective' measure of memory function which you can use for later comparison. Other short-term tests might include giving a list of five different objects and asking the individual to repeat these to you at certain times. You will also need to get an idea of long-term memory function – can the individual recall important personal dates (e.g. birthdays and anniversaries)? – although this is only useful if you have an objective source to check these with. Otherwise, use the dates of important historical events such as the dates of the Second World War, the death of Churchill, the date of the first moon landing, etc. You can sometimes ask for the names of five flowers, five animals or five capital cities. Short-term memory function deteriorates first in dementia syndromes, but all these memory tests may be affected in severe dementia or by mental retardation.

	30 seconds	1 minute	3 minutes	5 minutes
Number of address components	7/7	6/7	4/7	2/7

➤ **Cerebral lobe function:** If the cognitive screening has been normal up to now, it is probably not of use to probe further into cerebral lobe function, but if a dementia syndrome seems likely then some simple tests may be useful in determining whether there is frontal or parietal lobe damage.

A simple test for frontal lobe damage seeks to assess whether there are any perseverative tendencies. The patient is asked to copy a rhythmically changing line pattern. With some frontal lobe lesions the patient may perseverate as in Figure 1.2. Perseveration of actions such as in drawing or in speech is often linked with frontal lesions.

Other tests for frontal lobe function include verbal fluency, where the subject is asked to give as many words as possible in a minute beginning with the letter 'F', 'A', and then '5'. For the 'FA5' verbal fluency test normal subjects score >30 in total; a score of 20–30 denotes mild frontal dysfunction and a score <20 suggest large, frontal lesions or a dementing illness.

Interpreting proverbs is an example of abstracting ability and with frontal lobe lesions patients may interpret proverbs in a 'concrete' way. For example, in interpreting 'A rolling stone gathers no moss', a frontal lobe patient may say that 'The stone gathers no moss because it is moving too fast'.

Paper tests for parietal lobe damage may seek to assess whether there is a constructional apraxia. When asked to copy a line drawing of a house or a clock, the copy may be 'exploded', or there may be sensory inattention to one side of the diagram (*see* Figure 1.3).

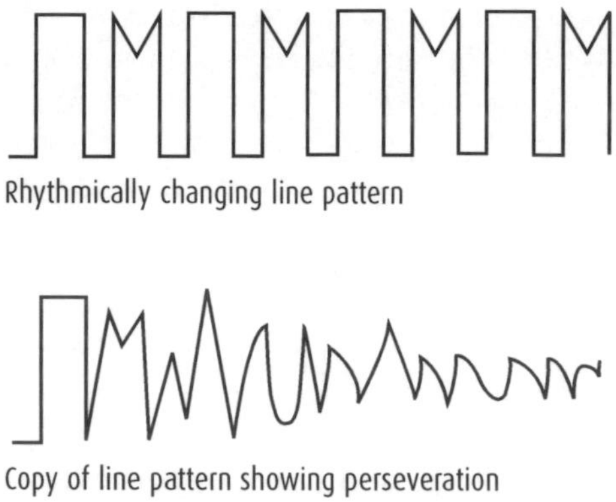

➤ **Abstract thought:** In schizophrenia, mental retardation and frontal lesions the capacity for abstract thinking may be reduced, so that concrete thinking is prevalent. Tests for abstract thought may therefore include asking for the meaning

Rhythmically changing line pattern

Copy of line pattern showing perseveration

Figure 1.2 In copying a regularly changing line pattern the patient with perseveration fails to change the pattern and continues in a zigzag fashion

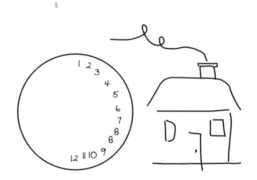

Figure 1.3 The results of asking a patient with unilateral spatial neglect to draw a clock face and copy a simple drawing of a house

of proverbs or for asking for similarities between things such as a banana and an apple (correct answer: 'both fruits' or 'both living things') or a car and a lorry, or for differences between things like a lake and a river or a child and a dwarf. Such tests may also provoke thought disorder in some predisposed individuals.

Insight

Finally, the interviewer assesses the patient's 'insight' into their illness – does the patient think they have any problems and if so are they due to ill health, do they think that the illness is treatable by doctors, and is it treatable by drugs? Psychotic illnesses often rob patients of insight so that they feel their voices are normal, or supernaturally derived, or attributable to some alien authority rather than being due to a treatable illness. If they make this assumption about their psychotic experiences and delusions, it would be illogical for the patient to think that doctors can help. Lack of insight may reduce or destroy the patient's compliance with treatment and, without outside intervention, condemn the mentally ill to permanent ill-health.

Insight is, therefore, about how the patient sees their predicament and is a complex construct.

PHYSICAL EXAMINATION AND INVESTIGATIONS

Psychiatrists are first and foremost doctors, trained in diagnosis and keen to exclude any treatable physical illness which may present with psychological symptoms. A routine physical examination of cardiovascular, respiratory, abdominal and nervous systems is, therefore, essential in all patients. Organic causes of psychiatric illness which may be picked up in this way might include: focal central nervous system (CNS) lesions, subdural haematomas, systemic lupus erythematosus (SLE), hyperthyroidism, hypothyroidism, diabetes mellitus, Addison's, Cushing's, hypertension, renal and liver failure, phaeochromocytomas, tuberose sclerosis, syphilis, bronchial and gastric carcinomas, stigmata of alcoholic liver disease, features of mental retardation syndromes, e.g. Down's or Fragile-X, and numerous others.

Similarly, investigations may usefully include a full blood count (various anaemias may present with dementia-like pictures, raised mean cell volume in alcoholism), liver enzyme tests (raised in alcoholism), thyroid function tests, serum B12 and folate, urea and electrolytes, syphilis screening tests, drug screening tests (street drugs may induce psychotic reactions), chest X-ray, skull X-rays, electroencephalogram (to detect focal lesions and epileptic phenomena), computed tomography / magnetic resonance scans, and more specialist tests, e.g. cortisol levels, homovanillic acid urine tests, or serum copper tests (for Wilson's disease).

Other investigations include social, occupational and psychological investigations. Social investigations (if consented to) may include discussions with family and friends, requests to schools for information on progress and abilities, home visits and the like. Occupational therapists may assist with rehabilitation as will functional assessments (how well people can manage their home life and plan their daily activities). Psychologists can sometimes help with specific neuropsychological tests of brain function and personality and IQ testing.

PUTTING THE INFORMATION TOGETHER

At the end of the assessment process the doctor pulls together the major findings from the history, mental state, physical examination and investigations into a summary. Sometimes the summary is built into a 'formulation', which also includes a differential diagnosis and a tentative management plan and prognosis. The differential diagnosis should include the most likely diagnoses, headed by the most likely of all, together with evidence extracted from the assessment interview to support or refute each diagnosis. Using the differential diagnosis you can then, and only then, reasonably construct a management plan and prognosis, which can be appended to the formulation.

In making your differential diagnosis you may wish to consider five 'levels of illness' in the diagnostic hierarchy or sieve. The first level to consider is organic; specifically ask yourself if there is any organic illness that might present with such features. This must be included in your differential diagnosis and steps taken to exclude treatable organic illness. It makes little sense to embark on psychological methods of treatment without treating underlying organic causes. The second level is psychotic or schizophrenic illness. The third level would

INSIGHT

One of the striking aspects of mental illness is its effect on insight. Patients with gross delusions often do not appreciate they are ill, or that their condition should have anything to with doctors or treatment.

Insight is important because it may affect whether people may accept treatment and their prognosis thus depends on it. Insight may also be linked to whether someone acts on a command hallucination or requires detention in hospital under the Mental Health Act.

The mental state examination includes a section where the doctor is supposed to assess insight. Simply saying that insight is 'good' or 'poor' does not convey much to the reader and so some people have devised ways to measure insight and help communication. Some of these are complicated and refer to various dimensions of insight. The following scale is designed to be simple and to focus just on the clinical setting.

Insight level	Insight level definition
0	Does not appreciate that any abnormal experience or abnormal belief that is present is unusual.
1	Appreciates that a personal experience (symptoms) or abnormal belief is different from that expected in usual range of experience/belief.
2	Attributes these symptoms (experiences, or beliefs) to an illness model + has insight at level 1.
3	Personally seeks help from a formal source for an illness producing these experiences + has insight at levels 1 and 2.
4	Appreciates need for a treatment for these symptoms (treatment can be psychological, social or physical) + has insight at levels 1, 2 and 3.
5	Complies (voluntarily) with agreed treatment plan + has insight at levels 1, 2, 3 and 4.
6	Appreciates need for continued compliance or follow-up from formal treatment provider + has insight at levels 1, 2, 3, 4, and 5.

The scale is designed as a hierarchy so that the interviewer considers each level from zero upwards and assesses whether that level is attained before moving any further up. For instance, if someone appeared to accept the need for continued follow-up and thus seemed to fulfil level 6, but they felt their symptoms were not due to an illness (requirement for level 3), their score would be less than 3, not 6. Some examples may illustrate this further.

INSIGHT RATING EXAMPLES

➤ Debbie is 25 and has a psychotic illness with second person auditory hallucinations and delusions that she is the mother of God. She believes she is God's mother because of the angelic voices. She does not accept that the voices are produced by her own mind and believes that they are genuine voices from the heavens. She has tried to jump off a building in response to the angels' 'invitations'. She is detained

> in hospital and receives treatment, but argues that this is unnecessary. Insight rating = 0
> ➢ Mark is 45 and has been hospitalised three times for bipolar affective disorder. He complains that he feels low in mood and seeks help from his community psychiatrist for this and takes the prescribed antidepressants. He wishes to see his psychiatrist more often than is possible. Insight rating = 6
> ➢ Daniel is 65 and depressed – he also has some overvalued ideas that his neighbour may be a terrorist. He sometimes thinks he can hear his neighbour through the wall – praying to God and denouncing Daniel in his prayers. Daniel knows he is low in mood, and accepts that some people might not understand his concerns about his neighbour, and that the idea his neighbour is a terrorist is an unusual idea. He feels he might have a depression but does not accept he needs treatment and will not even see the GP. Insight rating = 2.

be 'affective illness', by which we mean illnesses with affective features (such as mania or depression), which are not caused by gross organic disorder (such as delirium or intracerebral tumours or infarctions). The fourth level is 'neurotic' illness which encompasses anxiety disorders, phobias and eating disorders. Such illnesses may be very disabling, but they lack psychotic features. Finally, the fifth area to consider involves the personality. People's personalities differ to a greater or lesser extent. When those differences are marked, persistent and damaging to the individual or society, they are termed personality disorders. Some personality disorders may mimic other psychiatric illness but it is worth bearing in mind that just as all personality types can become physically ill, so all personality types can suffer from psychiatric illness. It would be unethical to deny treatment to someone purely on the basis that they had a personality disorder.

CLASSIFICATION

Classifying disease helps doctors to recognise clinically similar illnesses in people and enables research, particularly in terms of what causes those illnesses and what cures them. In psychiatry large groups have met to define illness categories and currently there are two broad classification systems in use.

The European and worldwide system is the International Classification of Diseases, 10th version, (ICD-10) and the American system is the Diagnostic and Statistical Manual, 4th version (DSM-IV).

There is substantial overlap between them. When you make a diagnosis according to the criteria for each disease in these classifications then other clinicians will be able to know what you mean when you diagnose schizophrenia.

Although one diagnosis may take precedence, remember that several diagnoses may be present, e.g. depression in a patient with residual schizophrenia or depression in a person with borderline personality disorder.

In the following section the main headings of ICD-10 are summarised. At this stage you may not be familiar with all the terms mentioned, but reference to the following chapters will help you.

ICD-10
F00–F09 ORGANIC MENTAL DISORDERS
Examples include:
➢ Dementia in Alzheimer's disease – may be early or late onset. Vascular dementia (includes acute, multi-infarct, and subcortical types).
➢ Dementia in the following: Pick's disease;

Creutzfeldt-Jakob disease; Huntington's chorea; Parkinson's disease; and HIV infection/AIDS.

➤ Delirium (an acute organic brain syndrome with disorientation and clouding of consciousness).

➤ Organic hallucinosis, e.g. caused by temporal lobe epilepsy, organic mood disorders, e.g. in Cushing's syndrome, organic anxiety disorders, e.g. in phaeochromocytoma.

➤ Organic personality disorder, e.g. frontal lobe tumours, which may disorganise personality; post-encephalitic syndromes and post-concussional syndromes.

F10–F19 MENTAL AND BEHAVIOURAL DISORDERS DUE TO PSYCHOACTIVE SUBSTANCE ABUSE

➤ This covers alcohol, opioids, cannabinoids, sedatives, hypnotics, cocaine, caffeine, amphetamines, other hallucinogens, tobacco, solvents and other drugs.

➤ May include harmful use, dependence, withdrawal states, psychotic disorders, e.g. delirium tremens and LSD experiences, amnesic syndromes, e.g. Wernicke-Korsakoff syndrome, and residual effects, e.g. LSD flashbacks.

F20–29 SCHIZOPHRENIA, SCHIZOTYPAL AND DELUSIONAL DISORDERS

➤ Schizophrenia (this may take the form of paranoid, hebephrenic, catatonic, undifferentiated, or residual types).

➤ Schizotypal disorder (this lacks the full psychotic features of schizophrenia – it is more of an extreme of personality featuring unusual or eccentric ideation; for instance, magical thinking).

➤ Persistent delusional disorders, e.g. monodelusional psychoses where the individual wrongly believes they are, say, infested by some insect, but no other psychotic features.

➤ Schizoaffective disorder – a rare category where the illness has marked features of both affective illness and schizophrenia.

F30–F39 MOOD (AFFECTIVE) DISORDERS

➤ Manic episode (which would include hypomania – a lesser form of mania and probably more common; mania without psychotic features; and mania with psychotic features).

➤ Bipolar affective disorder (this diagnosis requires evidence of both hypomanic or manic and depressive episodes at some stage in a person's life).

➤ Depressive episodes (which can be categorised as mild, moderate and severe without depressive symptoms and severe with psychotic symptoms).

➤ Recurrent mood disorders.

➤ Persistent mood disorders (cyclothymia – a varying series of low and high moods; dysthymia – a chronic, low mood not severe enough to fulfil the criteria for a depressive illness).

F40–F48 NEUROTIC, STRESS-RELATED AND SOMATOFORM DISORDERS

➤ Phobic anxiety disorders (such as agoraphobia, social phobias, specific phobias).

➤ Anxiety disorders (such as panic disorder, generalised anxiety disorder).

➤ Obsessive-compulsive disorder (involving obsessional thoughts or ruminations, compulsive acts and obsessional rituals).

➤ Reactions to severe stress and adjustment disorders.

➤ Dissociative (conversion) disorders – where some internal conflict or anxiety is converted into other symptoms like classical Freudian hysterical paralysis. Examples of dissociative disorders include dissociative amnesias, dissociative fugues, trance and possession states, dissociative convulsions and dissociative anaesthesia.

➤ Somatoform disorders – somatising anxiety into any physical symptom.

➤ Depersonalisation-derealisation syndrome.

F50–F59 BEHAVIOURAL SYNDROMES ASSOCIATED WITH PHYSIOLOGICAL DISTURBANCES AND PHYSICAL FACTORS

➤ Eating disorders (anorexia nervosa, bulimia nervosa and others).

➤ Non-organic sleep disorders (where organic causes have been excluded – insomnia, hypersomnia, somnambulism, night terrors, nightmares).

➤ Sexual dysfunction (not caused by organic disorder or disease) (includes: loss of sexual desire, sexual aversion, failure of genital response, orgasmic dysfunction, premature ejaculation, non-organic vaginismus, non-organic dyspareunia, excessive sexual drive and others).

➤ Mental and behavioural disorders of the puerperium.

➤ Abuse of non-dependence-producing substances (like laxatives, analgesics, antacids, vitamins etc.).

F60–69 DISORDERS OF ADULT PERSONALITY AND BEHAVIOUR

➤ Personality disorders (including paranoid, schizoid, dissocial, borderline, histrionic, anankastic, avoidant, dependent and other types).

➤ Enduring personality change after catastrophic experience or psychiatric illness.

➤ Pathological gambling, fire-setting, stealing, hair pulling.

➤ Transsexualism, dual-role transvestism. Sexual preference disorders – fetishism, exhibitionism, voyeurism, paedophilia, sadomasochism, etc.

➤ Factitious disorder (intentional feigning of symptoms or disabilities), sometimes also called Munchausen's syndrome.

F70–F79 MENTAL RETARDATION

➤ Mild, moderate, severe and profound.

F80–F89 DISORDERS OF PSYCHOLOGICAL DEVELOPMENT

➤ Developmental disorders of speech, receptive and expressive language disorders, specific arithmetical disorders.

➤ Childhood autism, Rett's syndrome, Asperger's syndrome.

F90–F98 BEHAVIOURAL AND EMOTIONAL DISORDERS WITH ONSET USUALLY OCCURRING IN CHILDHOOD AND ADOLESCENCE

➤ Hyperkinetic disorders, conduct disorders, emotional disorders, tic disorders, non-organic enuresis, non-organic encopresis, pica, stereotyped movement disorders, stuttering.

F99 UNSPECIFIED MENTAL DISORDER

LEARNING POINTS
PSYCHIATRIC ASSESSMENT

➤ A psychiatric assessment has four main components: history, mental state examination, physical examination and investigations (physical, psychological and social).

➤ The history is divided into presenting complaint, the history of presenting complaint, past psychiatric history, family history, personal history, psychosexual history, forensic history, social history, premorbid personality, corroborative history and summary.

➤ The mental state examination describes appearance, behaviour, and manner, speech, mood (including suicidal feelings), thought (form and content), cognition and insight.

SELF-ASSESSMENT
MCQs

1 Clinical features of depression typically include:

A psychomotor retardation

B diurnal mood variation

C early morning wakening

    D overactivity
    E constipation

2 Routine first line psychiatric investigations include:
    A full blood count
    B magnetic resonance imaging
    C serum copper
    D thyroid function tests
    E liver function tests

3 Types of personality disorder include:
    A schizoid
    B residual
    C blunted
    D borderline
    E hebephrenic

4 In the following mental state abnormalities:
    A echolalia is the copying of posture
    B tangentiality may occur in thought disorder
    C overvalued ideas are incorrect, unreasonable and bizarre ideas held with absolute conviction
    D word finding difficulties are a feature of early dementia
    E hallucinatory voices talking to the patient are third person auditory hallucinations

SHORT ANSWER QUESTIONS

1 What are the differences between a hallucination and an illusion?
2 What are the main features of a delusion? What different kinds of delusion are there?
3 What cognitive tests help to assess someone's attention and concentration? How do you perform these tests?

MCQ answers
1 A=T, B=T, C=F, D=T, E=T.
2 A=T, B=F, C=T, D=T, E=T.
3 A=T, B=F, C=T, D=F, E=F.
4 A=F, B=T, C=T, D=F, E=F.

EXPLORATIONS
CLASSIFICATION
www.who.int
Read up about the development of the World Health Organization's ICD-10 classification system and see how it classifies mental disorders.

PSYCHOPATHOLOGY
www.ncl.ac.uk/nnp/teaching/video
This Newcastle University website has some good webclips of interviews showing abnormal moods, hallucinations and delusions.

EXPERIENCE HALLUCINATIONS
This is an experiential task. Work in a group of three. Choose who will be the 'patient', the 'left hand voice', and the 'right hand voice'. The 'patient' sits in the middle and should be in a 'good mood' currently, that is to say in good health. The exercise has two parts to it: the patient needs to undergo both parts as the second is the antidote to the first. In part one the 'patient' closes his or her eyes and the 'left hand voice' makes negative comments such as 'You shouldn't live – you are a waste of space – jump off the tower – do it now' and the right hand voice makes similarly derogatory comments such as 'You're worthless – you smell – you stink – you did a bad thing'. Maintain this for a short time such as a minute, then ask the 'patient' what the experience felt like.

The next phase is hopefully an antidote to any gloom. The 'patient' again closes his or her eyes and the 'left hand voice' makes positive comments such as 'You are useful – you are worthwhile – study hard – you make me proud' and the 'right hand voice' makes comments such as 'You're brilliant – you smell nice – you look cool – you learned loads'.

(The exercise is meant to give the experience of second person auditory hallucinations. Some comments are like 'command' hallucinations and these are particularly problematic in clinical practice especially if the patient finds it difficult to resist them or has acted on them in the past. Hallucinations are experienced in external space and are as 'real' as normal perceptions. Imagine if you heard these kinds of voices in the exercise all day long. The second part of the exercise is designed to boost the person in the 'patient' role. Sometimes patients with hypomania experience similar positive voices and even miss them when they are treated.)

IDENTIFY RISKS

What are the risks in the two vignettes that follow? (There are at least two major risks in each.)

June is a 28-year-old woman with bipolar affective disorder. In the past she has severed both her legs on a railway line during a depressed phase. She has become depressed again in recent weeks with delusions of guilt and she has been hearing some voices telling her to 'cleanse' herself with fire.

Elspeth is aged 30 and abuses amphetamines and alcohol. She has a diagnosis of paranoid schizophrenia and accuses others of stealing her things. She assaults them on this basis. On her last admission she jumped on the ribcage of an elderly woman, breaking ribs and her sternum. Her current admission followed her stopping her medication, becoming ill and throttling her mother's pet cat.

AETIOLOGY

Aetiology is a way of looking at the causation of a case. Psychiatrists talk about precipitating, predisposing and perpetuating factors for an illness, but you can also think about the problem in biological, social and psychological terms.

As an awareness exercise, aim to gather a group of colleagues and get them all to set aside an hour or so for the following exercise. A flipchart or whiteboard would be useful.

1 Choose a possible diagnosis for a patient that you have seen and examined, e.g. someone with depression or anorexia nervosa.
2 One of the group should draw the following table on the flipchart or white board.

3 Consider factors that could fit into the nine cells: biological precipitating factors, psychological precipitating factors, and so on.

As an additional twist to the exercise, the group can research evidence for the factors.

	Biological	Psychological	Social
Precipitating			
Predisposing			
Perpetuating			

FURTHER READING AND REFERENCES

American Psychiatric Association. *Quick Reference to the Diagnostic Criteria from DSM IV TR*. APA; 1994.

American Psychiatric Association. *DSM IV TR Casebook*. APA; 2002.

Fish F. *Clinical Psychopathology*. Revised ed. London: Gaskell; 2007.

Green BH. Creating rapport. In: Green BH, editor. *Psychiatry in General Practice*. London: Kluwer Academic Publishers; 1994.

Jaspers K. *General Psychopathology*. (2 vols) Baltimore, Maryland: Johns Hopkins University Press; 1997.

Shea SC. *Psychiatric Interviewing*. Philadelphia: Saunders; 1998.

Sims A. *Symptoms in the Mind*. 3rd ed. London: Saunders; 2002.

World Health Organization. *The ICD-10 Classification of Mental and Behavioural Disorders*. Geneva: WHO; 1992.

GLOSSARY

Addiction: An organism's psychological or physical dependence on a drug, characterised by tolerance and withdrawal.

Adjustment disorder: A pathological psychological reaction to trauma, loss or severe stress. Usually these last less than six months, but may be prolonged if the stressor, e.g. pain or scarring, is enduring.

Affect: A person's affect is their immediate emotional state which the person can recognise subjectively and which can also be recognised objectively by others. A person's mood is their predominant current affect.

Agnosia: An inability to organise sensory information so as to recognise objects (e.g. visual agnosia) or sometimes even parts of the body (e.g. hemisomatoagnosia).

Agoraphobia: Fear of the marketplace literally; taken now to be a fear of public of public places associated with panic disorder.

Agraphia: Loss of writing ability.

Akathisia: An inner feeling of excessive restlessness, which provokes the sufferer to fidget in their seat or pace about.

Amnesia: A partial of complete loss of memory. *Anterograde* amnesia is a loss of memory subsequent to any cause, e.g. brain trauma. *Retrograde* amnesia is a loss of memory for a period of time prior to any cause.

Anorexia nervosa: Anorexia nervosa is an eating disorder characterised by excess control – a morbid fear of obesity leads the sufferer to try to limit or reduce his or her weight by excessive dieting, exercising, vomiting, purging and use of diuretics. Sufferers are typically more than 15% below the average weight for their height / sex / age. Typically, they have amenorrhoea (if female) or low libido (if male). 1–2% of female teenagers are anorexic.

Anxiety: Anxiety is provoked by fear or apprehension and also results from a tension caused by conflicting ideas or motivations. Anxiety manifests through mental and somatic symptoms such as palpitations, dizziness, hyperventilation, and faintness.

Asthenia: Asthenia is a weakness or debility of some form, hence neurasthenia, a term for an illness seen by doctors around the turn of the century, a probable precursor to chronic fatigue syndrome and myalgic encephalomyelitis (ME).

Bulimia nervosa: Described by Russell in 1979, bulimia nervosa is an eating disorder characterised by lack of control. Abnormal eating behaviour including dieting, vomiting, purging and particularly bingeing may be associated with normal weight or obesity. The syndrome is associated with guilt, depressed mood, low self-esteem and sometimes with childhood sexual abuse, alcoholism and promiscuity. May be associated with oesophageal ulceration and parotid swelling (Green's chubby chops sign).

Compulsion: The behavioural component of an obsession. The individual feels compelled to repeat a behaviour which has no immediate benefit beyond reducing the anxiety associated with the obsessional idea. For instance, for a person obsessed by the idea that they are dirty, repeated ritual handwashing may serve to reduce anxiety.

Confabulation: Changing, loosely held and false memories created to fill in organically derived amnesia.

Cyclothymia: A variability of mood over days or weeks, cycling from positive to negative mood states. The variability is not as severe in amplitude or duration as to be classified as a major affective disorder.

Déjà vu: Haven't you been here before? An abnormal experience where an individual feels that a particular or unique event has happened before in exactly the same way.

Delirium: An acute organic brain syndrome secondary to physical causes in which consciousness is affected and disorientation results; often associated with illusions, visual hallucinations and persecutory ideation.

Delusion: An incorrect belief which is out of keeping with the person's cultural context, intelligence and social background and which is held with unshakeable conviction.

Delusional mood: Also known as *wahnstimmung*, a feeling that something unusual is about to happen of special significance for that person.

Delusional perception: A normal perception which has become highly invested with significance and which has become incorporated into a delusional system, e.g. 'When I saw the traffic lights turn red I knew that the dog I was walking was a Nazi and a Mexican Nazi at that.'

Dementia: A chronic organic mental illness which produces a global deterioration in cognitive abilities and which usually runs a deteriorating course.

Depersonalisation: An experience where the self is felt to be unreal, detached from reality or different in some way. Depersonalisation can be triggered by tiredness, dissociative episodes or partial epileptic seizures.

Depression: An affective disorder characterised by a profound and persistent sadness.

Derealisation: An experience where the person perceives the world around them to be unreal. The experience is linked to depersonalisation.

DSM: DSM-IV is the American classification system for mental disorders. DSM stands for the Diagnostic and Statistical Manual. DSM has specific diagnostic criteria for each mental disorder. It also has a system of different axes to denote conditions that can co-exist such as mental illness and personality disorder.

Dyskinesia: Abnormal movements as in *tardive dyskinesia*, a late onset of abnormal involuntary movements. Tardive dyskinesia is conventionally thought to be a late side-effect of first generation antipsychotics, but some abnormal movements were seen in schizophrenia before the introduction of antipsychotics.

Dyspraxia: A dyspraxia is a difficulty with a previously learnt or acquired movement or skill. An example might be a dressing dyspraxia or a constructional dyspraxia. Dyspraxias tend to indicate cortical damage, particularly in the parietal lobe region.

Echolalia: A speech disorder in which the person inappropriately and automatically repeats the last words he or she has heard. Palilalia is a form of echolalia in which the last syllable heard is repeated endlessly.

Echopraxia: A movement disorder in which the person automatically and inappropriately imitates or mirrors the movements of another.

First rank symptoms: Schneider classified the most characteristic symptoms of schizophrenia as first rank features of schizophrenia. These included third person auditory hallucinations, thought echo, thought interference (insertion, withdrawal, and broadcasting), delusional perception and passivity phenomena.

Flight of ideas: In mania and hypomania thoughts become pressured and ideas may race from topic to topic, guided sometimes only by rhymes or puns. Ideas are associated, though, unlike thought disorder.

Frontal lobe syndrome: This follows frontal lobe damage or may be consequent upon a lesion such as a tumour of infarction. There is a lack of judgement, a coarsening of personality, disinhibition, pressure of speech, lack of planning ability, and sometimes apathy. Perseveration and a return of the grasp reflex may occur.

Hallucination: Sometimes very concisely defined as a percept without an object. It's an abnormal sensory experience that arises in the absence of a direct external stimulus. A hallucination has the qualities of a normal percept and is experienced as real and usually is experienced in external space. Hallucinations may occur in any sensory modality.

Hypomania: An affective disorder characterised by elation, racing thoughts, overactivity, and insomnia among other symptoms.

ICD: ICD stands for the International Classification of Diseases – a classification system, which includes mental disorders. The World Health Organization has maintained the system since 1948 when it was in its sixth version. From 1994 onwards the tenth version, ICD-10, has been in use. The system uses letters and numbers to designate various conditions. For instance F32.1 is a moderately severe depressive episode. The first ICD version, the International List of Causes of Death, was created in 1893.

Illusion: An abnormal perception caused by a sensory misinterpretation of an actual stimulus, sometimes precipitated by strong emotion, e.g. fear provoking a person to imagine they have seen an intruder in the shadows.

Insight: In psychotic mental disorders and organic brain syndromes a patient's insight into whether or not they are ill and therefore requiring treatment may be affected. In depression a person may lack insight into their best qualities and in mania a person may overestimate their wealth and abilities.

Jamais vu: An abnormal experience where an individual feels that a routine or familiar event has never happened before. (*See* Déjà vu.)

Korsakoff's syndrome: A syndrome of amnesia and confabulation following chronic alcoholism. Short-term memory is particularly affected. Named after the Russian psychiatrist Sergei Korsakoff.

Made experiences: *See* 'Passivity phenomena'.

Mania: An affective disorder characterised by intense euphoria, overactivity and loss of insight.

Neologism: A novel word often invented and used in schizophrenic thought disorder.

Neuroleptic malignant syndrome: A syndrome ascribed to neuroleptics. The syndrome includes hyperpyrexia (temperature over 39 degrees

Celsius), autonomic instability and muscular rigidity. The syndrome is not dose related and appears to be related to a very wide variety of substances including antidepressants, antipsychotics and lithium. There is a significant risk of mortality. Whether the syndrome is a variant of the lethal catatonia syndrome (described before the advent of modern neuroleptics) is a debated point.

Obsession: An unpleasant or nonsensical thought which intrudes into a person's mind, despite a degree of resistance by the person who recognises the thought as pointless or senseless, but nevertheless a product of their own mind. Obsessions may be accompanied by compulsive behaviours which serve to reduce the associated anxiety.

Parietal lobe signs: Parietal lobe signs include various agnosias (such as visual agnosias, sensory neglect, and tactile agnosias), dyspraxias (such as dressing dyspraxia), body image disturbance, and hemipareses or hemiplegias.

Passivity phenomena: In these phenomena the individual feels that some aspect of themselves is under the external control of another or others. These may therefore include 'made acts and impulses' where the individual feels they are being made to do something by another, 'made movements' where their arms or legs feel as if they are moving under another's control, 'made emotions' where they are experiencing someone else's emotions, and 'made thoughts' which are categorised elsewhere as thought insertion and withdrawal.

Perseveration: Describes an inappropriate repetition of some behaviour or thought or speech. Echolalia is an example of perseverative speech. Talking exclusively on one subject might be described as perseveration on a theme. Perseveration of thought indicates an inability to switch ideas, so that in an interview a patient may continue to give the same responses to later questions as he did to earlier ones. Perseveration is sometimes a feature of frontal lobe lesions.

Schizophasia: A severe form of thought disorder.

Seasonal affective disorder (SAD): A form of depressive illness only occurring during winter months, associated with overeating and sleepiness. Responsive to antidepressants and phototherapy. Little researched and scientifically controversial.

Tardive dyskinesia: An abnormal involuntary movement disorder which may manifest as lip-smacking bucco-lingual movements or grimacing, truncal movements or athetoid limb movements.

Thought blocking: The unpleasant experience of having one's train of thought curtailed absolutely, often more a sign than a symptom.

Thought broadcasting: The experience that one's thoughts are being transmitted from one's mind and broadcast to everyone.

Thought disorder: A disorder of the form of thought, where associations between ideas are lost or loosened.

Thought echo: Where thoughts are heard as if spoken aloud, when there is some delay these are known as *echo de la pensée* and when heard simultaneously, *Gedankenlautwerden*.

Thought insertion: The experience of alien thoughts being inserted into the mind.

Thought withdrawal: The experience of thoughts being removed or extracted from one's mind.

Word salad: A severe form of thought disorder.

CHAPTER 2
Organic psychiatry

The body's homeostatic mechanisms strive to create a supportive environment for the brain. These mechanisms regulate blood pressure so that the brain is adequately perfused with blood rich in glucose and oxygen. If threats to the brain arise, such as metabolic disease, infection or starvation, other body systems will often be denied in order to preserve the life of the brain. However, if these pressures are too severe, these homeostatic mechanisms will be overwhelmed and brain function will suffer.

The presentation of this organic illness may well be through psychological symptoms, but clinical management involves identifying the organic cause of the cerebral disorder and to treat this where possible. Failure to treat the underlying cause increases the risk of death.

CONTENTS

A REVIEW OF BRAIN FUNCTION

The brain consists of a cluster of neural structures which have evolved over time. Some structures such as the brainstem are relatively ancient in evolutionary terms and perform necessary but rudimentary functions such as coordinating respiratory rhythm and fulfilling basic aims of life such as consciousness. Higher, later structures such as the white matter allow the functions of association and learning. Relatively new structures such as the cortex allow the integration of sensations, ideas and movements and form the core of sentient cognition. Forebrain structures in the frontal lobes of the brain allow higher functions still such as judgement, insight and detailed planning.

Psychological symptoms may be produced by lesions, which affect any or all brain components.

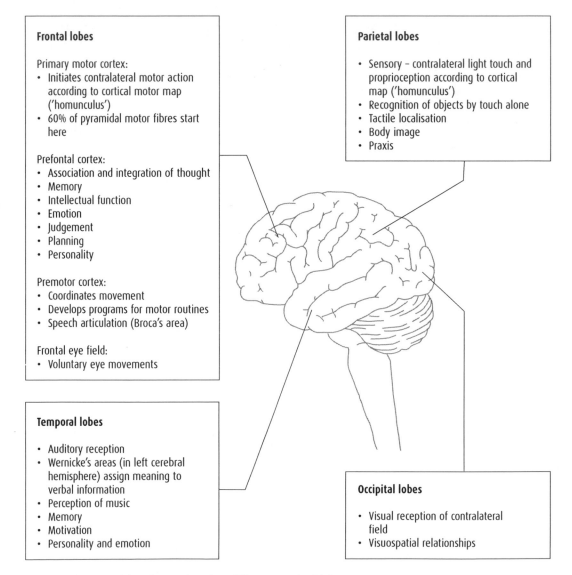

Frontal lobes

Primary motor cortex:
• Initiates contralateral motor action according to cortical motor map ('homunculus')
• 60% of pyramidal motor fibres start here

Prefontal cortex:
• Association and integration of thought
• Memory
• Intellectual function
• Emotion
• Judgement
• Planning
• Personality

Premotor cortex:
• Coordinates movement
• Develops programs for motor routines
• Speech articulation (Broca's area)

Frontal eye field:
• Voluntary eye movements

Temporal lobes

• Auditory reception
• Wernicke's areas (in left cerebral hemisphere) assign meaning to verbal information
• Perception of music
• Memory
• Motivation
• Personality and emotion

Parietal lobes

• Sensory – contralateral light touch and proprioception according to cortical map ('homunculus')
• Recognition of objects by touch alone
• Tactile localisation
• Body image
• Praxis

Occipital lobes

• Visual reception of contralateral field
• Visuospatial relationships

Figure 2.1 Normal functions related to different cerebral lobes

Figure 2.1 shows how various functions correspond to different areas of the cerebral cortex. Left and right hemispheres also appear to have different roles. In over 90% of people the left hemisphere houses the language centres and controls handedness. Certain functions are shared out between the hemispheres via the integrative ability of the corpus callosum. Figure 2.2 indicates the differing functions of left and right hemispheres.

General conditions, such as hypoglycaemia or hypoxia, alter the function of all parts of the brain, i.e. producing a global impairment. Effects on the frontal lobe may produce disinhibition and impaired judgement. Effects on the temporal lobe may lead to hallucinatory experiences, and effects on general neural activity may result in diminished consciousness, so that the hypoxic older patient may appear drowsy, but also experience frightening hallucinations and be unable to distinguish what is real and what is unreal about him or her.

Specific space-occupying lesions such as tumours or abscesses may produce symptoms only in the brain areas they impinge upon. Early symptoms of a frontal lobe tumour may involve fairly subtle changes in personality – a slight coarseness of manner in a previously urbane and polite character. Figure 2.3 shows how lesions in various cerebral lobes may present. Depending on the size and type of the lesion none, some or all of these symptoms and signs may occur.

Appreciation of how organic disease can affect brain function helps provide a link between the symptoms of a psychiatric disease such as senile dementia and the neuropathology that underlies it.

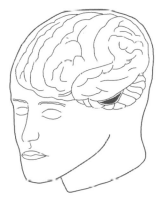
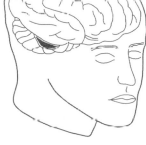

Left
- Language
- Handedness
- Movement of right side of body
- Sensory information from right side of body
- Visual reception of right visual field
- Verbal memory
- Bilateral auditory reception
- Processing of verbal sound
- Visuo-verbal processing

Right
- Movement of left side of body
- Sensory information from left side of body
- Visual reception of left visual field
- Non-verbal memory, e.g. pictures, patterns
- Bilateral auditory reception
- Processing of music, noise
- Visuo-spatial processing
- Emotional processing

Figure 2.2 Functions of the right and left sides of the brain

CAUSES OF CEREBRAL DISORDER

In general we might think of causes in terms of *vulnerability* and *stress*. If the stress is sufficient any brain will cease to function correctly – so a young adult who acquires malaria may suffer from *delirium* (an acute organic brain syndrome). Some brains are more vulnerable and may succumb to lesser stresses. A general anaesthetic may prove harmless to a young adult brain, but to the more vulnerable brain of an otherwise fit 90 year old, the stress of general anaesthesia may result in temporary disorientation post-operatively. Accumulated brain cell death, diminished cardiovascular

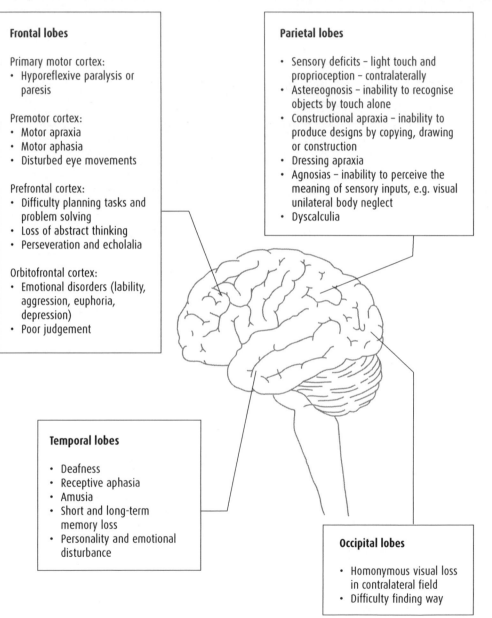

Frontal lobes

Primary motor cortex:
• Hyporeflexive paralysis or paresis

Premotor cortex:
• Motor apraxia
• Motor aphasia
• Disturbed eye movements

Prefrontal cortex:
• Difficulty planning tasks and problem solving
• Loss of abstract thinking
• Perseveration and echolalia

Orbitofrontal cortex:
• Emotional disorders (lability, aggression, euphoria, depression)
• Poor judgement

Parietal lobes

• Sensory deficits – light touch and proprioception – contralaterally
• Astereognosis – inability to recognise objects by touch alone
• Constructional apraxia – inability to produce designs by copying, drawing or construction
• Dressing apraxia
• Agnosias – inability to perceive the meaning of sensory inputs, e.g. visual unilateral body neglect
• Dyscalculia

Temporal lobes

• Deafness
• Receptive aphasia
• Amusia
• Short and long-term memory loss
• Personality and emotional disturbance

Occipital lobes

• Homonymous visual loss in contralateral field
• Difficulty finding way

Figure 2.3 Symptoms and signs related to lesions in different cerebral lobes

performance and other factors such as pigment deposition, neurofibrillary tangles and senile plaque formation all contribute to an increased vulnerability for older brains. Chronic degenerative disease in older brains may lead to a chronic brain syndrome called *dementia*.

Stresses that can produce brain dysfunction are listed in Table 2.1 on p. 34.

DELIRIUM AND DEMENTIA
DELIRIUM

Delirium is an *acute* brain syndrome. Key features that help distinguish it from traditional psychiatric illnesses are that it involves disorientation (in time, place or person) and a reduced level of consciousness. The level of consciousness may fluctuate with the underlying physical illness. The patient may also misinterpret the environment. Illusions are common. Hallucinations may occur. Delirium often occurs suddenly and is more likely to occur in vulnerable brains. *Delirium tremens* (or DTs) is an acute organic brain syndrome which may occur three to five days after alcohol-dependent people stop drinking; that is, shortly after they have been admitted to hospital. The DTs are characterised by fearful illusions or occasionally hallucinations, classically of small creatures or figures (so-called Lilliputian hallucinations after the little people of Lilliput in *Gulliver's Travels*). The DTs is associated with a considerable mortality of 10% and requires careful medical management.

DEMENTIA

Dementia is a *chronic* brain syndrome. Disorientation is a likely feature, but not essential. The key feature is a history of progressive global cognitive decline over weeks and months. Inability to learn new material (loss of short-term memory) is seen as a hallmark of dementia. Dementia may be caused by a variety of cerebral and systemic diseases.

Dementia is often caused by Alzheimer's disease (accounts for 50–60% of cases) or dementia with Lewy bodies (accounts for 15–20%). Dementia caused by a succession of strokes is called multi-infarct dementia (accounts for 20–25% of cases).

In younger patients dementia may be produced by inherited conditions such as Huntington's chorea and Wilson's disease, infections such as HIV or the consequences of alcoholism.

A new case of dementia deserves a very full medical assessment to exclude treatable causes of dementia including a full history, thorough physical examination, blood and other investigations and additional assessments such as occupational therapy. Some clinical features tend to distinguish between causes – Alzheimer's is characterised by short-term memory loss, relentless progression, dysphasia, dyspraxia and behavioural changes such as wandering; Lewy body dementia involves Parkinsonism, marked sensitivity to antipsychotics and fluctuating alertness; vascular dementia shows a stepwise progression and is often associated with previous hypertensive disease. Huntington's disease presents early in the third to fifth decades and may be associated with unusual movements and psychotic symptoms. Prion diseases may have a very early onset and be rapid in their progression to death.

CEREBRAL DISORDER AND ORGANIC PSYCHIATRY: LEARNING POINTS

➤ Psychological symptoms may be caused by general stressors such as metabolic disease or specific stressors such as cerebral tumours.
➤ Some brains are made more vulnerable to stressors through neuronal loss or disease. A stressor may therefore produce cerebral dysfunction in one person that does not in another.
➤ Specific stressors produce symptoms according to the site of the lesion. There are some syndromes associated with certain cerebral lobes.
➤ Frontal lobe syndrome includes changes in personality, poor judgement, social

Table 2.1 Stresses that can induce cerebral disorder

Cerebrovascular insufficiency	Heart failure, e.g. rhythm disturbance or myocardial infarction
	Pneumonitis
	Obstructive airways disease
Infections	Direct CNS infections
	Viral, e.g. Epstein-Barr, Varicella zoster, HIV
	Bacterial, e.g. tuberculosis
	Fungal, e.g. cryptosporidium
	Protozoal, e.g. Entamoeba histolyticum
	Toxins produced by distant infection
Tumour	Primaries (such as meningiomas) and Secondaries (e.g. breast and lung)
Metabolic	Hypoglycaemia
	Hyperglycaemia
	Electrolyte disturbance, e.g. hyponatraemia
Endocrine	Hypothyroidism
	Hyperthyroidism
	Addisonian crisis
	Cushing's syndrome
	Parathyroid instability
Epilepsy	Auras and post-ictal phenomena
	Temporal lobe epilepsy
	Epileptogenic foci
Iatrogenic	Digoxin
	Histamine blockers
	Diuretics
	Beta-blockers and many other drugs in therapeutic and excess dosage
Other CNS	Space-occupying lesion, e.g. subdural haematoma
	Encephalitis
	Multiple sclerosis
	Huntington's disease
	Parkinson's disease

Note: Alcohol withdrawal and delirium tremens should always be considered as causes of delirium.

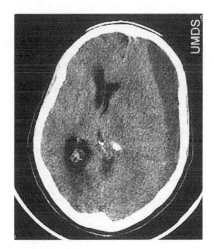

Figure 2.4 CT brain scan of patient showing crescent-shaped chronic subdural haematoma (Image courtesy of AC Downie, Victoria Infirmary, Glasgow)

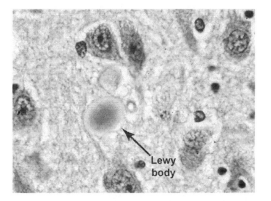

Figure 2.5 Micrograph of brain tissue with Lewy Body (Image courtesy of Kondi Wong, Armed Forces Institute of Pathology)

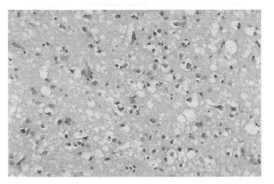

Figure 2.6 Micrograph of brain tissue showing spongiform appearance of Creutzfeldt-Jakob Disease (CJD) (Image courtesy of Centres for Disease Control and Prevention, National Centre for Infectious Diseases (NCID))

Table 2.2 Potential causes of apparent dementia

Neurodegenerative disorders	Senile dementia of the Alzheimer's type (SDAT)
	Lewy body dementia
	Creutzfeldt-Jakob disease and other prion diseases
	Pick's disease
	Parkinson's disease
	Huntington's disease
Vascular causes	Multi-infarct dementia
	Strokes
	Subdural haematoma
Auto-immune and inflammatory	Systemic lupus erythematosus (SLE)
	Multiple sclerosis
Head injury	Repeated head trauma, e.g. in boxers
Infection	Neurosyphilis, Lyme disease, HIV, post-encephalitis
Metabolic and nutritional	Chronic uraemia
	Wilson's disease
	Liver failure
	Hypoxia
	Anaemia (iron, vitamin B12 and folate insufficiency)
Endocrine	Hypothyroidism
	Cushing's syndrome
	Hypopituitarism
	Adrenal insufficiency
Anatomical/space occupying lesions	Primary tumours
	Normal pressure hydrocephalus
	Cerebral secondaries
Toxic	Carbon monoxide
	Heavy metals
	Alcohol and organic solvents
	Organophosphates

ESSENTIAL NOTES

Delirium	Acute, fluctuating level of consciousness associated with disorientation in time, place, person and misperceptions such as illusions or abnormal experiences such as visual or somatic hallucinations. May be associated with fear and anxiety. Patients may attempt to escape from upper floor windows, moving cars, etc.
Dementia	Chronic brain syndrome producing global cognitive changes – loss of recognition, memory, spatial perception and skills and so on. Problems with disinhibited behaviour, mood changes, hallucinations, etc. may also occur.
Pick's disease	Dementia in 50+ age group associated with atrophy of frontal and temporal lobes – producing personality change, nominal aphasia, perseveration and memory problems. 'Knife-blade' atrophy of gyri and Pick's bodies important to pathology.
Huntington's disease	Autosomal dominant condition affecting chromosome 4 – onset aged 30+, so often after they have started families. Genetic testing possible. Occasional sporadic cases.
Alcohol withdrawal	Onset often within 12 hours after stopping alcohol. Tremor, anxiety, sweating, nausea and withdrawal fits may occur.
Delirium tremens	Onset three to five days after stopping alcohol. Visual hallucinations prominent. Disorientation. Mortality 10%+. Support using benzodiazepine, rehydration, management of electrolyte disturbances, addition of thiamine and high dose vitamin therapy. Monitor for development of any seizures.
Creutzfeldt-Jakob disease	Early onset prion-related dementia with aggressive 'new variant' since mid-1990s associated with bovine spongiform encephalopathy (BSE). Spongiform histology of brain tissue in humans too. Median CJD age of onset 68 years, variant Creutzfeldt-Jakob disease (vCJD) about 28. Some teenage cases of vCJD described. EEG may show characteristic changes in some cases. Death more rapid than in other dementias (six months to two years). CJD as a whole responsible for 50–100 deaths per year in UK. www.cjd.ed.ac.uk/
Normal pressure hydrocephalus	Treatable cause of dementia. Occurs in 70+ age group. Dilatation of ventricular system seen on CT. Unsteady gait, nystagmus and urinary incontinence may be associated. Treatment involves ventriculoperitoneal shunting.
Korsakoff's syndrome	Late chronic complication of alcohol abuse and concomitant thiamine deficiency. Sometime called Wernicke-Korsakoff syndrome or amnesic syndrome. Loss of short-term memory, but without global cognitive decline or altered consciousness. Haemorrhages in the mamillary bodies and in walls of the third ventricle.
Wernicke's encephalitis	Acute complication of thiamine deficiency in alcohol abuse. Delirium-altered consciousness with disorientation, confabulation, nystagmus, glove and stocking neuropathy, ophthalmoplegia/lateral nerve palsy, ataxia.

(continued)

Neurosyphilis	Syphilis is a sexually transmitted disease (STD) caused by the bacterium *Treponema pallidum*. The old term, general paralysis of the insane (GPI), encompassed a chronic grandiose psychotic illness (associated with later cognitive decline) which, pre-antibiotic therapy, may have accounted for up to 10% of old asylum inpatients. Characteristic signs include Argyll-Robertson pupils. Neurosyphilis may present to psychiatrists. Early neurosyphilis has also been seen in HIV patients. Screening tests include Rapid Plasma Reagin (RPR) and Venereal Disease Research Laboratory (VDRL) tests. Treatment is Penicillin G iv every four hours or continuously for 14 days. The incidence of new cases of syphilis has been rising every year since 2000. Incidence of congenital syphilis is also rising.
Cerebral SLE	SLE is nine times more common in women than men. SLE may account for 1% of new cases of psychosis. May present with depression and hallucinations.
Thyroid disorder	Hypothyroidism can cause a partially reversible dementia – associated with depression, psychomotor slowing, deafness, dry and thinning hair, loss of eyebrows, hypothermia, heart failure, bradycardia, slow reflexes and other symptoms and signs. Hyperthyroidism can be associated with mania and persecutory psychosis, tachycardia, exophthalmos, weight loss, heat intolerance, atrial fibrillation, etc. In both conditions the need for psychiatric medication may continue even after thyroid hormone level correction.
Addison's disease	Depression, weight loss, malaise and apathy, loss of body hair, vitiligo.
Cushing's disease	Paranoid psychosis and depression, 'lemon-on-sticks' appearance, purple striae. Increased glucocorticoid levels.
HIV	Can present with features of encephalitis, and AIDS dementia. Opportunistic and other infections (Cryptococcus, fungi, Toxoplasma) may also trigger untoward referral to psychiatry.
Porphyria	Acute presentations may present with depression, mania and psychosis. Delirium, vomiting and constipation may help doctor spot that psychiatric presentation is unusual. Vincent van Gogh and George III may have suffered.
Wilson's disease	Also known as hepatolenticular degeneration. Abnormal copper metabolism leads to copper deposition in liver, cornea (leading to classic brown Kayser-Fleischer rings) and brain (basal ganglia deposition producing abnormal movements). Dementia and personality deterioration noted. Treatment with lifelong use of chelating agents such as D-penicillamine or trientine hydrochloride.
Multiple sclerosis	Demyelination may occur in CNS white matter with intellectual decline, mood abnormalities such as euphoria or depression and frank psychosis.

SCREENING FOR DEMENTIA: MINI-MENTAL STATE EXAMINATION

The Mini-Mental State Examination (MMSE) is a screening test for dementia. The MMSE generates a score out of 30. The normative scores vary according to sex and age over 65. Scores lower than the predicted 'normal' scores indicate possible cognitive problems.

Mean normative scores on MMSE in population without dementia					
Age	65–9	70–4	75–9	80–4	85+
Male	28	28	27	27	26
Female	28	28	27	26	25

Function area	Test item	Item description	Insert patient score	Available points
Orientation	1	What is the year?		1
		Season?		1
		Date?		1
		Day?		1
		Month?		1
	2	Where are we?		
		State?		1
		County?		1
		Town or city?		1
		Hospital?		1
		Floor?		1
Registration/ Memory	3	Name three objects, taking one second to say each, then ask the patient to name all three after you have said them. Give one point for each correct answer. Repeat the answer until patient learns all three.		3
Attention and Concentration	4	Serial 7s. Give one point for each correct answer. Stop after five answers. Alternatively, spell WORLD backwards.		5
Recall	5	Ask name of three objects learned in q. 3. Give one point for each correct answer.		3

(continued)

Language	6	Point to a pencil and a watch. Have the patient name them as you point.	2
	7	Have the patient repeat 'No ifs ands or buts'.	1
	8	Have the patient follow a three-stage command: 'Take a paper in your right hand. Fold the paper in half. Put the paper on the floor.'	3
	9	Have the patient read and obey the following: 'CLOSE YOUR EYES'. (Write it in large letters.)	1
	10	Have the patient write a sentence of his/her choice. (The sentence should contain a subject and an object and should make sense. Ignore spelling errors when scoring.)	1
	11	Enlarge the design printed here to 1.5 cm per side and have the patient copy it. (Give one point if all sides and angles are preserved and if the intersecting sides form a quadrangle).	1

Total out of 30

Reproduced with permission from JC Anthony, L Le Resche, U Niaz, MR Von Korff and MF Folstein. Limits of the 'Mini mental State' as a screening test for dementia and delirium among hospital patients. *Psychological Medicine*. 1982; **12**: 397–408.

disinhibition, lability of mood, poor planning and loss of abstract thought. It may mimic psychiatric illness like hypomania.

➤ Delirium (acute organic brain syndrome) is an acute brain dysfunction which involves impaired consciousness, disorientation and misperception of the world around the person.

➤ Dementia (chronic organic brain syndrome) is a chronic global deterioration of cognitive abilities occurring in clear consciousness.

➤ Features which should alert the doctor to organic brain syndromes are disorientation, fluctuating or impaired consciousness, illusions, visual hallucinations and intermittent periods of lucidity.

➤ Treatment of organic brain disease is by establishing the cause rather than sedation. Delirium may herald the patient's imminent demise – so beware.

CASE HISTORY 1

The family doctor was summoned by Mrs Jones' daughter at two o'clock in the morning. The daughter met the doctor at the front door of her mother's house. She told the doctor how her 78-year-old mother had been unwell for the past week with flu. In the last two days her mother had stayed in the bedroom all day, but had become agitated as night drew on. Mrs Jones had phoned her daughter (who lived two roads away) at 2 am the previous day complaining that a burglar was trying to get into bed with her. When her daughter and son-in-law hurried round to help they found that there was no sign of a burglar and no sign of a break-in. Mrs Jones had appeared confused and called her daughter by her own sister's name. She had been very restless through the night, but as dawn came she appeared less disturbed.

The daughter had called the doctor in the early hours of this morning because her mother had phoned her at midnight saying that a black mass was being held in the house opposite. When her daughter arrived she saw that Mrs Jones was talking about a man working on his car in the garage across the road. Mrs Jones described the lights in the garage as 'candles held by witches', who she said were 'chanting swear words'. The daughter had to wrestle her frightened mother back into bed.

The daughter was very worried because her mother had never been like this before and had never seen a psychiatrist in her life.

What are the key features that point towards an acute organic brain syndrome?
The history gives a probable stressor – a recent infection – possibly a bacterial infection superimposed on influenza. Mrs Jones' age makes her brain more vulnerable and as her consciousness fluctuates she becomes disorientated and misperceives reality. She perceives the man working on his car across the road as a 'black mass'. This is an example of a misinterpretation and may suggest an *illusion* rather than a hallucination.

What are the main points to consider in this patient's management?
If there is an underlying bacterial infection this will need treatment, but the doctor will need to exclude other physical illnesses as well. A physical examination and investigations such

as a chest X-ray, full blood count, urea and electrolytes, random serum glucose and ECG would all be useful. Admission to hospital would be appropriate.

CASE HISTORY 2

Mr Dowling, 65, was brought to the accident and emergency department early one Saturday morning. He had been depressed for several weeks and had been talking about the pointlessness of life. Late on Friday night he had begun confusing his wife with his sister and talking about events that had happened 20 years ago as if they were only yesterday. He had suddenly become very frightened and said that a man with very long legs was standing in the living room beckoning him. His wife had been alarmed because she was in the room at the time and couldn't see what her husband was staring at. The psychiatry registrar was called to see the patient and took a careful history. The most important point in the history as far as the registrar was concerned was the fact that Mr Dowling had just been put on a tricyclic antidepressant by his family doctor.

Is this severe depression or delirium? What features are not typical of a severe depression and more typical of delirium?
Although it is possible for people with depression to become psychotic and have hallucinatory experiences, it is important to distinguish a psychotic depression from a delirium overlying a long-standing depression. The important points are the sudden change in the illness – Mr Dowling suddenly begins to be disorientated (mistaking his wife for his sister) and suddenly begins to have visual hallucinations. Visual hallucinations are strongly suggestive of an organic state. Taken together with the prescription of a drug that day would suggest a possible link between the two.

What is the likely cause of the delirium?

Tricyclic antidepressants affect various neurotransmitter systems including noradrenergic, serotonergic, histaminergic and cholinergic systems. The effects on cholinergic systems can induce hallucinatory experiences. It is obviously important to distinguish the delirium from a depressive psychosis, because in the former you would discontinue the antidepressants whereas in the latter you would continue them (and probably perpetuate the delirium).

CASE HISTORY 3

Emma, 19, came to see her family doctor because occasionally she had episodes where she felt very unwell. The episodes started with rumblings in her stomach and palpitations. She often felt very frightened because these would go on for a few minutes, then she would see a blinding flash of light. Once she had heard someone talking to her for a few seconds. The voice had said, in a very strong voice, 'FEAR IS THE KEY!' She had been so frightened that she couldn't tell anyone and had gone on regardless, hoping that it wouldn't happen again. Unfortunately, the voice came back two weeks later after she had been out all night at a party. This time it said, 'It is nobler to suffer silently.' After these extraordinary experiences Emma felt very tired and often found that she could not concentrate on her school work. Her family were worried because her university exams were coming up and they said that sometimes she seemed so 'vague'. Emma was very worried she was 'going mad'.

What pointers are there to an organic illness?

There is a fluctuating history. Most of the time Emma is well, but the illness happens to her in discrete episodes. The episodes begin with autonomic symptoms like palpitations and gastro-intestinal rumbling, focus in brief visual or auditory hallucinations, and are followed by a variable period of lassitude and reduced consciousness. This episodic history is not like the mainly continuous symptoms in schizophrenia, but is more suggestive of epilepsy. Temporal lobe epilepsy (TLE) often produces symptoms suggestive of schizophrenia, but in this episodic way. Like other epilepsies, TLE is more common when people are psychologically stressed (Emma is coming up for her exams) and when they are physiologically stressed (e.g. when Emma is tired or maybe even hypoglycaemic after the party and alcohol).

There is also a possibility that Emma may have been experimenting with drugs, and drug-induced experiences would have to be excluded by a careful history and a relevant drug screen.

Emma's management would include a physical examination, routine blood investigations and an electroencephalogram (EEG) to try to confirm the diagnosis of TLE. Sometimes TLE is a difficult diagnosis to confirm and a referral to a neurologist would be appropriate. If the diagnosis of TLE appears to be correct, advice about lifestyle and prescription of an antiepileptic drug like carbamazepine may be effective.

CASE HISTORIES: LEARNING POINTS

➤ The management of organic brain syndromes relies upon a full history, physical examination and a range of investigations. Several causes may be present simultaneously.

➤ A careful drug history may reveal items that depress consciousness or act on specific neurotransmitters that may provoke cerebral disorder (e.g. dopamine agonists or anticholinergics).

➤ Temporal lobe epilepsy may induce various psychotic symptoms including hallucinations. The course of the history is usually episodic rather than continuous. An EEG may help in the diagnosis. Antiepileptic drugs are the treatment of choice.

EPILEPSY

Epilepsy involves a recurrent tendency to brain seizures – abnormal paroxysmal electrical discharges. Seizures can be focal or generalised without focal onset. Focal seizures can include simple motor or sensory seizures which do not impair conscious or complex partial seizures which do affect consciousness and may go on to generalise. Generalised seizures may include absence seizures or the classic tonic-clonic seizures.

Seizures may be preceded by an aura – particularly temporal lobe partial seizures. These auras may involve olfactory, gustatory, auditory, visual or somatic hallucinations, including epigastric 'churning'. Other disturbances of experience can occur such as *déjà vu*, *jamais vu*, depersonalisation and derealisation. Occasionally, affective changes such as fear, rage or intense euphoria may occur. The patient may then go on to fit, but usually only the aura is remembered by the patient. A post-ictal phase of confusion, tiredness and listlessness may follow.

Between fits, patients with epilepsy are statistically more prone to depression, deliberate self-harm and suicide.

Epilepsy is usually managed by the neurologist, but psychiatrists may sometimes be involved. Psychotropic drugs alter the fit threshold and care must be exercised when choosing antidepressants or other drugs in patients prone to epilepsy. Similarly, anti-epileptic drugs may alter the metabolism of drugs used in psychiatry.

HEAD INJURY

The late effects of acquired brain injuries, say resulting from closed head injuries from road traffic accidents or assaults, may present to neuropsychiatrists. Acquired brain injuries can affect cognitive performance, affective stability and personality with devastating consequences for the individual and their family.

The functional implications of a brain injury can be assessed by considering the duration of the post-traumatic amnesia (PTA) – that is,

the time between the injury and the return of normal day-to-day memory – reasonable functional return occurs when the PTA is up to a few days. Longer than this and there may be severe consequences for psychological functioning. Complications may arise if there was any concomitant brain hypoxia and a dementing process may begin after such injuries.

After the head injury an initial agitated phase of delirium with misidentification of people around may occur, followed by resolution of delirium and the onset of more chronic effects such as depression, anxiety, irritability, poor concentration and insomnia (post-concussional syndrome). Lasting cognitive impairment may follow frontal injury with disinhibition, loss of drive and difficulty in planning and sequencing events (dysexecutive syndrome). Post-traumatic stress disorder (PTSD) can also present.

SELF-ASSESSMENT
CASES

Read through the three cases that follow. As you read them ask yourself which illnesses might fit with these clinical presentations. Ask yourself how you would investigate these cases.

The answer section gives the actual diagnoses.

1   Mrs Alberta, 60, had been finding it difficult to concentrate on books and newspapers for a few weeks. Her thinking somehow felt different to her – less clear – and she was becoming much more forgetful. Her daughter had noticed how tired and sluggish Mrs Alberta had become. From being an active pensioner who had helped in the local church coffee shop every day, Mrs Alberta had become a tired old lady who preferred to sit alone at home by the fire.

2   Mr Williams, 46, was admitted to hospital after his wife had to call the police to their home. That day he had refused to get dressed and had been running naked

around the house making unwanted sexual advances to his wife. His comments to her had been uncharacteristically coarse, harsh and threatening. When the police arrived he stood naked before them, shouted swear words at them and tried to sexually assault the woman police officer. In the preceding month he had lost his job as a bank manager because of some bad loan judgements he had made and some indiscreet comments to a female customer. His wife was bewildered and distraught because her husband of 20 years had always been such a mild-mannered and polite man. It was as if his whole character had changed.

3 Jemima, 26, a staff nurse, had three short-lived episodes of auditory hallucinations. Each time had been when she was working a double shift at the nursing home she helped run. Each time she had been on duty for over 12 hours without rest or a food break. The voices she had heard were marked auditory hallucinations, which had lasted for only a few minutes, but had really frightened Jemima. Before these episodes she reported feeling faint for a few minutes and also experiencing the sensation of *déjà vu*.

MCQs

1 Recognised features of frontal lobe lesions include:
   A perseveration
   B disinhibition
   C visual agnosia
   D homonymous hemianopia
   E receptive aphasia

2 Organic causes that may induce depressed mood include:
   A hypothyroidism
   B hyperthyroidism
   C Cushing's disease
   D bronchial carcinoma
   E cerebrovascular accident

3 Dementia-like syndromes can be caused by:
   A hypothyroidism
   B vitamin B12 deficiency
   C acute alcohol withdrawal
   D neurosyphilis
   E Huntington's chorea

Cases answers

1 Hypothyroidism. (Hypothyroidism is a reversible cause of dementia. Physical symptoms such as tiredness, constipation, mental and physical slowness and cold intolerance are suggestive of the illness.)
2 Frontal lobe tumour. (There are features of the frontal lobe syndrome – a description of personality change, coarsening of behaviour and disinhibition. Hypomania would be a reasonable differential diagnosis.)
3 Temporal lobe epilepsy. (There is a history of discrete short-lived psychotic episodes occurring when the patient is tired and possibly hypoglycaemic. *Déjà vu* is a common TLE symptom.)

MCQ answers

1 A=T, B=T, C=F, D=F, E=F.
2 All true.
3 A=T, B=T, C=F, D=T, E=T.

EXPLORATIONS

Use the suggested reading and references to find out how to answer the following:

LINKS WITH MEDICAL HISTORY

➤ Who was Phineas Gage? What horrific accident helped lead to the theory of cerebral localisation?
➤ Who were Broca and Wernicke? What were their contributions to our understanding of speech? How did they make their discoveries and how did they analyse them?
➤ What venereally transmitted infectious disease was responsible for many of the chronically mentally ill patients of the 19th century? What symptoms did they have and how was the neuropathology related to these symptoms?

LINKS WITH MEDICINE

- ➤ What are the main clinical features of systemic lupus erythematosus (SLE)?
- ➤ What is the underlying pathology in SLE?
- ➤ How does the pathology link with the clinical features?
- ➤ What percentage of patients with SLE have psychiatric symptoms?
- ➤ How does the pathology of SLE link with these symptoms?

LINKS WITH GENETICS

- ➤ What inherited condition may present with psychosis in the third and fourth decades?
- ➤ How is it inherited?
- ➤ What can be done in terms of genetic counselling for relatives?
- ➤ How might relatives of the patient be affected by learning the results of predictive genetic testing?

LINKS WITH PAEDIATRICS

- ➤ How common is schizophrenia in children?
- ➤ If you were to assess a 10-year-old boy who had a sudden onset of visual hallucinations and who had tried to fly out of a first floor window, what would you suspect as the cause?
- ➤ What questions would you ask the boy and the boy's parents?

LINKS WITH PUBLIC HEALTH AND OCCUPATIONAL MEDICINE

- ➤ What heavy metals can affect brain function?
- ➤ What public health initiatives aim to reduce the exposure of children to heavy metals?

- ➤ Workers in which industries may suffer CNS effects from heavy metals?
- ➤ Which workers may suffer cognitive effects from organophosphates?
- ➤ Which causes of dementia are transmissible diseases? How are they transmitted?

LINKS WITH NEUROLOGY

- ➤ During the physical examination of a patient, what features on examination of the nervous system might suggest a cerebral lesion?

LINKS WITH PSYCHOLOGY

- ➤ What psychological tests might predict the presence of, and site of, brain lesions?

FURTHER READING AND REFERENCES
TEXTS

Arnadottir G. *The Brain and Behaviour: assessing cortical dysfunction through activities of daily living.* St Louis: CV Mosby; 1990.

Asbury AK, McKhann GM, McDonald WI, Goadsby PJ, McArthur JC, editors. *Diseases of the Nervous System: clinical neuroscience and therapeutic principles.* 3rd ed. Cambridge: Cambridge University Press; 2002.

Gleitman H. *Psychology.* 3rd ed. New York: WW Norton; 1993.

Lindesay J, Macdonald A, Starke T. *Delirium in the Elderly.* Oxford: Oxford University Press; 1990.

Lishman WA. *Organic Psychiatry.* 3rd ed. Oxford: Oxford Medical Publications; 1998.

PAPER

Adams F. Emergency intravenous sedation of the delirious medically ill patient. *Journal of Clinical Psychiatry,* 1988; **49**(Suppl. 12): 22–6.

CHAPTER 3

Mood disorders

Mood disorders (sometimes called affective disorders) involve severe and persistent disturbances of mood that endure despite the influence of external events.

CONTENTS

CLASSIFICATION OF MOOD DISORDERS

Everybody's mood varies according to events in the world around them. We are happy when we achieve something or when we are enjoying a friend's company. We are saddened when we fail a test or lose something. When people are sad they sometimes say that they are 'depressed', but the clinical depressions that are seen by doctors differ from the low mood brought on by everyday setbacks. Clinically, important disturbances of mood are known as mood disorders (or affective disorders). Mood disorders are more severe and more persistent than simple sadness or happiness.

In mood disorders our normal emotions are polarised into more severe forms. Happiness can become mania and sadness can become profound despair or depression. This polarisation can be called a bipole, with mania at one extreme and depression at the other.

Patients who suffer with repeated episodes of depression have recurrent depressive disorder. When patients suffer manic episodes and depressive episodes they are said to have bipolar disorder (*see* Figure 3.1).

The American classification system (DSM) echoes Kraepelin's original idea that the psychotic disorders broke down into either schizophrenia or manic depression. Based on reviews of available research, the DSM system recognises a bipolar (I) disorder and a bipolar (II) disorder. Bipolar (I) disorder involves recurrent episodes of depression (without hypomania) and bipolar (II) disorder involves recurrent episodes of mania and depression. The nomenclature using numbers as differentiators is clumsy, however, and somewhat removed from the conditions it seeks to describe.

However you classify bipolar mood disorder, its episodic nature may mean that it is diagnosed only long after it has started and long after its devastating effects on careers and relationships have begun. Some research suggests that firm diagnosis by professionals may be delayed until five years after the disorder's onset.

Depressive episodes can be classified into mild, moderate and severe types and classified as being with or without psychotic symptoms.

A condition where the mood is persistently low, but which does not quite fulfil all the criteria for a depressive episode, is sometimes called *dysthymia*.

Major depression is relatively common. Community studies have found prevalence rates of between 5 and 20%. About 10% of people aged over 65 have a major depressive episode at any one time. The incidence of depression seems to be higher in women than men and in urban rather than rural settings. Figure 3.2 shows how many cases of depression

MOOD DISORDER IN HISTORY

Concepts about what mental illness is do change with time, but physicians have always recognised there have been mood disorders like melancholia and mania, even if they disagreed about the nature of those illnesses. Writing before Christ was born, Aretaeus of Cappadocia noted that mania and depression might follow one another. In 1850 Falret of the Salpêtrière Hospital in Paris lectured about '*la folie circulaire*', an alternating pattern of mania and melancholia. For a while after this there was a unitary concept of psychosis – that all psychoses were essentially the same disorder.

When trying to classify mental illness on a scientific analysis of a range of symptoms from hundreds of patients it was the German psychiatrist Emil Kraepelin (1856–1926) who differentiated schizophrenia from mood disorders. Interestingly, Kraepelin tended to categorise mania and depression into one disorder – manic depression.

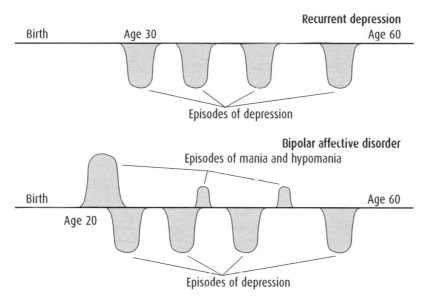

Figure 3.1 The lifetime course of affective disorders

there are in a small general practice of 3000 patients. You can also see how much of these illnesses are detected by family doctors and how many are treated by psychiatrists.

COST BURDEN OF AFFECTIVE DISORDERS

Mental ill health has been estimated to cost about £8.4 billion a year in terms of absenteeism alone. Presenteeism (which is the term for the costs of inefficiency by employees at work) associated with mental illness may cost a larger sum, estimated at £15.1 billion a year. This is without adding in other costs such as healthcare, benefit costs and so on.

The overall cost of depression in 2000 was estimated to be about £9 billion. Most of this was occupational and social cost. The NHS costs were £8 million for primary care attendances, £51 million for secondary healthcare and £310 million for medication. The costs of bipolar disorder was £2.1 billion in 1999/2000. Ten per cent of the costs was due to healthcare and 86% was due to unemployment.

DEPRESSION

Depression is often accompanied by slowing of thought and biological features of depression altogether unlike everyday sadness.

Crying is a frequent symptom, although some individuals are reluctant to admit this, and others feel so depressed it is as if they have 'gone beyond crying'.

Suicidal ideas occur in most depressed people, and asking about these is a crucial aspect of their assessment. Depressed patients often find it a relief to talk about these ideas with their doctor. Asking about suicidal ideas is a sequential process, beginning with questions about the severity of the low mood, then asking about if the patient has ever felt that life is not worth living, following this by enquiring whether the patient has ever felt like ending their own life, and finally assessing whether the patient has any particular plans in mind.

On mental state examination depressed patients may appear unkempt or untidy. Depressed people feel bad about themselves and also lack the motivation to care for their appearance. The normally appearance conscious person may have stopped combing their

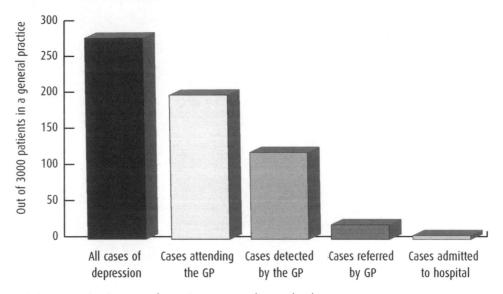

Figure 3.2 Depression in general practice: one year's case load

hair and washing as often as before. Women may stop using make-up and men may stop shaving. When you interview someone who is depressed they may sit dejectedly, gazing down at the floor. You may notice that they do not make eye contact with you and that they fail to smile in response to greetings and jokes, but are preoccupied and serious in manner. Their movements may be minimal or slowed to such an extent that they are prepared to sit alone brooding in a chair, or lying in bed for hours during the day. They may appear unusually thin, having lost weight, because of a poor appetite. Occasionally, the typical picture of psychomotor retardation may be replaced by a restless agitation and distraught displays of weeping.

Their speech may be minimal, monosyllabic, or they may even be mute. Depressed speech lacks spontaneity and variety and be spoken in a monotone. The facial expression may show sadness, anxiety, or sometimes a masklike absence of emotion sometimes described as flattened affect.

When you ask about thoughts and preoccupations the depressed patient may describe a catalogue of worries about money, close relationships or the health of themselves or others.

Rarely, they may say that there are almost no thoughts in their head because their thoughts have slowed down so much. Depressed people think little of themselves, their abilities or their achievements. They feel guilty over past misdemeanours; helpless and hopeless; that the world is a bad place and that the future is exceptionally bleak. Occasionally, depression becomes so severe that it takes on a psychotic quality so that hallucinations and delusions, consistent with low mood, manifest themselves. Hallucinations are characteristically unpleasant. Auditory hallucinations, usually in the second person, are derogatory, e.g. 'You're a fat cow!', 'You're so evil you should be put to death'. Auditory hallucinations are more common than hallucinations in other modalities. Sometimes olfactory hallucinations occur, e.g. a patient smelling rotting flesh, but such hallucinations may suggest an underlying organic cause which should be excluded such as a frontal lobe tumour. Abnormal sensory experiences are rare, however, and it is more usual for sensory experiences to be diminished if anything, so that the world becomes grey and unpleasantly quiet, and food seems uncharacteristically bland.

If present, delusions are usually secondary to low self-esteem, guilt, anxiety, fear or hallucinations. Delusions of guilt are sometimes extreme: 'I am responsible for the AIDS epidemic'. Delusions of ill health, sometimes called hypochondriacal delusions, may involve a conviction that the individual is riddled with cancer, when there is no objective evidence of carcinoma. Often there is a theme of deserved punishment to such delusions: 'My face is rotting away with venereal disease because of what I did when I was young.' An extreme bodily delusion is the nihilistic delusion, e.g. 'I have no bowels' or 'My head is emptied of its brains'. Delusions of poverty and infestation are other examples of depressive delusions.

Cognitive testing is often problematic. Depressed people find concentration particularly difficult, and although they are grossly orientated to time, place and person, tests of attention (such as serial 7s and the months of the year reversed) are poorly performed. Memory testing may suggest a short-term memory defect, but the apparently poor memory is often due to problems with registration and concentration rather than recall. Depression in the elderly can mimic dementia. This kind of problem is called a pseudodementia, and the apparent memory defect usually resolves once the depression has been treated.

CASE HISTORY 1

Janet Gordon was aged 35 when she lost her job as a manageress of a department store. At first she looked on her period of unemployment as an opportunity to try out activities she hadn't had time for before. She went hill walking and painting every day. Two months later she had lost interest in these things and was convinced that she would never work again, although she had an exemplary work record. Her sleep at night was poor and she had started going to bed during the day. Janet cried almost daily and had lost interest in the food she cooked. All food tasted bland, she said to her mother (who was concerned when she saw how much weight Janet had lost). At her mother's suggestion Janet went to her family doctor where she complained about how tired she always felt and asked for some sleeping tablets to help her sleep at night.

What biological features of depression are present?

Two clear features are Janet's lack of appetite (anorexia) and weight loss. We are told that her sleep was poor, but we need to know exactly what the sleep problem was before we can say whether this was early morning wakening.

What precipitated the depression?

Adverse life events such as exam failure, bereavement and job loss may precede the onset of depression. In Janet's case the onset of depression is gradual, coming on some weeks after the loss of her job. Sometimes the onset of depression is so gradual that it is difficult for the depressed individual to date exactly when the illness started and it is as if the depression has crept up on them, in which case it may only be apparent to others. Because the depression has become a way of life to the depressed person, only outsiders can see the illness for what it is. In Janet's case it is her mother who asks her to seek help.

How does Janet present her problem to her doctor?

Some people are wary of taking psychological symptoms to their doctor. They know that something is wrong with them, but consciously or unconsciously choose to take the symptoms that they feel doctors will be most interested in. Janet chooses to present her fatigue as her main problem and asks for sleeping tablets. Other depressed people will take bodily symptoms of anxiety and depression to their doctor – headaches, muscular aches and pains, tremors and palpitations for instance. Depressed people may be very concerned about their health and seek multiple physical investigations because they are sure there is some morbid physical cause for the wretched way they feel. In these cases the doctor must be very certain that there is no underlying physical problem before dismissing the depressed individual's concerns. It is possible for people to be depressed and physically ill. It is well documented that about a quarter of medical inpatients have some depressive symptoms.

CASE HISTORY 2

Alan Benson was a 52-year-old man who was brought to the accident and emergency department by his son. Alan had tried to hang himself from the stair banisters at the family home, but fortunately the clothes line that he had chosen to hang himself with had broken under his weight. When he was seen by the psychiatrist, Alan had a red ligature mark around his throat from the noose. He was staring at a fixed point on the floor. Every now and then he would groan deeply and whisper to himself. He kept repeating the words 'I'm for it . . . I'm for it now'. He would not make eye contact with the doctor and initially refused to answer questions.

His son said that the previous week Alan had stopped going to work as a bailiff after he found out that his wife was having an affair. He had watched her obsessively for two days, not letting her out of his sight. Then a few days ago he had taken to his bed, and lain there for hours and hours not moving, not speaking, not eating and not drinking. He had talked about how everything was his fault and had at times appeared to be pleading with an unseen person to forgive him. He felt that he must have committed some unpardonable crime and that he should now be punished.

Armed with this information the psychiatrist talked to Mr Benson again. This time

---

Mr Benson replied, albeit only briefly. He said that God was telling him that his wife had had to find another man because her husband had been so evil. He confessed that he had once had an affair himself many years before, and that God had told him in the last week that He had punished Mr Benson with a slow-growing syphilis. His wife could be spared from the syphilis only if he killed himself. Once he was dead his wife could begin a clean life with another man.

What evidence is there that this is a psychotic illness?

There is evidence of severe psychomotor retardation in the history where Mr Benson takes to his bed and lies there immobile. The retardation is so severe that Mr Benson sounds almost stuporose. Still more characteristic of psychosis are the references to auditory hallucinations (pleading with an unseen person; God telling him about his guilt and punishment), and a secondary delusion of ill-health (syphilis). The patient's insight has been lost.

How high is the risk of this patient attempting suicide again?

The risk is very high indeed, because the psychotic depression is still unchecked and Mr Benson's insight is lacking. The hallucinations he hears tell him that his wife will only be saved if he dies, and since he has just tried to hang himself he obviously finds it impossible to resist these ideas. Without adequate treatment another suicide attempt seems exceedingly likely. If Mr Benson were to attempt to leave the hospital it would be necessary to detain, assess and treat him under the relevant mental health legislation. While he was in hospital he would need to be watched very carefully (close or 1:1 observations) in case he tried to kill himself again on the ward.

LEARNING POINTS: DEPRESSION

➤ Depressive illness affects 5–10% of the adult population.

> Depressive illness in the community is largely untreated, because patients generally do not seek medical help, and of those that do seek help only about 60% of those that see their family doctor are recognised by them as suffering from depression.

> Depressive illness is treatable – over 80% of cases can be resolved with adequate treatment.

> Treatment may include antidepressants (selective serotonin re-uptake inhibitors: SSRIs) or tricyclic antidepressants for moderate to severe depression, ECT (for severe or delusional depression) or cognitive behavioural therapy (CBT) for mild to moderate depression.

> *Always* ask depressed patients about suicidal ideation and suicide plans.

MANIA

Elation, overactivity and insomnia are the classical features of mania. Society has never tolerated the mentally ill very well, and perhaps because society finds manic patients particularly disruptive, such patients may reach the attention of the police or other civic agencies relatively early. Even so there may be a delay before people begin to realise that illness is playing a part. People can acquire convictions and a series of failed relationships before a doctor is ever involved to even start to make a diagnosis.

Mania implies the presence of a bipolar disorder and somewhere along the line depressive episodes are likely to affect the sufferer, with an increased risk of suicide.

Less severe presentations of mania are termed hypomania, and these are more common. The diagnosis of mania is reserved for the more severe case.

Mania has an earlier age of onset than depression (late adolescence/early adulthood) and more often has a family history. If one of a pair of identical twins suffers with bipolar disorder there is an 80% lifetime chance that the other twin will eventually suffer with the same illness, indicating a strong genetic component.

Mania can occur for the first time late in life, but it is then vital to exclude other physical causes such as hyperthyroidism or frontal lobe damage (perhaps due to a stroke).

A mnemonic proposed to guide the diagnosis of bipolar disorder is DIGFAST:

> **d**istractibility
> **i**ndiscretion and insomnia
> **g**randiosity
> **f**light of ideas
> **a**ctivity increase
> **s**peech pressure
> **t**houghtlessness

('I' could also stand for irritability).

Just as there is a persistent form of low mood termed *dysthymia* (not amounting to clinical depression), there is a mild form of alternating mood that corresponds to bipolar affective disorder. This persistent instability of mood involves many short-lived episodes of depression and elation and is called *cyclothymia*, from the cycling nature of the mood. A few weeks' period of happiness and high productivity is replaced by a few weeks of low mood, low self-confidence and social withdrawal. Cyclothymia does not tend to come to medical attention, because of its mild nature.

CASE HISTORY 3

Elizabeth was a 27-year-old doctor who worked as a trainee in primary care. She had always been very conscientious about her work and was keen to progress in her chosen career. Her practice colleagues had noticed a slight change in her over the previous days. She had seemed very cheerful indeed and full of good humour, but one patient had complained to the receptionist that 'the young lady doctor was giggling when I told her about my infection'. Her colleagues assumed that perhaps Elizabeth was in high spirits, because she was due to go on an all-expenses-paid conference at the weekend.

At the conference she made friends very freely and seemed very attached to a young doctor she had never met before. People in the audience around her were unnerved by the loudness of her laugh, however, and became embarrassed when she seemed to laugh rather too long after one speaker's presentation. Someone next to her whispered to her to be quiet. Elizabeth put out her tongue at this colleague and flounced out of the lecture room, slamming the door behind her.

That night she was sighted in the bar, drinking heavily and leering at a salesman who was running his hand up her thigh. They disappeared off to her room, but she was seen an hour later talking intimately to a different man in the coffee lounge. Her voice was loud and she was making very suggestive remarks that could be heard by the whole company.

The next day she was not to be seen in the conference room. Some delegates wondered what had become of her, and made some cruel remarks about her.

The lecture by the local Professor of Primary Care (a gentleman that Elizabeth was hoping to get an important research post with) was presenting a talk on 'Screening for Diabetes in Primary Care'. The first slide of his computer presentation was just onscreen when a naked figure rushed from the side of the stage and hugged the eminent professor. There was a slight struggle while he tried to disentangle himself from Elizabeth. By this time she had removed the lapel mike from him and shouted into it: 'It's not screening in primary care you want, but screaming in primary care' – and so saying she began to scream into the microphone to the discomfort of the bewildered audience. A quick-thinking friend from Elizabeth's medical school days rushed onto the stage and, wrapping her in a coat, coaxed her offstage, and later took her to the hospital.

What features of mania did Elizabeth have?

The onset of the illness was during the week before the conference. Her patients noticed that she was less sympathetic to them, and even laughed at their troubles, suggesting a degree of disinhibition.

Her colleagues noticed that she was overly happy, but wrongly ascribed it to her forthcoming leave. At the conference itself Elizabeth becomes progressively disinhibited: talking loudly during presentations and later disrupting them by appearing naked. There is irritability (she storms out of the lecture theatre at one point) and some suggestion of promiscuity. An informant might be able to tell you about Elizabeth's normal behaviour, but her approach to strangers sounds both unusual and potentially dangerous.

What risks does Elizabeth run?

Elizabeth's judgement is impaired because she is disinhibited. Her sexual approaches to strangers leave her vulnerable to abuse, assault, rape, unwanted pregnancy, venereal disease and HIV infection. We may assume that such approaches are not her normal behaviour.

Her physical safety is of primary importance, but there are other risks – her unusual behaviour prior to the conference may lead her to lose her professional standing in the practice (a patient might make a formal complaint about her manner or actions) and her bizarre behaviour at the conference could destroy her long-term career hopes. It is not unusual for people with affective disorders to lose their jobs or their marital partners long before a diagnosis of mental illness is made and treatment begun. Although in this vignette we are not told whether Elizabeth has grandiose ideas, it is common for manic people to feel wealthier than they in fact are. Manic individuals may make rash business decisions and overspend, for instance ordering a new car when they have no real means of paying, or running up huge credit card bills.

Psychiatrists, with their knowledge of mental illness, must act to protect such ill individuals from the consequences of their temporarily impaired judgement.

CASE HISTORY 4

Mr Unwin, 56, presented to casualty having assaulted a police officer and having caused a disturbance in an Internet café. The doctor who was going to assess Mr Unwin heard him shouting and swearing loudly even before opening the door of the assessment room. The trainee psychiatrist introduced himself: 'Hello Mr Unwin? My name is Dr Brown . . .'

Mr Unwin interrupted, 'Brown, green, blue – what you going to do?' He paced the room, watched by the police constable who had escorted him to hospital. 'I've no time to waste, so make haste. I've got a hundred and one things to do, Dr Blue. A hundred and one Dalmatians to give to the nations. The nation's going to the dogs. I have a plan to make a million before supper and I will not put up with the likes of you Dr Blue. Come on, come on, speak up!' Mr Unwin himself spoke very rapidly indeed – so rapidly that it was hard to make out what he was saying. It was difficult for the doctor to get Mr Unwin to focus on any one issue, because he was so distractible. At one point the sound of an aeroplane coming from outside made the patient pause. 'It's not easy,' he said. 'Five hundred people on that jumbo. Rajah Airways – and I'm responsible for everyone. I'm responsible for keeping the plane in the air. It's so difficult being God – having to keep touch with everyone and everything – you can't even go to sleep.'

It transpired that Mr Unwin had not slept for three days. He had not been drinking, but had been found in a telephone box, beating the receiver against the glass. He had become frustrated after the television station that he had been phoning hung up on him. 'If they'd let me on the television I could have stopped the war in Africa,' he said.

What features of this case suggest a manic illness?

Mr Unwin speaks rudely to the doctor (he is disinhibited); he speaks rapidly (pressure of speech) and displays flight of ideas. He uses rhyming associations. There is ample evidence of grandiosity (he believes he can stop the war in Africa and is deluded that he is God). He also displays some irritability.

What might the differential diagnoses be?

The illness sounds like an acute one, but if there was evidence of personality change over time you might need to exclude a frontal lobe tumour or an endocrine cause like hyperthyroidism. Head injuries and toxic states due to drugs or infection might present atypically in this way. In older men with hypertension and no past psychiatric history the possibility of a cerebral infarction should be excluded. The trainee psychiatrist should therefore be alert for any signs of an altered level of consciousness.

What lines of enquiry would help you decide what the diagnosis was?

A past psychiatric history might reveal previous episodes of bipolar affective illness. An informant history would cover drug or alcohol use, physical ill health and recent personality change. A drug history might reveal whether lithium carbonate or antipsychotics have been used in the past, and whether poor compliance with medication is a cause of relapse or not.

What management issues are important?

Mr Unwin probably has poor insight given that he has been acting on his grandiose ideas (phoning up television stations) and may not believe that he is ill. If he does not believe that he is ill he may well refuse to come into hospital. Mental health law may need to be used to compel him to be admitted. Once admitted he will need a full physical examination and relevant investigations. Treatment with antipsychotics may be necessary to control his manic symptoms in the short term and a mood stabilising drug started in the medium term. Suitable mood stabilisers might be lithium or sodium valproate. These would help prevent relapse or recurrence of the illness. While he was in hospital, staff would need to protect Mr Unwin from the consequences of his illness (e.g. overspending behaviour and suicidal mood swings).

MOOD DISORDER IN LITERATURE

Literature and films can sometimes yield interesting descriptions that accurately reflect mental disorders and at other times they can unhelpfully caricature the disorder, patients and their psychiatrists. Harry Thompson's novel *This Thing of Darkness* (2006) concerns the life of Captain FitzRoy. FitzRoy was the captain of HMS *Beagle* during Charles Darwin's world-changing voyage in the southern hemisphere. He was also later Governor of New Zealand and the founding father of meteorology, through which he saved many sailors' lives, but also acquired many enemies (since sailors would not sail when the shipping weather forecasts were bad and this was resented by ship owners). Thompson's fictionalised description of FitzRoy is fascinating as he portrays him as having episodes of deep depression and frank hypomania, when he felt inspired by God and thought he had various special missions. FitzRoy did kill himself with a razor eventually and this much is historical fact.

I've selected two passages from his book. One from early on in FitzRoy's career describes a switch from an elated phase into a phase of depression and very cleverly describes the sense of loss FitzRoy experiences as he moves from an earlier expansive mood where he felt he glimpsed some God-directed mission into a sense of shame and social withdrawal.

The inside of the cabin was dark and silent. A faint rattling and creaking indicated that the ship was still at anchor. FitzRoy stirred. The worst of the night's terror had drained away now. Fear and dread had come in the dark, had choked him and mocked him, tugging his emotions this way and that, playing with him like a bird of prey with a mouse. But now they were gone, and shame and embarrassment flooded his mind, together with a terrible, crushing disappointment that the tiny glimpse he had been given, of something infinitely strange and wonderful, was now snatched away from him forever. He opened half an eye and the grimy skylights blurred into focus. He realised that a blanket had been laid over the outside to keep his cabin dark. How long had he been lying there? How long had his madness lasted? The events of the previous days came flooding back now in all their hideous detail. *Dear Lord, what sickness possessed me? Please God, what damage have I done?*

The second passage about FitzRoy is from later in the book. FitzRoy has accompanied Darwin round the world on HMS *Beagle* and although FitzRoy is a very practical and scientific man, he is a strong Christian and has argued terribly with Darwin about the whole concept of evolution. He attends a debate in Oxford about evolution after Darwin's book *On the Origin of Species* has caused a sensation (in contrast, FitzRoy's own book about the *Beagle* voyage caused hardly a ripple). In the course of the debate he starts to suffer with symptoms of hypomania – his senses become intense, his thoughts run quickly, he becomes incoherent and his judgement is seemingly badly affected.

The rush of arguments in his head became a landslide, an avalanche, each irrefutable fact tumbling incoherently over the others. The inability of natural selection to account for the origin of life itself. The unsatisfactory reduction of the aesthetic, the emotional and the spiritual to mere epiphenomena. The falsity of Darwin's fossil narrative, which had been constructed on foundations that were geologically poles apart. The failure of natural selection to explain the development of complex organs, such as the eye, and their coordination in bodily systems. The presence of advanced creatures in the earliest strata of the fossils, and of the most primitive creatures alive today. He felt both excited and agitated, and aggrieved by this sudden inarticulacy. Before he knew what he was doing, he had grabbed a bible from one of the priests in the audience and was waving it above his head. 'I implore you all to believe in God, rather than man!' he heard a voice shouting, and realised that it was his own. The chorus of jeers drowned him out.

On the dais, Professor Henslow had recognised him, and was trying to record his interruption in some sort of official status. 'Please, ladies and gentlemen Captain FitzRoy wishes to contribute to the debate! Pray silence for Captain FitzRoy!'

Nobody paid any heed.

FitzRoy tried to tell them that he had been there with Darwin, that he observed the same things, that *the origin of species* was not a logical arrangement of the facts that he had witnessed, but his throat was constricting in the most alarming way, and he found that he couldn't speak. He could only wave the borrowed bible above his head. Bizarrely he became aware he could distinguish each individual voice that made up the surrounding, could follow each and every line separately, as if they were the instruments of an orchestra. He looked at Hooker seated on the platform, handsome and fine boned, his wire-rimmed pebble spectacles perched elegantly on the bridge of his long nose, an amused smile on his face and he realised that he could make out the waxy quality of the man's skin as if it were but an inch away, could see each of its tiny downy hairs, his sight had become as crystal clear as his other senses, each of them intensified to a strength that only God Himself could possibly know. He could even feel the warmth of the little gas jets on the walls. Electrical sensations ran up and down his limbs, and played across the surface of his skin. So intense were all these feelings, so wonderful and terrifying, that he thought perhaps he should try to fend some of them off, to find order amid the chaos, but they would not be deflected. It just kept coming, kept overwhelming. And all the while this man, this Captain FitzRoy, who was him and yet who seemed to stand apart from him, stood paralysed and holding aloft a borrowed bible making incoherent noises.

Somewhere deep within himself beneath a whirling, unpredictable hurricane of sensations, a tiny spark of self-preservation remained. It told him to get out, to leave now before something unimaginably awful happened. Captain FitzRoy heard this in a voice, as if from a great distance and remarkably he listened to it. He put down his head and bulldozed his way to the exit, shouts and laughter reverberating in his ears. Driving himself ever onward he did not stop until he reached the station, where he noticed, he was still tightly clutching the borrowed bible.

LEARNING POINTS: MANIA

➤ Key symptoms of mania include overactivity and insomnia coexisting with either elation or irritability.

➤ Key signs of mania include restlessness, distractibility, irritability, pressure of speech or thought and disinhibition.

➤ Mania usually implies a bipolar affective illness and episodes of mania may be followed by episodes of depression.

➤ Despite elation and grandiose ideas the hypomanic patient may switch into a depressed or suicidal state.

➤ Doctors should endeavour to protect manic patients against the consequences of their poor judgement.

➤ Mania is much less common than depression.

➤ Mania has an earlier age of onset than depression.

➤ Acute treatment may include neuroleptics; prophylactic treatment may involve lithium or carbamazepine therapy.

THE TREATMENT OF MOOD DISORDERS

Prior to effective physical treatments being invented in the 20th century, patients with severe mood disorders might find themselves as inpatients in asylums for long periods of time. Kraepelin described inpatient episodes of mood disorder in the 19th century lasting years.

The first effective treatment was probably electroconvulsive therapy invented by Ugo Cerletti, an Italian, in the 1930s. Early treatments involved generalised bilateral tonic clonic fits induced by electric current. These were without muscle relaxants or anaesthetics and the fits were sometimes so strong that the patient's own contracting muscles might cause fractures. The treatment was 'modified' by the introduction of muscle relaxants such as suxamethonium and short-acting anaesthetics. The procedure is now so smooth that the fits may not be visible and only be detected on EEG monitors. A course of 8–12 treatments with two treatments a week might be typical in a severe case of depression. The treatment is a life saver where the depression is profound and there is food refusal or delusional ideation. Efficacy rates equal or surpass antidepressant therapy, but the procedure is uncommon and unpopular, partly because of how the media presents ECT. Memory problems are associated with the treatment, but we lack good studies on how long-term affective disorders affect memory anyhow. Relapse rates are high once ECT treatment has stopped so concomitant antidepressants may be required to maintain recovery after ECT.

Observations that the drug isoniazid improved mood in tuberculosis sufferers led to the development of drugs that boosted monoamines such as noradrenaline and serotonin. These early antidepressants in the 1950s included the monoamine oxidase inhibitors such as phenelzine and tranylcypromine. The inhibitors acted irreversibly, however, and if the patient took in substantial amounts of tyramine in the diet then hypertensive crises could occur. Patients carried cards warning them not to eat food rich in tyramine such as pickled herrings or drink Chianti wine. Next emerged the tricyclic antidepressants like imipramine and amitriptyline. They had useful sedative properties (by acting on histaminergic receptors), but were cardiotoxic in overdose and were associated with completed suicides. The 1980s saw the development of safer selective serotonin reuptake inhibitors (SSRIs) such as fluoxetine and sertraline. These had gastro-intestinal side-effects, but were less cardiotoxic. Later antidepressants include the SNRI venlafaxine and mirtazapine. Courses of 6–12 months are often required to avoid relapse.

In the 1990s research evidence accumulated that cognitive behavioural therapy (CBT) was effective in mild and moderate severity depression. The treatment is relatively cost effective requiring, say, 8–10 sessions and is popular as it does not involve taking medication. However, despite its recommendation by various bodies,

COGNITIVE BEHAVIOURAL THERAPY IN PREVIOUS CENTURIES

The invention and development of cognitive behavioural therapy is generally recognised to have been in the 20th century by Aaron Beck, based on other 20th-century work, for example that of Ellis. However, there are historical examples of the use of cognitive therapy in previous centuries. One such example is incorporated in Daniel Defoe's *Robinson Crusoe*, arguably the first English novel. The book was published in 1719.

The cognitive therapy is delineated in a table of 'evil' or negative thoughts which are countered or reframed in a sequence of corresponding 'good' thoughts. The purpose of this exercise in written self-therapy is to 'deliver my thoughts from daily poring upon them and afflicting my mind' and to 'master my despondency'. This is a fair description of intrusive depressive thinking.

The table set out by Defoe is as follows:

Evil	Good
I am cast out upon a horrible desolate island, void of all hope of recovery.	But I am alive, and not drown'd as all my ship's company was.
I am singled out and separated as it were, from all the world to be miserable.	But I am singled out too from all the ship's crew to be spared from death; and he that miraculously saved me from death can deliver me from this condition.
I am divided from mankind, a solitaire, one banish'd from human society.	But I am not starv'd and perishing on a barren place affording no sustenance.
I have not clothes to cover me.	But I am in a hot climate, where if I had clothes I could hardly wear them.
I am without any defence or means to resist any violence of man or beast.	But I am cast on an island, where I see no wild beasts to hurt me, as I saw on the coast of Africa. And what if I had been shipwreck'd there?
I have no soul to speak to or relieve me.	But God wonderfully sent the ship in near enough to the shore, that I have gotten so many necessary things as will either supply my wants, or enable me to supply my self even as long as I live.

An evaluation of the self-therapy is given thus 'let this stand as a direction from the experience of the most miserable of all conditions in the world, that we may always find in it something to comfort our selves from, and to set in the description of good and evil, on the credit side of the accompt.'

The principles of CBT seem to have existed in Defoe's mind when he was writing *Robinson Crusoe*. The notion that rational argument could be used to treat his fictional hero's depressed mood is clearly evident.

the demand exceeds supply and waiting lists of over six months in the UK preclude its usefulness in someone who is acutely depressed.

CBT follows on from the work of psychiatrists like the American Aaron Beck who thought that depressives tend to make various *cognitive errors* such as minimising positive events or self-attributes and maximising negative events or negative self-qualities to the point of catastrophisation. He noted a cognitive triad in depressed patients of a negative view of the self, the world and the future. CBT seeks to help the patient detect and correct such errors in their thinking. For instance, a patient might say, 'Everything I do ends in failure.' The CBT therapist would ask the patient to challenge the notions behind the words 'everything' and 'failure', perhaps focusing on something that had been a success, to outline the error inherent in the depressing statement 'everything I do ends in failure' by pointing out that some things can be a success.

CBT can help protect the depressed patient from relapse, but it requires constant practice, and initial enthusiasm about the treatment is beginning to be tempered by a realisation that in a recurrent illness such as a mood disorder CBT has a short- to medium-term efficacy and may need to be repeated after a year or so.

We lack data on the long-term efficacy of all treatments on the course of mood disorder.

Mood stabilisers are useful in recurrent mood disorder. Lithium has been in use since the 1960s to help prevent recurrent mania. Its is excreted renally and the therapeutic range is narrow before toxicity supervenes so blood monitoring is essential It may produce foetal abnormalities (e.g. Fallot's tetralogy) in the offspring of pregnant women who take it and it has other adverse effects such as hypothyroidism. Valproate can be useful in mania and depression, but has its own side-effect profile. Lamotrigine is useful in preventing recurrent depression, but must be started gradually because of potential Stevens Johnson syndrome in 1/1000 cases. Carbamazepine has fallen out of use because of its propensity to cause rashes, impair concentration and interact with other drugs' hepatic metabolism.

Antipsychotics such as risperidone or quetiapine have been found useful in controlling early behavioural problems with mania and psychotic symptoms in both depression and mania. Sometimes they are prescribed long term in mood disorders too.

SELF-ASSESSMENT
MCQs
1 Depression:
   A is more common in men than women
   B is usually treated by a psychiatrist
   C is often extremely difficult to diagnose
   D usually responds well to appropriate antidepressant therapy
   E is rare after the age of 70

2 Patients who are manic:
   A are best treated in their own home
   B may show irritability rather than elation
   C usually have their first episode of mania after the age of 40
   D may overspend
   E classically have paranoid delusions

3 Common symptoms of depression include:
   A nihilistic delusions
   B ideas of self-harm or suicide
   C disturbed sleep
   D derogatory auditory hallucinations
   E poor concentration

4 Biological (or somatic) features of depression include:
   A early morning wakening
   B mood worse in the mornings
   C psychomotor retardation
   D anorexia
   E loss of libido

SHORT ANSWER QUESTIONS
1 What are the clinical features of mania and hypomania?

2 What kinds of delusions are associated with psychotic depression?

3 What is the prevalence of depression?

4 How can episodes of depression be treated and subsequently prevented from recurring?

MCQ answers

1. A=F, B=F, C=F, D=T, E=F.
2. A=F, B=T, C=F, D=T, E=F.
3. A=F, B=T, C=T, D=F, E=T.
4. A=T, B=T, C=T, D=T, E=T.

EXPLORATIONS

LINKS WITH MEDICINE

Many endocrine disorders are associated with affective illness, such as hypothyroidism and Cushing's disease.

➤ What other endocrine disorders are associated with affective illness?

➤ What could the links between physical illness and psychological symptoms be?

Find out what the symptoms of adult growth hormone deficiency are.

➤ What happens to growth hormone production during normal ageing?

➤ What is the age of onset of adult depression and how does this fit with growth hormone production decline?

➤ Using MEDLINE, explore whether there are any studies linking growth hormone production and mood disorder.

LINKS WITH OBSTETRICS AND GYNAECOLOGY

➤ What reasons could there be for an apparent excess of depression in females?

➤ What endocrine hypotheses exist for post-natal depression and pre-menstrual syndrome?

➤ What evidence is there for these hypotheses?

➤ Following childbirth what percentage of mothers experience the 'baby blues'?

➤ When are the 'baby blues' most likely to occur?

➤ How do the 'baby blues' differ from post-natal depression?

➤ Is post-natal depression a true affective disorder?

LINKS WITH MEDICAL STATISTICS

Can moods be measured? Look out scales that propose to measure depression and mania such as the Beck Depression Inventory (BDI-II), Young Mania Rating Scale (YMRS) and the Mood Swings Questionnaire (MSQ).

➤ Try to find out how they are used and also how statistically reliable and valid they are.

➤ How are such scales researched to see if they actually measure what they are supposed to measure?

LINKS WITH SURGERY

Adverse life events are often associated with depression. Redundancy and bereavement are well-established risk factors for depression. Some surgical procedures such as mastectomy are associated with depression.

➤ Which other surgical procedures do you think would be particularly associated with later depression?

➤ What factors about such operations and diagnoses may provoke depression?

➤ What could services do to minimise suffering from depression after such operations?

LINKS WITH GENERAL PRACTICE

Ten per cent of all elderly people suffer with depression. Only about 5% of these cases of depression are treated.

➤ What can family doctors do to detect and treat these cases of depression?

➤ Loneliness, lack of satisfaction with life and bereavement are key risk factors for such depressive illness in the aged. What can be done to prevent depressive illness?

LINKS WITH PROFESSIONAL VALUES/ ETHICS

➤ What percentage of junior and senior hospital doctors suffer with depression?

➤ In what way might depressed doctors underperform?

➤ How could you recognise depression in colleagues or yourself?

➤ What would you do about it?

Look at the Firth-Cozens paper mentioned below for further information and references.

LINKS WITH EPIDEMIOLOGY

Figure 3.3 shows a graph of adult (ages 15–59) inpatient NHS admissions for depressive episodes in England between 2002 and 2007. Note the downward trend.

➤ What could be an explanation for this decrease?

➤ Why do female admissions outnumber male admissions?

➤ What are the barriers to admission, i.e. what has to happen before cases of depression are recognised, referred and admitted?

➤ What happened to the total number of mental illness beds in the NHS during this time?

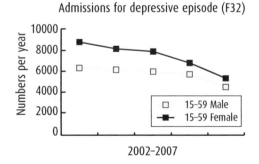

Admissions for depressive episode (F32)

Figure 3.3 Admissions for depressive episode (F32)

FURTHER READING AND REFERENCES
TEXTS

Brown G, Harris T. *The Social Origins of Depression*. London: Tavistock; 1978.

Defoe D. *Robinson Crusoe*. (1719). Edition quoted from: Penguin Classics; 2001. pp. 53–4.

Ellis A. *Reason and Emotion in Psychotherapy*. New York: Lyle Stuart; 1962.

Parker G. *Bipolar II Disorder: modelling, measuring and managing*. Cambridge: Cambridge University Press; 2008.

Storr A. *Churchill's Black Dog and other Phenomena of the Human Mind*. London: Fontana; 1990.

PAPERS

Beck AT. Cognitive therapy: nature and relation to behaviour therapy. *Behaviour Therapy*. 1970; **1**: 184–200.

Chambers R. Avoiding burnout in general practice. *British Journal of General Practice*. 1993; **43**: 442–3.

Das Gupta R, Guest J. Annual cost of bipolar disorder to UK society. *British Journal of Psychiatry*. 2002; **180**: 227–33.

Dinan TG. Glucocorticoids and the genesis of depressive illness. *British Journal of Psychiatry*. 1994; **164**: 365–71.

Firth-Cozens J. Doctors, their wellbeing and their stress. *British Medical Journal*. 2004; **326**: 670–1.

Green BH, Copeland JRM, Dewey ME, *et al*. Risk factors for depression in old age. *Acta Psychiatrica Scandinavica*. 1992; **86**(3): 213–17.

Piccinelli M, Wilkinson G. Outcome of depression in psychiatric settings. *British Journal of Psychiatry*. 1994; **164**: 297–304.

Roy A. Early parental separation and adult depression. *Archives of General Psychiatry*. 1995; **37**: 987–91.

Sclare P, Creed F. Life events and the onset of mania. *British Journal of Psychiatry*. 1990; **156**: 508–14.

Thomas C, Morris S. Cost of depression among adults in England in 2000. *British Journal of Psychiatry*. 2003; **183**: 514–19.

Weissman MM, Klerman GL. Sex differences in the epidemiology of depression. *Archives of General Psychiatry*. 1977; **34**: 98–111.

Young MC, *et al*. A rating scale for mania: reliability, validity and sensitivity. *British Journal of Psychiatry*. 1978; **133**: 429–35.

AFFECTIVE DISORDERS IN LITERATURE
The Bell Jar by Victoria Lucas (Sylvia Plath).
   London: William Heinemann; 1964.
This Thing of Darkness by Harry Thompson.
   London: Headline Review; 2005.

AFFECTIVE DISORDERS IN CINEMA
Vincent Van Gogh seems to have had episodes of psychotic depression, although it is difficult to retrospectively allocate contemporary diagnoses. Some writers have wondered whether Van Gogh suffered from bipolar affective disorder or even an organic disorder such as porphyria.
Van Gogh (1992) directed by Maurice Pialat.
Vincent (The Life and Death of Van Gogh) (1989)
   directed by Paul Cox.

RESOURCES
Fellowship of Depressives Anonymous (or just FDA)
A national self-help association with local groups and open meetings.

Box FDA, Self Help Nottingham, Ormiston House, 32–6 Pelham Street,
Nottingham NG1 2EG
Information Line: 0870 774 4320
Fax: 0870 774 4319
www.depressionanon.co.uk/

MDF The BiPolar Organisation
MDF (Manic depression fellowship) The BiPolar Organisation is a user led charity working to enable people affected by bipolar disorder/manic depression to take control of their lives.

MDF The Bipolar Organisation, Castle Works, 21 St George's Road, London SE1 6ES
Tel: 0845 634 0540
www.mdf.org.uk/

The Samaritans
The Samaritans has hundreds of local branches manned by some thousands of volunteers and takes millions of calls for help per year. It now offers an email service whose electronic mail box is read regularly. It has expanded its mission to schools and prisons.

The Samaritans, The Upper Mill, Kingston Road, Ewell Surrey KT17 2AF
Telephone service for suicidal: 0845 790 9090
Otherwise: 020 8394 8300
Fax: 020 8394 8301
www.samaritans.org.uk/
Email service for suicidal and despairing:
jo@samaritans.org
Otherwise: admin@samaritans.org

MIND
22 Harley Street, London W1N 2ED
Tel: 020 7637 0741

POST-NATAL DEPRESSION
Post-natal depression is now generally regarded by psychiatrists as an episode of affective disorder, but because of the circumstances it requires tailored management which takes account of various risks to the child and the need for adequate support and treatment for the mother.

Association for Post-Natal Illness
145 Dawes Road, Fulham, London SW6 7EB
Tel: 020 7386 0868
www.apni.org/

National Childbirth Trust
Alexandra House, Oldham Terrace, Acton, London W3 6NH
Tel: 0870 444 8707
www.nct.org.uk/

BEREAVEMENT
CRUSE – Bereavement Care
Cruse has over 100 local branches and provides individual and group counselling.

CRUSE – Bereavement Care
Cruse House, 126 Sheen Road, Richmond, Surrey TW9 1UR
Tel: 0870 167 1677
www.cruse.org.uk/

Foundation for the Study of Infant Death
Cot Death Research and Support
Artillery House, 11–19 Artillery Row, London SW1P 1RT
Helpline: 020 7233 2090
General: 020 7222 8001
www.sids.org.uk/

OTHER WEB PAGES WITH MOOD DISORDER RESOURCES

www.nimh.nih.gov/
www.pendulum.org/
www.psycom.net/depression.central.html
www.bbc.co.uk/health/
www.rcpsych.ac.uk
http://nimhe.csip.org.uk/
www.Blackdoginstitute.org.au

CHAPTER 4

Anxiety disorders

Anxiety disorders are a group of disorders with neurotic symptoms such as anxiety, panic or fear. Somatic sensations such as dry mouth, nausea, dizziness and urinary frequency often accompany the anxiety. Psychotic symptoms are absent. Anxiety disorders (neuroses) are relatively common and as such represent an important source of morbidity in the community. For their sufferers, anxiety disorders are often both long lasting and disabling. Anxiety disorders cause a lot of time lost from work.

CONTENTS

GENERALISED ANXIETY DISORDER

Generalised anxiety disorder (anxiety neurosis) is an illness with two components – psychological and somatic. Psychological symptoms of anxiety include a fearful preoccupation with the future, but with a free-floating anxiety. In other words, the anxiety cannot be pinned down to any particular event or person. The somatic symptoms include tachycardia, palpitations, essential tremor, muscular tension, hypertension, dizziness, sweating, hyperventilation, and epigastric discomfort. Anxiety is often a presenting symptom of depressive illness, and it can be difficult to distinguish the two. Anxiety may also be the presenting symptom of physical disorders. Several physical causes of anxiety are listed in Table 4.1 on p. 67. Generalised anxiety disorder is twice as common in females and affects up to 5% of the general population.

PANIC DISORDER

In panic disorder the anxiety is felt in separate recurrent bouts (panic attacks) – somatic symptoms of palpitations and dizziness may predominate and the sufferer may feel that they are about to die. Depersonalisation and derealisation may accompany the attack. The sufferer tends to avoid the places where such attacks have occurred in the past. A series of panic attacks may precipitate agoraphobia. Sometimes sufferers overcome their fear by misusing alcohol (Dutch courage).

Panic disorder can affect up to 1 to 3% of the population and often begins in adolescence or the early twenties.

In Figure 4.1 (p. 67) you can see the reciprocal relationship between panic and somatic symptoms, such that panic begets somatic symptoms and these trigger further fears, e.g. that palpitations herald imminent death, stimulating further layers of panic. Psychological treatment may be to focus the patient's attention from the internal environment to the outside world. The method of threes is one such treatment method.

It is important to exclude organic causes for anxiety and panic disorders. Thyrotoxicosis often presents with anxiety and mitral valve prolapse and cardiac arrhythmias are associated with panic attacks.

PSYCHOLOGICAL DEFENCE MECHANISMS

Anxiety and tension are uncomfortable and the mind tries to keep such feelings at bay, sometimes by using defence mechanisms. These unconscious mechanisms exist to try to keep psychological conflicts at bay. An example might be *denial* where an uncomfortable fact such as debt or a bad diagnosis is isolated out of consciousness and the individual behaves as if the distressing incident never happened. It was Sigmund Freud and his daughter Anna who worked on defining the defence mechanisms – such as *projection* where personal attributes or motives (e.g. anger or jealousy) are projected onto another individual. Anna Freud also described *displacement, rationalisation, reaction formation,* and *repression*

Melanie Klein, another psychoanalyst, described *splitting*.

Defence mechanisms act against true insight and can be destructive.

A less destructive and more sophisticated defence mechanism is *sublimation* where individuals may suppress internal conflict by focusing on other activities such as art, music . . . or healing others.

Table 4.1 Some physical causes of anxiety

Metabolic disorders	e.g. hypoglycaemia
CNS disorders	e.g. temporal lobe epilepsy
Endocrine disorders	e.g. hyperthyroidism, Addison's disease
External causes	• alcohol withdrawal
	• benzodiazepine and other drug withdrawal
	• theophylline and aminophylline
	• caffeine
	• experimental infusion of sodium lactate
	• some bronchodilators, e.g. salbutamol
other sympathomimetic drugs	

PHOBIAS

Phobias have been recognised for thousands of years and were certainly described by Hippocrates (c. 460–370 BC). A phobia is an excessive and irrational fear of some object or situation which is usually so disturbing to the individual that it leads them to avoid that object or situation (avoidance behaviour).

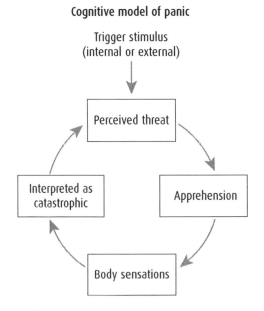

Cognitive model of panic

Trigger stimulus
(internal or external)

Perceived threat

Apprehension

Body sensations

Interpreted as catastrophic

Figure 4.1

Avoiding the feared thing only makes further contact with it more anxiety-provoking. Psychological treatment is therefore based on two principles: reducing the anxiety associated with the feared object and practising exposure to the feared object or situation.

About 10% of the general public have some kind of phobia.

AGORAPHOBIA

Agoraphobia is literally a fear of the market place, but covers a fear of crowds, fear or travelling on public transport, an avoidance of social situations and a marked tendency to stay at home, rarely, if ever, venturing outside. Often panic attacks in shops and crowds may herald the avoidance behaviour of agoraphobia. Three-quarters of sufferers are women.

SPECIFIC PHOBIAS

Most people have fears of things like the dark or spiders or mice, but rarely do they dominate our existence. When the fears become preoccupying and the individual takes special steps to avoid the feared thing (like asking a neighbour to read through all her magazines first to ensure that there are no pictures of spiders) then a minor fear of some particular thing becomes a specific phobia. Only about one in 10 sufferers is male. Table 4.2 shows some specific phobias.

Table 4.2 Some specific phobias

> Birds
> Spiders
> Dogs
> Cats
> Mice and rats
> Moths
> Wasps
> Thunder
> Heights
> Darkness
> Flying
> Lifts
> Closed spaces
> Dentistry
> Doctors

SOCIAL PHOBIA

This involves the fear of meeting people, or the fear of behaving in an out of the ordinary way in company. Whereas the agoraphobic is frightened of people in the mass, the social phobic is also often afraid of one-to-one interactions with others. Alcohol or benzodiazepines are often abused to reduce anticipatory anxiety ahead of the event. The anticipation causes anxiety, which impairs performance in the feared situation leading to reduced confidence and more anxiety before the next meeting and so on.

OBSESSIVE-COMPULSIVE DISORDER (OCD)

Obsessive-compulsive disorder was first described by Sir Aubrey Lewis, an English psychiatrist (born Australia in 1900, died London 1975), in 1935.

Obsessional ideas are repeated thoughts that come into a person's mind, and which have some undesirable quality to that person. The ideas may be nonsensical, violent or obscene. The sufferer often tries to resist dwelling on the ideas, to little avail. The ideas may be distressing, such as ideas about harming a baby in a new mother or swear words in a priest. Obsessional ideas are sometimes called intrusive thoughts. Patients may describe them as being *like* a conversation in their head. The key points to distinguish these intrusive thoughts from hallucinatory voices are that they:

> lack the real quality of a voice
> are experienced inside the sufferer's head (i.e. not experienced as external)
> and are recognised as a product of the sufferer's own mind.

The intrusive thoughts are not delusional either because, although the thoughts are sometimes incorrect, they can usually be challenged or the patient will volunteer how absurd the thoughts are, but that they are tormented by them all the same.

Compulsive acts or rituals may be performed to reduce the anxiety associated with obsessional thoughts. For example, the person who continually fears contamination may wash and re-wash their hands many times a day. The compulsions therefore are thought to ward off some undesirable event.

Performance of these rituals may interfere with everyday life. A patient who repeatedly spends two hours cleaning his hands after a toilet break at work may lose their job.

There is an overlap with depressive illness (since depressive illness may have obsessional features) and with obsessional personality (sometimes called anankastic personality). Obsessional personalities are essentially meticulous and perfectionistic workers who, if given a deadline will work to it, but who may expend great effort in getting things just right. Their attention to detail may infuriate those around them.

The lifetime prevalence of OCD is 2%.

Most sufferers have obsessions and compulsions; 25% have just obsessions and 5% just compulsions.

Some 5% have coexisting Tourette's syndrome, 25% have coexisting motor tics.

There is a high hereditability. The concordance rate for dizygotic twins is 47% and for monozygotic twins this rises to 88%.

Treatments include SSRI antidepressants and cognitive behavioural therapy. Response prevention (e.g. preventing compulsive acts), exposure therapy (e.g. exposure to contamination) and anxiety management techniques are also often employed.

DISSOCIATIVE DISORDERS

Imagine the mind has many layers of awareness. In clear consciousness we are aware of our surroundings and our inner thoughts at all levels. A thought which occurs at one level is apparent throughout the system. The sensation of hunger at one level is accompanied by fantasies of food and plans of how to get that food at other levels. At other levels of the mind memories of past meals and events might be triggered too. Somehow the thoughts, memories and sensations on all these levels are integrated.

In dissociation disorders we might imagine that somehow the layers are not being integrated properly, so that there are discrepancies or dissociations between thought activity at different levels. Some people speak of a 'splitting of the stream of consciousness'. An example of this dissociation might be that some memories are seemingly unavailable to the conscious individual. Hypnotic or trance-like states, and depersonalisation states, are other examples.

When something extremely unpleasant happens dissociation may be a way of coping. Children who are being abused often feel *as if* the abuse is not happening to them, but to somebody else. They feel removed from it all. When the abuse is not happening it may be difficult for them to access the memories and feelings they had while they were being abused. Sometimes these split-off memories may only be acknowledged by the abused individual years later. The information about the unpleasant event is not lost, but is stored at some relatively inaccessible level to protect the sufferer from hurt. A further example of dissociation is the phenomenon in battle where a soldier running across a battlefield is shot at, but continues running oblivious of the bullet that has entered him. Only when he returns to safety can he begin to feel the pain and acknowledge the wound he has sustained.

The lack of integration caused by dissociation may produce a number of related disorders.

Sigmund Freud described a variety of cases, then diagnosed as hysteria, but which now attract the diagnosis of *dissociative conversion disorders*. An example might be a young patient who has no physical abnormality, but who is adamant that they are unable to walk. The patient may undergo many diagnostic tests, but no abnormality is found. Other patients may present with atypical pains that defy our knowledge of human anatomy, or a sudden inability to talk (*aphonia*). *Catharsis*, an emotional return to the original traumatic event, via psychotherapy, hypnosis, or drug abreaction (provoked by intravenous diazepam, say), may release the patient from their symptom. Often the symptoms have some symbolic meaning, so that a child who is frightened to speak out against the abuser may develop an aphonia, i.e. the trauma is 'converted', hence the term *conversion disorder*.

Other dissociative disorders include dissociative amnesia (where important recent events are not recollected, but there is no organic cause). The amnesia usually revolves around recent bereavement, or traumatic accidents, and is selective. Closely related to dissociative amnesia are dissociative fugues (wandering away from home couple with amnesia and sometimes the assumption of a new identity) and dissociative stupor (psychomotor retardation in the absence of a history of depression, or loss of consciousness, often following some adverse event).

SOMATISATION

Not all patients have the ability to formulate psychological distress in psychological or emotional terms. They may present their inner conflicts and distress as physical symptoms. At a basic level this may be 'a way in' to discussing their problems with their doctor, but at another level the patient may be quite unable to accept a psychological basis for their illness at all.

Somatising patients may take their 'physical' symptoms from doctor to doctor in a vain attempt to find some test, investigation or cure that has not been offered elsewhere. Many negative investigations and therapies may have been tried by past doctors to no avail. Symptoms may involve any bodily system and include gastric pain, belching, vomiting, nausea, itching, burning, tingling and numbness among others.

Somatisers place doctors in a real dilemma. There is a temptation to pursue countless costly investigations to get a diagnosis, based on the knowledge that rare syndromes can sometimes present in such unorthodox ways. There is also a temptation to do nothing and wash one's hands of such difficult patients. Usually, there is a deal of anxiety about when to stop physical investigations and begin psychological therapies. Patients usually have a deal of depression and anxiety themselves and specific antidepressant therapy may be warranted.

Confronting somatisers with 'the truth' is rarely helpful. They have usually received multiple reassurances that there is no physical explanation for their symptoms and resent the implication that they are not telling the truth. Attempting to help the patient make a link between the development and fluctuation of symptoms to life events and circumstances may produce results. However, the patient must 'own' the link themselves. It is no good for the doctor to present the entire theory out of the blue. It will not be accepted. Somatisation in an extreme form can sometimes present as a conversion disorder. Here a serious stressor, e.g. a traumatic event such as sexual abuse, may be held at bay (dissociated) into the unconscious and converted into a physical symptom, e.g. a hysterical inability to speak – aphonia.

Psychiatric disorders occur in about 15% of general medical outpatients, and in almost a third of medical outpatients and primary care attenders there is some degree of somatisation.

ADJUSTMENT DISORDERS

When something unpleasant happens to someone – like a car accident or a bereavement, or bad news about a physical illness – it takes time to adapt to this event. The individual will initially feel numb, and may deny the situation before accepting that what has happened *has happened*, and then becoming emotionally distressed. The distress usually affects the individual's ability to carry on their social and occupational roles. For a short time the individual may be unable to face work or friends. Ultimately, the individual may come to terms with what has happened and may form some means of coping with their changed life.

The time used to turn life round after an adverse life event can be referred to as a period of adjustment, and the condition itself an adjustment disorder. The onset of the disorder is within a month of the event and the duration of symptoms is usually less than six months. If the disorder persists the diagnosis may be that of a depression.

POST-TRAUMATIC STRESS DISORDER

After severe life-threatening accidents or traumas, victims may suffer with a post-traumatic stress disorder (PTSD). PTSD is common in soldiers and it has been described in various wars. During the First World War it was known as 'shell shock'. Symptoms of PTSD include episodes of reliving the trauma.

Reliving may occur in *flashback* sequences during the daytime or as *vivid recurrent dreams* during sleep. Other symptoms include hyperarousal, insomnia, social withdrawal, numbness, fear and avoidance of cues that trigger memories of the event. Reliving the trauma may be associated with anxiety, fear and aggression.

Depression may coexist with the disorder. Patients may also self-medicate with alcohol, and substance abuse problems are often associated with the disorder.

Antidepressant therapy may be helpful. Counselling as a matter of course is often offered to victims of disasters and those who witness them (e.g. stadium fires, crowd disasters). However, counselling can make PTSD worse in some people. The psychotherapy of choice is cognitive behavioural therapy.

CASE HISTORY 1

Alex would not shake hands when he came in to see the doctor. He looked at the two chairs in the doctor's room and chose the one that he thought looked least dirty. He perched on the very edge of the seat and folded his hands.

Alex told his doctor that he was sleeping badly and that his degree work at the university was suffering. When the doctor asked about his sleep Alex told him that he would lie awake worrying whether he had switched off all the lights or pulled out all the electric plugs in the living room or locked all the doors. He would get up to check not once, not twice, but at least 10 times. If he did not get up to check these things, he was overwhelmed with anxiety until he did so. In addition he was washing his hands up to 20 times a day to rid himself of germs. Whenever he went out of the house he always had to shower on his return and put on clean clothes.

He had always been a neat person and a meticulous worker. All his essays at university were word-processed and laced with detailed references. However, in the last two months he had fallen behind on the deadlines for his essays, because he had been checking and rechecking every sentence for mistakes. He was troubled by thoughts that he had become contaminated by other people. He had stopped seeing his girlfriend because he could not bear her to touch him lest she give him germs. He knew that the idea was illogical, but he could not stop thinking about contamination.

His father had anxiety problems and over-used alcohol. His mother had had anorexia nervosa as a teenager.

Is Alex suffering with a neurotic or a psychotic illness?

This is a very disabling illness – his relationships and work are being impaired. Despite this there are no psychotic symptoms. The thoughts of contamination coming into his head are not delusional (he knows that they are irrational) and the thoughts are clearly 'owned' by him (therefore ruling out thought insertion). These are examples of intrusive thoughts. Since there are no psychotic symptoms this disorder is more typical of a so-called neurotic illness.

What is the most likely diagnosis?

The intrusive thoughts and associated anxiety are typical of obsessional thought. The repeated checking behaviour which Alex does to reduce his anxiety is an example of compulsive behaviour. Alex feels compelled to check the light switches and plugs or else he is tormented by anxiety. Similarly, his obsessional fears about contamination are the basis for his compulsive hand washing. The most likely diagnosis is obsessive-compulsive disorder. Careful questioning would be justified to exclude a delusional basis for the obsessions, e.g. that alien beings were deliberately conspiring to cover him with alien spores. Schizophrenia can sometimes present with some obsessive-compulsive behaviour.

Nevertheless, as given above, the story is consistent with obsessive compulsive disorder, not schizophrenia.

What treatments can be offered?
Some antidepressants with serotonergic activity are used to treat obsessive-compulsive disorder – namely fluoxetine and clomipramine. Either of these drugs may produce an improvement within a few weeks.

Psychological treatments include thought stopping, response prevention and systematic desensitisation. Thought stopping involves the patient voluntarily trying to distract him or herself from obsessional ruminations – by flicking a rubber band on the wrist, say. Response prevention may be carried out by a co-therapist attempting to prevent the patient from responding to obsessional impulses, say, by stopping Alex from washing his hands and helping him seek alternative ways to reduce his anxiety. For fears of contamination the therapist may 'model' more adaptive behaviour, e.g. exposing him or herself and the patient to a graded hierarchy of increasingly dirty objects, say working from dirty pullovers to dirty dishcloths and ultimately handling the contents of a waste basket. The patient follows the therapist's lead and models behaviour on the therapist, because the therapist handles the objects first.

> ### CASE HISTORY 2
> Elaine, 60, was a passenger in a car in a road traffic accident. She sustained a broken pelvis and spent some months in hospital. When she was discharged Elaine could not face travelling in a car again.
>
> She went to her family doctor complaining of poor sleep with early morning wakening. She was also troubled with recurrent nightmares about the crash. During her waking hours she was haunted by sudden visual images of the accident coming into her mind. 'It's as if it's all happening again,' she said. 'I am there in the car again. I can see the other car coming towards us. I can hear the crashing metal. I can't get the smell of petrol out of my mind.' Anything on the television to do with cars brings the unwanted pictures and sensations back into her mind. Since television programmes and advertisements repeatedly feature cars, Elaine has stopped watching television altogether.

Aetiology: Alex

	Precipitating	Predisposing	Perpetuating
Biological		Family history	
Psychological		Obsessional personality	Avoids contamination
Social	University pressure		

Figure 4.2 Aetiology matrix for Alex

What additional features of Elaine's history would you want to know about?

A full history and examination would be essential in any psychiatric assessment, but her past psychiatric history and pre-morbid history are of special relevance. Has Elaine a history of recurrent depressions or is this her first psychiatric presentation?

Her pre-morbid personality will give an indication of how well we can expect Elaine to be when she is well again. We also need to know about any other biological features of depression, suicidal ideation and any related alcohol abuse.

What are the main differential diagnoses?

The recurrent nightmares and daytime intrusive visual imagery (almost like being back in the accident) are fairly typical of post-traumatic stress disorder. The poor sleep is suggestive of a depressive illness, though, and a full history from Elaine and an informant would help us in our diagnosis.

How could Elaine be treated?

Antidepressants can be helpful in treating the depressive component of the disorder. Elaine's avoidance of certain stimuli (cars, television) could be reduced by using behavioural techniques, for instance by a programme of desensitisation to cars.

CASE HISTORY 3

Olivia, 42, had been married for 22 years and had two teenage daughters. According to Olivia, the family is a very close one.

One day while shopping in town Olivia had a panic attack. She described it as 'being like a wave of anxiety that rolled my breath away. I stood there in the street shaking and staring.' She managed to get to a public telephone and called her husband at work. He came to pick her up and took her home.

Ever since then Olivia has been unable to leave the house alone. If her husband or one of her daughters accompanies her, she can walk to the corner supermarket to buy small items of food. Even accompanied by other people she cannot face the weekly shopping trip to the hypermarket, or venture into town. Unless her old friends call and see her she does not see anybody but her immediate family.

Her husband's career is a demanding one, but is beginning to pay dividends. He is being asked to head overseas sales trips on the company's behalf. He is very worried that Olivia's problem will mean he has to stay at home with her and he does not wish to lose his job.

In desperation her husband asked the family doctor to make a home visit to see Olivia. When the doctor arrives he finds Olivia is tearful and guilty about the 'burden' she 'imposes on the family'. Even so she is adamant that she will never be able to go out alone again.

What are the likely diagnoses?

The low mood that Olivia displays could be a result of a depressive illness. The episode of illness begins with what sounds like a panic attack in the town centre. The attack seems to have been so frightening that Olivia has become sensitised to the place where she had the attack. She avoids similar places in case another attack is triggered. She has been conditioned to certain stimuli. The avoidance and fear of places like shopping centres is an example of agoraphobia. Whether the agoraphobia is part of the depression or vice versa is not known yet.

Panic attacks are sometimes caused by physical disorders such as thyrotoxicosis, epilepsy or mitral valve prolapse. These would need to be excluded.

What is the interaction between the illness and the family?

The illness requires the adaptation not only of the individual, but of the family as well.

Everybody in the family has to adapt their lifestyle to help Olivia. This in itself provides some 'reward' for Olivia's behaviour and helps maintain the illness in one way. Olivia would not admit consciously to using her illness to control the family. Nevertheless this is the effect of the illness. At one level Olivia may be very worried about her husband's job and may perceive his success and trips abroad ultimately as a threat. Exploring the state of the marriage and the family dynamics would be important in helping the patient and her family. Sometimes illness is a form of communication. It may be too difficult for Olivia to say outright that she does not want her husband to travel abroad, or conversely she might know that he would not listen to such a message. He does though take account of her illness behaviour. However, 'blaming' Olivia for the illness will not help matters and any therapeutic initiative with the family must be carefully negotiated.

CASE HISTORY 4

Diarmuid was taken to the children's hospital with a suspected spinal fracture during a hockey match. He had suddenly lost the ability to walk. His parents were distraught. He spent three weeks on the children's medical ward. His brain scans and muscle electrophysiology were normal, however. He was transferred to the child psychiatry ward, much against his parent's wishes. They were sure that the doctors had missed some crucial diagnosis. Their son still remained in a wheelchair and maintained he could not move or feel his legs. Nursing staff, however, were sure that they saw him occasionally tapping his feet in time to music on the ward.

What condition might Diarmuid have?

There are no organic causes for his sudden inability to feel or move his legs. Diarmuid has astasia abasia – sometimes defined as an inability to walk through a defect of will.

Astasia abasia was familiar to 19th-century psychiatrists like Freud, who labelled these kind of illnesses *hysteria*. Interestingly, astasia abasia was described before Freud by the 19th-century novelist Dostoevsky, who also was able to describe the psychological conflicts that could provoke it and the kind of magical healings that could end it.

What psychological conflict has caused this in Diarmuid?

Diarmuid was never able to explain what severe stress he had been under. Throughout his stay at the hospital he maintained he was physically ill and that there was 'nothing wrong at school or home'. His parents took him home and to a Christian healing ministry where he was just as suddenly cured as he had suddenly become ill.

He refused to go back to school, however, and was schooled at home from then on.

Two years later he was seen in an accident and emergency unit after an overdose. In subsequent psychotherapy he disclosed that he had been sexually abused by the school hockey teacher.

What function did the symptom of astasia abasia serve?

The astasia abasia provided Diarmuid with a let out from the intolerable situation of being abused at school. The astasia abasia meant Diarmuid did not have to go to school, without having to name the situation he was in. It gave him some control in a situation where he was otherwise powerless.

SELF-ASSESSMENT
MCQs

1 Features of panic disorder include:
   A chronic low-grade anxiety
   B palpitations
   C passivity phenomena
   D episodic feelings of fear or panic
   E insomnia

2 Obsessive-compulsive disorder:
   A usually involves intrusive ideas, images or impulses
   B is much more common in women than men
   C usually has its onset in late life
   D often involves intrusive hallucinations
   E may involve rituals that involve checking or cleanliness

3 Specific phobias:
   A are usually accompanied by generalised anxiety
   B usually manifest in middle age
   C often involve avoidance behaviour
   D may include a morbid fear of AIDS
   E can be treated with desensitisation

SHORT ANSWER QUESTIONS

1 What is somatisation?
2 What treatments can be used for obsessive-compulsive disorder?
3 What investigations would you consider in a middle-aged woman presenting with anxiety?

CASE VIGNETTE

Paul, a 34-year-old man, presents to his family doctor with feelings of panic associated with a dread of a forthcoming office party. He works as a porter in a large, local firm, responsible for sorting and distributing the mail. He has only just got the job after years of unemployment. His boss is expecting all the workers to be at the party, but Paul has always avoided any social gathering with friends or family. In social situations he finds that he blushes and stammers and that people make fun of him. In the last few days he has begun drinking heavily which he finds calms his anxiety a bit. He smells of alcohol to his doctor.

1 What problems does Paul describe?
2 What might the differential diagnosis be? What other information would you need to confirm a diagnosis?

3 What investigations might the doctor consider?
4 What management or treatment might the doctor suggest?

MCQ answers
1 A=F, B=T, C=F, D=T, E=F.
2 A=T, B=F, C=F, D=F, E=T.
3 A=T, B=F, C=T, D=T, E=T.

EXPLORATIONS
LINKS WITH PHYSIOLOGY

➤ What are the physical or somatic components of anxiety?
➤ How are the physical effects of anxiety mediated?
➤ What physiological systems are involved?
➤ How can this somatic component of anxiety be reliably measured?

LINKS WITH PHARMACOLOGY

➤ Which neurotransmitter systems are responsible for producing somatic symptoms of anxiety?
➤ How can these effects be blocked?
➤ What adverse effects can occur through blockade?
➤ What mechanisms at the synapse underlie tolerance and addiction?

LINKS WITH PSYCHOLOGY

Watch a copy of *There Will Be Blood*, the Oscar-winning 2008 film, and watch out for examples of defence mechanisms in play. Identify **two** scenes where *projection* is in play and **two** scenes where *displacement* is at play.

FURTHER READING AND REFERENCES

Angst J, Vollrath M. The natural history of anxiety disorder. *Acta Psychiatrica Scandinavica*. 1991; **84**: 446–52.
Batelaan N, Smit F, de Graaf R, van Balkom A, Vollebergh W, Beekman A. Economic costs of full-blown and subthreshold panic disorder. *Journal of Affective Disorders*. 2007; **104**(1–3): 127–36.

Croft-Jeffreys C, Wilkinson G. Estimated costs of neurotic disorder in UK general practice. *Psychological Medicine*. 1989; **19**: 549–58.

Cuijpers P, Smit F, Oostenbrink J, de Graaf R, ten Have M, Beekman A. Economic costs of minor depression: a population-based study. *Acta Psychiatrica Scandinavica*. 2007; **115**(3): 229–36.

Freud A. *The Ego and the Mechanisms of Defence*. London: Hogarth Press and Institute of Psycho-Analysis; 1937.

Freud S. *Introductory Lectures on Psychoanalysis*. Volume 3. Penguin Books Edition; 1915–17.

Freud S, Breuer J. *Studies on Hysteria*. Volume 1. Penguin Books Edition; 1895.

Gask L, Goldberg D, Porter R, Creed F. The treatment of somatisation: evaluation of a training package with general practice trainees. *J Psychosom. Res*. 1989; **33**: 697–703.

Green BH. Diagnosis and treatment of somatisation. *The Practitioner*. 2003; **247**: 704–10.

Green B. Pain and somatisation. Psychiatry On-Line; 2007. www.priory.com/psych/pain.htm

Kaaya S, Goldberg D, Gask L. Management of somatic presentations of psychiatric illness in general medical settings. Evaluation of a new training course for general practitioners. *Med Educ*. 1992; **26**: 138–44.

Kirmayer IJ, Robbins JM. Three forms of somatisation in primary care. Prevalence, co-occurrence and sociodemographic characteristics. *J Nerv Ment Dis*. 1991; **179**: 647–55.

Pawlikowska T, Chalder T, Hirsch SR, Wallace P, Wright DJM, Wessely SC. Population based study of fatigue and psychological distress. *BMJ*. 1994; **308**: 763–6.

Valliant GE, Bond M, Valliant O. An empirically validated hierarchy of defence mechanisms. *Archives of General Psychiatry*. 1986; **43**: 786.

Van Hemert AM, Hengeveld MW, Bolk JH, Rooijmans HG, Vandenbroucke JP. Psychiatric disorders in relation to medical illness amongst patients of a general medical outpatient clinic. *Psychological Medicine*. 1993; **23**: 167–73.

NEUROTIC SYMPTOMS IN LITERATURE

Dostoevsky F. *The Brothers Karamazov*; 1880.
du Maurier D. *Rebecca*. London: Gollancz; 1938.
Flaubert G. *The Temptation of St Anthony*; 1874.
Hodgson-Burnett F. *The Secret Garden*; 1911.
Murdoch I. *The Good Apprentice*. London: Chatto & Windus; 1985.
O'Doherty B. *The Strange Case of Mademoiselle P*. London: Chatto & Windus; 1992.

RESOURCES

Anxiety Alliance
1 Taylor Close, Kenilworth, Warwickshire
CV8 2LW
Tel: 0845 296 7877
www.anxietyalliance.org.uk

National Phobics' Society
339 Stretford Road, Hulme, Manchester
M15 4ZY
Tel: 0844 477 5774
www.phobics-society.org.uk

Relaxation for Living Institute
1 Great Chapel Street, London W1F 8FA
Tel: 020 7439 4277
www.relaxationforliving.co.uk

NO PANIC
93 Brands Farm Way, Telford, Shropshire
TF3 2JQ
Tel: 0808 808 0545 (Helpline)
www.nopanic.org.uk

Social Anxiety UK
www.social-anxiety.org.uk

CHAPTER 5

Schizophrenia

Schizophrenia is a psychotic disorder that primarily affects thought and behaviour. Abnormal perceptions such as hallucinations are characteristic, as are abnormal beliefs such as delusions. The disorder is often chronic and relapsing. Usually, it can be well controlled with antipsychotic drugs (sometimes called neuroleptics).

CONTENTS

THE ONSET OF SCHIZOPHRENIA

CASE HISTORY 1

The consultant on call was asked to make an emergency visit to the vicarage of St Mary's church. The patient's father, the vicar, explained that Jane was a sixth form pupil at a local private school. She had always done well at school and had achieved high grades in her fifth form exams. She was hoping to go to university. Over the last few months, though, her behaviour had changed. She had started refusing to go to school, but had declined to give any reason why. She spent her days writing in her room, and had not eaten for the last three days. She would not let her parents in to see her and had barricaded the door. There was no history of drug abuse.

The consultant talked to her through the door, and finally persuaded her to trust him sufficiently to let him into her room. He found that Jane was a tall, thin girl with a pale face. The room smelt of urine, and the walls had been covered in a fine, spidery writing. When the consultant tried to read what it said, she shouted at him. Jane looked at him suspiciously, and at times seemed to be conferring with an unseen person as to how trustworthy the doctor was. The doctor could see scratch marks on her neck where Jane had cut herself with the blade of a pair of scissors. She said that this was 'to let the bad blood out'. Jane appeared alert and knew the day and the time. When asked about her refusal to eat, Jane mumbled about her parents trying to poison her, because, she said, 'My mother offered me an Arrowroot Thin biscuit . . . that would make me thin . . . and she offered me some cabbage . . . that would turn me into a cabbage.'

The doctor felt that Jane's health was at risk because she had been harming and starving herself, and that there was evidence of a mental disorder which warranted admission to hospital for further assessment.

What evidence is there that Jane is suffering from a psychotic disorder?

Firm evidence includes the asocial speech (muttering to unseen and unheard persons) which may well mean she has auditory hallucinations, and the concrete thoughts in her statement that eating thin biscuits would make her thin and eating cabbage would turn her into a cabbage. Circumstantial evidence includes the social withdrawal, self-neglect, suspiciousness, and marked alteration in her normal behaviour.

What evidence suggests that this is not an acute organic psychosis?

Jane is in clear consciousness (she is alert and is orientated). The onset of the illness is relatively insidious – her behaviour has changed over months, gradually becoming more bizarre and chaotic.

What are the diagnostic features of schizophrenia in this case?

Perceptual disorder (hallucinations) and thought disorder in a clear consciousness, together with 'negative' symptoms of social withdrawal, and significant and consistent change in her personal behaviour. Jane was a conscientious student, but through illness has become self-absorbed and apathetic. Features of the illness have been present for months. Her suspiciousness of the consultant and her fear that she was being poisoned suggest a degree of paranoia, and hospital assessment would probe whether there were further persecutory delusions. Certainly, there are enough grounds to make *paranoid schizophrenia* the primary differential diagnosis.

How would Jane be assessed in hospital?

The consultant might well suspect that his key differential diagnosis (paranoid schizophrenia) was correct, but because this is the first presentation of psychiatric illness in a young person especial care must be taken to ensure the diagnosis is correct. Organic illnesses can mimic schizophrenia and some have specific cures (such as hyperthyroidism and neurosyphilis or general paralysis of the insane). Reasonable care must be used to exclude these. Table 5.1 shows some other causes of schizophrenia-like illnesses.

Assessment would therefore include a full history and mental state examination, a physical examination and various investigations. Physical investigations would include a full blood count, urea and electrolytes, thyroid function tests, urine and blood drug screen and a screen for sexually transmitted diseases, specifically including syphilis. Besides blood tests, physical investigations should include an electroencephalogram (EEG) which would help identify any epileptic activity or focal lesions, and some form of cerebral imaging (CT scan or MRI scan) to rule out cerebral lesions such as a pre-frontal meningioma.

Why does schizophrenia often appear to begin in adolescence?

Jane appears to have had a normal childhood according to her father, and has always done well at school. The onset of schizophrenia at her age is a devastating event, which may well disrupt her career and the rest of her life, but why should it arise now, when her development up to now has been apparently going so well?

Usually, there is a prodromal phase to schizophrenia, and people who later develop the illness are noticed to be unusual in their interests or absence of friends. Their premorbid personality is sometimes described as *schizoid* – aloof, cold, no friends, withdrawn, no sexual partners, and with unusual religious or scientific interests. Jane appears to be different from this stereotype. Some research has suggested that even in such relatively normal people there are 'soft' neurological signs present before the overt mental state features are noticed – slightly abnormal gaits in childhood, dysgraphaesthesia and proprioceptive errors. Current opinion is that schizophrenia originates perinatally, from whatever cause (genetic and/or environmental), but classical

Table 5.1 The differential diagnosis of schizophrenia

- Affective psychoses
- Schizoid personality
- Schizotypal personality
- Severe obsessional compulsive disorder
- Drug-induced psychosis (LSD, cannabis, ecstasy, cocaine, steroids etc.)
- Thyrotoxicosis
- Cerebral tumour
- Temporal lobe epilepsy
- Huntington's chorea
- Cushing's disease
- Porphyria
- Hypothyroidism
- HIV – opportunistic cerebral infections
- Neurosyphilis

schizophrenia only manifests later during adolescence or early adulthood.

LEARNING POINTS

➤ Schizophrenia mainly affects thought and behaviour, as opposed to affect. It is often a chronic disorder in that there are multiple acute episodes and between these residual effects.

➤ The diagnosis of schizophrenia is usually made with the help of a longitudinal view of the patient, i.e. the form of the illness is as important as the content of the illness in making a diagnosis.

➤ Schizophrenia affects up to 1% of the population (up to 600 000 people in the UK). Given that it is often a chronically disabling condition it is therefore responsible for a great deal of the population's morbidity. It has an incidence of 18–20 cases per 100 000 per year. Its peak age of onset differs for men and women. The average age of onset for men is 20–25 and the average

age of onset for women is 25–30. In social terms, chronic illnesses generally consume much of the total health budget. The cost of psychiatric healthcare has trebled in the last 20 years. In the United States schizophrenia consumes $35–40 billion per year in direct and indirect costs. In the UK, direct and indirect annual costs total £3.5 million.

CLINICAL FEATURES

Concepts about schizophrenia have changed over time. Different names and different criteria have been used to make the diagnosis at different times. This may be because the disease itself changes with time, or because we are actually witnessing a phenomenon with several different causes presenting a common picture, i.e. a picture involving disturbances of thought and behaviour. In the 19th century, patients with general paralysis of the insane (GPI) caused by *Treponema pallidum* were classed in with schizophrenic-like patients. About 10% of asylum cases of psychosis may then have been neurosyphilis. It may be that what we term schizophrenia today is still a heterogeneous group of diseases with different causes.

Research has shown that poor insight, auditory hallucinations, ideas of reference, suspiciousness, blunted affect and persecutory delusions are statistically the most common symptoms. The clinical features are closely linked in with the conceptualisation of schizophrenia and so some consideration of the history of the illness is warranted.

THE CONCEPT OF SCHIZOPHRENIA

An illness like schizophrenia has been variously described over the years. The Greek physician Aretaeus gave recognisable descriptions of a schizophrenia-like psychosis in the 2nd century AD. Kahlbaum in 1863 described a psychosis beginning in the young called *hebephrenia*. Hecker in 1871 described a psychosis with onset in the young and associated with a downhill course. *Catatonia* (a movement disorder) and *paranoia* were also recognised entities. Morel used the term *dementia praecox* in 1852 and Kraepelin in 1893 considered *dementia praecox* further and said there were four types: simple, paranoid, hebephrenic and catatonic, depending on the clinical presentation. He believed it was a biological illness. Simple dementia praecox involved a slow social decline, with apathy and withdrawal rather than florid psychotic symptoms – such people became drifters or tramps. Paranoid dementia praecox involved fear and systematised persecutory delusions. The hebephrenic type was silly and facetious. (Such terms enter common usage, with their meaning slightly shifted – hebephrenia was misappropriated by the public and corrupted to the phrase 'heebie-jeebies'.) Catatonic patients were those with predominant motor symptoms – increased muscle tone, preservation of posture (patients could be manipulated like passive mannequins into unusual postures which they would maintain for hours), waxy flexibility, and fear. Despite their persistent immobility such catatonic patients were acutely aware of their surroundings. Before suitable pharmacological treatments arrived, unless the catatonic episode aborted spontaneously, the patient would die through starvation or thirst unless carefully nursed.

Bleuler, in 1908, criticised the use of the term dementia praecox, because he said that there was no global dementing process. He first used the term *schizophrenia* and said that there were four characteristics (the four As):

➤ blunted affect
➤ loosening of associations
➤ ambivalence
➤ autism.

Eugen Bleuler (1857–1939) invented the term *schizophrenia* from schizein (split or shattered) and phren (mind), replacing the term dementia praecox. He also coined the terms *autism* (1910) and *ambivalence* (1911).

Regarding the four As, blunted affect referred to a restricted range of affect. Loosening of associations referred to the thought disorder present in schizophrenia. Ambivalence, or an inability to make decisions, was often seen in untreated cases were patients might hover for hours on the threshold of a doorway, uncertain whether to come in or go out (sometimes called ambitendence). Autism referred, not to the childhood condition, but to a retreat into an inner world, incomprehensible to the outsider.

The four diagnostic criteria of Bleuler have been revised over the years. Kurt Schneider listed the so-called 'first rank features' of schizophrenia in 1959. One of these, in the absence of organic disease, persistent affective disorder, or drug intoxication was sufficient for a diagnosis of schizophrenia:

➤ third person auditory hallucinations (running commentaries on the patient's actions or thoughts, or arguments about the patient)
➤ thought echo (*écho de la pensée*), thoughts spoken out loud (*gedankenlautwerden*)
➤ passivity phenomena (made actions, made emotions, made impulses)
➤ thought insertion, withdrawal, broadcasting
➤ delusional perception.

However, the criteria were criticised for being too narrow and only looking at a 'snapshot' of a patient at one point in time.

ICD-10 clinical guidelines from 1992 state:
➤ 'A minimum requirement is one of the following symptoms: thought echo, insertion, withdrawal, broadcasting, passivity phenomena, delusional perception, third person hallucinations, and persistent delusions – all in clear consciousness.
➤ Other symptoms used to make the diagnosis (two must be present) include persistent hallucinations in any modality, thought blocking, thought disorder, catatonic behaviour, negative symptoms, loss of social function.'

Symptoms should have been present for at least one month. This emphasis on the *form* of the illness helps exclude patients with transient psychotic symptoms or signs. Affective disorder should have been excluded. Symptoms should be present in the absence of overt brain disease, drug use, or epilepsy (which can all mimic schizophrenia).

ICD-10 lists the following types: paranoid, hebephrenic, catatonic, residual (a chronic state) and simple.

Latterly people have presented other concepts about the illness. One such is the division of symptoms into positive or negative types. Positive symptoms are the florid ones such as hallucinations and delusions and negative ones are the defect states such as blunted affect or apathy. Young men with early onset schizophrenia may show more negative symptoms, and these may be associated with more obvious brain changes on brain scans. Another concept developed by Liddle in 1987 is the analysis of symptoms into three cluster types – disorganisation, reality distortion and psychomotor poverty. Some people have likened these to the old concepts of hebephrenia, paranoia and catatonia.

CASE HISTORY 2

J Albert Arthur Andrew Churchill Chamberlain was a man who went under several aliases and had a career as a small time con-man. Some days he was Albert Chamberlain and some days he was Andrew Churchill.

He presented to his general practitioner with feelings of 'great sadness and loss of sincerity', as he put it. His general practitioner found his speech difficult to understand, but his main concerns seemed to be about his ex-wife. He claimed that his ex-wife was plotting with the British Security Forces to remove his 'sincerity and personality'. The GP noted down some of his speech verbatim: 'My divorced wife has an albigisty of conscience which she has terpolated with the Security Forces. They're debating my existence even now. They're saying we will drain his face of emotions, put our emotions into him and alter what the doctor's writing on the page to alter the circumstance and the circumcision of the truth.'

On further questioning the patient seemed wholly convinced that a transmitter had been inserted into his neck – he said he could actually feel it there – and that the transmitter was designed to put his wife's thoughts into his head. He could distinctly hear conversations between his wife and agents of the British Security Forces commenting on his thoughts and actions.

What Schneiderian first rank features does this patient exhibit?

He clearly describes multiple third person auditory hallucination giving a running commentary on his thoughts and actions (his wife and agents of the British Security Forces). In addition, his wife's thoughts are inserted into his mind (thought insertion), and he feels that his emotions are being replaced by those of another (made emotions – a passivity phenomenon).

What is the significance of his using words like 'albigisty' and 'terpolated'?

These are examples of *neologisms*, embedded here in thought-disordered speech. Neologisms are sometimes a feature of schizophrenic thought disorder, although neologisms are not pathognomonic of schizophrenia.

What kind of schizophrenia is this?

In view of the persecutory delusions which have been elaborated into a delusional system it would seem that Mr Chamberlain has paranoid schizophrenia.

CASE HISTORY 3

Shakil, 32, was brought to casualty by his brother. His brother had found him in a nearby seaside town, by accident. Shakil had been missing from home for several years. By chance his brother had seen Shakil walking down the road and had followed him home. Home had turned out to be ramshackle flat above an empty sewing machine shop.

His brother had been disgusted to find the remains of Shakil's last meal, an unplucked, ungutted and uncooked pigeon. Shakil said he had put the bird in the oven for half an hour to cook it, but since the electricity supply had been long since discontinued, the attempt had been pointless.

Shakil had been unwilling to draw unemployment benefit, because he said the money should be sent to the third world instead. A god, called Abu-Lafram, living in the bathroom, had told Shakil that he should deny himself for the benefit of the third world.

Shakil had little furniture left – he had sold most of it to buy bread and aluminium tin foil. He had used the tin foil to line the walls of the flat, to protect Abu-Lafram from the evils of Western civilisation that seeped through the walls. His brother had been most upset when he had told Shakil the bad news that his mother had died while Shakil had been away from home. Shakil had started to laugh.

On interview in casualty Shakil was unkempt and dressed in a grimy boiler suit, to which adhered blood and feathers. A large pentagram was daubed on the breast pocket. Shakil giggled at times and appeared to be listening to some voice that other people could not hear. He was mildly thought disordered and distractible, pacing about casualty, preaching the gospel of Abu-Lafram to other patients, using various neologisms. When he was asked how he felt about the death of his mother, Shakil grinned and said that his mother was a 'white cloud in a darkening and prejudiced sky'. He claimed to be a prophet of Abu-Lafram, and that he had been chosen as his first earthly disciple. Abu-Lafram talked to him throughout the day in a sonorous male voice, 'realer than the realest reality'. The thoughts he had had since knowing Abu-Lafram were 'the purest of purée' and were broadcast out of Shakil's head by Abu-Lafram for 'the benefit of all mankind'. Shakil did not believe that he was ill, but was adamant that he was a 'chosen one'.

What evidence is there to support a diagnosis of schizophrenia?

There is a history of declining social functioning and withdrawal. Shakil is observed to be hallucinated, and says that he hears the voice of Abu-Lafram, a god, who talks only to him (second person auditory hallucination). Shakil has a variety of secondary delusions based on this hallucinatory voice – that he is the chosen one and a prophet. The delusions have a markedly grandiose flavour. Shakil also has an inappropriate affect (laughing when first told of his mother's death). There is a complete lack of insight into his condition – he is able to live with the apparent paradox of being a 'chosen one' and living in squalor

What is the relevance of the patient's lack of insight?

If Shakil does not accept that he is ill he will be less likely to accept hospital treatment. There is good evidence that, without treatment, his lifestyle alone is likely to lead to harm to his health. Compulsory admission and treatment may be necessary.

THE COURSE OF THE ILLNESS

The onset in men is earlier than in women (onset in men in the age range 20–25 compared with 25–30 in women). Before the illness can be recognised there is often a prodromal phase in late teenage with social isolation, interest in fringe cults, social withdrawal (e.g. living alone in their bedroom with minimal contact with family, and no friends). Patients with schizophrenia often have 'neurological soft signs' – dysgraphaesthesia, clumsiness, movement

disorders and the like. Recent research has indicated that such soft signs, dyskinesias and gait disturbances may be detectable in childhood, before the onset of florid psychotic symptoms. (Such work has investigated home movies of American children who later developed schizophrenia, and compared these with home movies of children who have not developed the disease in later life. The movies were rated by neurologists 'blind' to the subsequent diagnosis.) The presence of such a 'soft sign' in childhood is not pathognomonic of schizophrenia, but such signs are seen significantly more often in children at risk for schizophrenia. So, symptoms and signs may pre-date (by many years) the next phase, which is the 'active' phase of the illness, characterised by positive symptoms such as hallucinations, delusions, thought insertion and the like. The active phase coincides with the 'obvious' onset of the illness. Table 5.2 shows positive and negative features of schizophrenia.

The active phase may last forever if untreated or may resolve spontaneously without treatment (although this would be very rare). Most active phases can be aborted by antipsychotic medication. After an active episode of schizophrenia there may be a complete return to normal function and no further episode may happen. It is more likely that there will be several episodes through life, and that function and personality may be damaged. This impairment of function/personality may be progressive. Often the active phase with its positive features is replaced by a residual phase characterised by 'negative' features such as blunted affect or poverty of thought.

What happens to people in the years after a first episode of schizophrenia? About 20% of patients have only one episode and had no impairment of function or personality. Thirty-five per cent go on to have several episodes with no impairment between. About 10% have multiple episodes of schizophrenia with a static level of functional and personality impairment between. Thirty-five per cent have multiple episodes with increasing levels impairment

Table 5.2 Positive and negative features of schizophrenia

Positive features	Negative features
Hallucinations • second person auditory 75% • third person auditory 58% • visual 49%	Affective blunting 96%
Delusions • persecutory 81% • religious 31% • grandiose 35% • of reference 49%	Alogia (impoverished thinking) 53%
Bizarre behaviour • clothing 20% • sexual 33%	Avolition/apathy 95%
Formal thought disorder 50%	Anhedonia/asociality • few interests 95% • little sexual interest 69% • few friends 96%
Thought dysfunction • broadcasting 23% • insertion 33% • withdrawal 27%	

between, as shown in Figure 5.1 (p. 85).

In a study which looked at the 35 year outcome of schizophrenia, 20% of those with a first episode in the 1940s were well, 45% were incapacitated by their illness, 67% had never married and 58% had never worked since their first episode.

About 10% of people with schizophrenia die by their own hand, often in response to psychotic symptoms such as command hallucinations – second person auditory hallucinations telling them to kill themselves. The public often associates schizophrenia with the perpetration of violence. In fact people with schizophrenia are more than 14 times more likely to be the victims of violence rather than perpetrators. However, schizophrenia is more likely to be associated with the perpetration of violence if risk factors such as command hallucinations, persecutory delusions, morbid jealousy, substance misuse or a past history of violence are present.

Features that predispose to a bad prognosis in schizophrenia include:

➢ insidious onset
➢ neurological soft signs
➢ past psychiatric history
➢ history of violence
➢ long duration of first illness
➢ emotional blunting
➢ social withdrawal
➢ poor psychosexual functioning.

In summary, a minority of a fifth of patients with a first episode of schizophrenia have a good prognosis. The majority have multiple episodes, and about half have chronic impairment of function affecting their ability to form relationships and work. Schizophrenia can therefore be seen as a chronically disabling disorder with important family and social consequences.

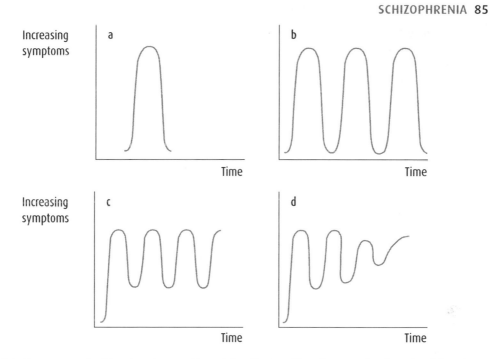

Figure 5.1 The course of schizophrenia over time: (a) patients with only one episode 20%; (b) patients with several episodes with no impairment 35%; (c) patients with multiple episodes with some static level of impairment between 10%; and (d) patients with multiple episodes and increasing

AETIOLOGY

Kraepelin delineated 'functional psychoses' from 'organic psychoses'. Organic psychoses included dementias and epilepsy. Kraepelin was well aware of the pathology of the brain in such illnesses. The brain, however, looked normal at the post-mortems of affective and schizophrenia sufferers. Hence Kraepelin called affective disorder and schizophrenia 'functional psychoses', implying there was no gross pathology to be seen in the brain. Modern neuroimaging though has found organic abnormalities in affective and schizophrenic disorders and so the term 'functional psychosis' is not so useful.

For a long time, when schizophrenia was seen as a 'functional' disorder, there were doctors who advocated that the whole concept of schizophrenia was untrustworthy, and not an illness, but a sociological phenomenon – i.e. that patients with schizophrenia were normal people driven insane by an insane world.

Some pointed to the role of the mother and said that some mothers' parenting behaviours were 'schizophrenogenic', i.e. that the mother's brought up their children incorrectly and induced schizophrenic thought patterns in them. They did this by using a 'double bind', e.g. asking the child to do something, but giving a contrary non-verbal message. Other doctors and psychologists have suggested that mental illness is a 'myth'.

The efficacy of antipsychotic drugs, and recent advances in biological research, have countered these anti-psychiatry concepts, but difficulties with the concept of schizophrenia remain. It is possible that the people who have schizophrenia are a heterogeneous group with different areas of their brains affected to varying degrees by neurochemical imbalances, neurodevelopmental problems, genetic defects, viral infections, or perinatal damage among other causes. Continuing research is essential. A treatable cause for a percentage of patients is worth hunting for. Prior to this century, between 10 and 30% of schizophrenia-like patients probably had neurosyphilis. Without the knowledge of neurosyphilis that we now have, this group of treatable patients would merely be a subgroup of an even larger population of undifferentiated schizophrenia.

Recent research has continued to search for a gene for schizophrenia. No specific gene has yet materialised and this would be the case for a heterogeneous illness. Some 'susceptibility' gene candidates have been proposed such as neuregulin which is involved in neuronal and glial cell growth and synaptic plasticity and dybindin which controls symptom function and signalling.

Other recent research has linked schizophrenia to early cannabis use (Arseneault *et al.* 2004) and maternal influenza.

FAMILIES AND SCHIZOPHRENIA
GENETIC ASPECTS
If one family member has schizophrenia, the closer you are to that individual in genetic terms, the more likely you are to get schizophrenia too. In twin studies if one twin of a dizygotic pair gets schizophrenia (the case is called 'the proband'), the other twin has a 14% chance of also getting schizophrenia in his or her lifetime (lifetime risk). In a monozygotic pair the twin of the proband has a 50% lifetime risk. This shows that the higher the proportion of genetic material in common, the greater the chance of developing schizophrenia. Table 5.3 shows the lifetime risks of developing schizophrenia for different individuals.

Spectrum disorder
Relatives of patients with schizophrenia have been noted to have mild features of the illness themselves to a certain degree. Relatives may have some mild loosening of associations in their everyday speech, but not to such a degree that it could be described as thought disorder. This has resulted in the idea that schizophrenia may be one extreme of a spectrum of schizophrenia-related disorders, which

Table 5.3 Lifetime risks of developing schizophrenia

● Member of the general public	1%
● Children who have one parent with schizophrenia	12%
● Children of parents who both have schizophrenia	46%
● Siblings of a patient with schizophrenia	8–14%
● Parents of a patient with schizophrenia	5–10%
● Second degree relatives of a patient with schizophrenia	2.5%

include language disturbance and personality differences – such as schizoid or eccentric behaviour.

THE FAMILY ENVIRONMENT
The emphasis on community care has meant that instead of sufferers being removed to large asylums for most of their lives, they can be accommodated in the community, within a family setting. There are advantages and disadvantages for the sufferer and the family. Some research has indicated that certain types of family environment may be harmful to the patient, but that with help characteristics of this environment can be altered to help the individual remain within the family. The environment which promoted a greater frequency of relapses is called *a high expressed emotion environment.* High EE environments involve a lot of negative criticism towards the patient, over-involvement by certain members of the family, expressed hostility, and greater than 35 hours per week face-to-face contact. Education programmes for the family seek to explain features of the illness to the family, reduce the amount of hostile criticism, and 'ration' contact. Such programmes have been shown to reduce EE and reduce relapse rates.

Table 5.4 Evidence of a physical basis for schizophrenia

Family and twin studies	
EEG abnormalities	• abnormal theta and delta waves
Neurological soft signs (in 75% of patients)	
PET scanning	• reduced glucose metabolism in frontal lobes (so-called hypofrontality responsible for negative symptoms)
CT/NMR scanning	• cortical thinning
	• lateral ventricular enlargement
	• sulcal enlargement
	• cerebellar atrophy
	• reduction in temporal lobe and hippocampal volume (Abnormalities almost exclusively in early onset young men)

ORGANIC EVIDENCE FOR SCHIZOPHRENIA

Table 5.4 outlines some of the current biological evidence that there is a physical basis for schizophrenia.

Current opinion favours an organic aetiology based on the neurodevelopmental hypothesis. According to this hypothesis an early brain insult affects brain development, leading to abnormalities which are expressed in the mature brain. There are animal precedents for such delayed effects. If the satiety centre of the rat hypothalamus is experimentally damaged in rat neonates no effect can be discerned on eating behaviour until day 40, when rats suddenly become anorexic. The onset of the anorexia seems to coincide with the rat adolescence. Similarly, if small areas in the ape frontal lobe are experimentally damaged no effect on behaviour can be discerned until age eight when the ape begins its adolescence. It is argued from these animal models that it is possible that in schizophrenia the effects of the pre- or perinatal insult lie dormant until late adolescence and the onset of positive symptoms. Some people have proposed that these perinatal insults involve hypoxia or birth trauma. Others have suggested that maternal viral infections damage the developing brain *in utero*.

Some schizophrenia family pedigrees have been linked to markers on chromosome No. 5, but this work is disputed.

TREATMENT

CASE HISTORY 4

Michael and his father were brought to casualty by the police. He had tried to set light to his father's bedroom. When his father had smelt smoke and tried to stop his son, Michael had hit him with a table lamp. While his father was having his wounds tended by the accident and emergency doctor a psychiatrist was called to see Michael. Michael was so disturbed that it took three policemen to keep him in casualty. He shouted that the devil was after him and that the policemen were demons.

The psychiatrist who saw him noted that Michael was in his early twenties and dishevelled in appearance. There were smuts over his face from the fire he had tried to light. She was only able to speak to him briefly. He was very frightened that he would be killed by the police and had auditory and visual hallucinations. He was responding to 'the angel of death' which he said was standing in the corner of the room. The psychiatrist checked that he was in clear consciousness and asked whether Michael had been taking any street drugs. It seemed that he was grossly orientated and that he had not been abusing drugs (according to Michael and his father). Although he could respond to closed questions, his answers became more thought disordered if he was allowed to continue. Once he referred to the devil putting 'demon thoughts' into his head.

Michael was so disturbed that a detailed history was impossible. Shortly after the psychiatrist arrived to see him, Michael lashed out at her with his fists saying that the angel had told him she was the 'whore of Babylon'. He was desperately trying to wriggle free of the policemen's grasp in order to leave the accident and emergency department.

What is the differential diagnosis?

Michael's presentation is marked by fear, and he has various persecutory hallucinations and secondary delusions. He acts on these fearsome hallucinations – for instance he tries to attack the psychiatrists because a voice tells him she is the 'whore of Babylon'. There is no doubt that this is a psychotic illness, but what is the cause? If the illness was of a very sudden onset, with a previously 'normal' pre-morbid personality, an acute organic psychosis due to drugs might be top of the differential diagnosis in a young man. Drugs like ecstasy, cocaine and amphetamine may all lead to such an acute presentation. However, if the illness had a more insidious onset (days or weeks) then paranoid schizophrenia would be a likely candidate. It is worth bearing in mind that Michael and his father deny any drug history and that Michael seems orientated. If there was no drug history and he was in clear consciousness, paranoid schizophrenia would be the main diagnosis. However, it is possible for drugs users to deny their habit, and Michael would need further

assessment (full history, physical examination and investigations including a drug screen), before a final diagnosis could be made.

Michael presents a management problem. He is not in hospital voluntarily, and he has allegedly assaulted his father and allegedly tried to set a fire. How could he be managed?

There are two immediate problems: firstly, he is mentally disordered and violent and, secondly, he is not giving consent to remain and be treated so that there are legal issues to be dealt with. There is a clear requirement for emergency sedation so that the psychiatrist can gain control of the situation. Mental Health legislation or common law usually provides for a one-off emergency treatment. To sedate a young, highly aroused male safely would require an adequate dose of an antipsychotic such as zuclopenthixol or haloperidol given via a suitable route. Oral medication may be too slow in this situation and an intramuscular injection might be required. An example might be 10 mg haloperidol IM. Intravenous chlorpromazine could promote a dangerous arrhythmia and kill the patient. *Intravenous* sedation with benzodiazepines might be an adjunct for quick control (e.g. diazepam 5–10 mg given via a slow intravenous injection) – however, attempting to find a vein in a writhing patient can be an impossible and hazardous task. It is important from a safety point of view to have adequate numbers of people restraining the individual before, during and after the injection is given. It may take some time before the intramuscular injection works. Such restraint should not be excessive and must avoid damage to chest or abdomen.

Mental Health legislation usually covers cases where mentally disordered people are removed by the police from private property or public places to what is termed a 'place of safety', such as casualty or a police station. To admit him to hospital for assessment, however, further legal steps may be required.

How is chlorpromazine metabolised?

Chlorpromazine is metabolised by the liver. There is a substantial first-pass metabolism, so that almost 80% of the oral dose is removed before entering the general circulation.

Liver enzymes become induced over time and so proportionately less drug reaches the CNS. (*See* Chapter 13 for further information on antipsychotic drugs.)

What is the function of procyclidine?

Procyclidine is an example of an anticholinergic, often prescribed with antipsychotics to overcome acute movement disorders like dystonia and other cholinergic side-effects.

Such anticholinergics should not be prescribed automatically with antipsychotics, but on a more rationalised basis.

What negative features of schizophrenia does Julian have?

Social withdrawal, hyposexuality, blunted affect, and apathy.

How else might Julian be managed?

Julian's symptoms conflict with his treatment in that his hallucinations affect his compliance – he has to constantly resist a voice telling him to stop taking his tablets. The exacerbations of schizophrenia which occur when he stops his maintenance treatment of chlorpromazine are unpleasant and potentially avoidable. If Julian would agree to regular injections of depot antipsychotics (e.g. flupenthixol 40 mg every fortnight) these would relieve him of the burden of constantly having to remember to take his tablets and would enable the community nurse who gives the injections to monitor his mental state and compliance.

Another way of looking at the problem might be to say that Julian still has untreated positive and negative symptoms of his schizophrenia. These seem to be resistant to conventional treatments. If an alternative could be found that effectively removed the auditory hallucinations, perhaps compliance would not be a problem. About 20% of schizophrenia cases prove to be resistant like this. A proportion of these resistant cases may respond to an atypical antipsychotic called clozapine. Clozapine might occasionally be used as an alternative to traditional antipsychotic agents, because of its different mode of action. Clozapine is not available as a depot injection. It can produce white blood cell dyscrasias so the blood count must be very carefully monitored. Despite the risk of dyscrasia in about 1% of clozapine treated patients, the benefit of treatment may outweigh the potential risk.

SERVICES FOR SCHIZOPHRENIA
ENTRY TO SERVICES

Best practice is that initial diagnosis is by the psychiatrist who may become involved when the patient presents to casualty for the first time, or via outpatient referral from the GP, or via an the acute / crisis psychiatry team for an assessment in the patient's home, or via calls to police stations to assess people in the police cells. Diagnosis must rule out treatable organic causes, e.g. temporal lobe epilepsy, and other organic causes (e.g. Huntington's chorea, drug-induced psychosis). Assessment includes family, psychological and social assessments and corroborative histories.

INITIAL SERVICE OPTIONS

Once a firm diagnosis is made (excluding other treatable organic causes) some cases can be managed in the community with sufficient outpatient resources provided by the community mental health team or crisis team and may involve monitoring of antipsychotic medication at home by a home treatment team or attendance at a clinic or day hospital. This is possible when the diagnosis is clear-cut and where the illness is 'mild'. First episode cases may also be seen by a specialist team who provide early interventions in schizophrenia – providing education about the condition and beginning family work.

In cases where there is profound loss of insight, refusal of treatment, and perhaps violent behaviour (based on, say, delusions or hallucinations) towards the self or others, then inpatient assessment or treatment is usually required. If consent to admission is not forthcoming, then depending on the circumstances, compulsory admission under mental health legislation may be needed.

The absolute mainstay of treatment is oral antipsychotic medication, with a move to maintenance treatment with IM depot antipsychotic injections as an option. Sometimes violent or particularly disturbed patients may require emergency sedation of rapid tranquillisation with intramuscular benzodiazepines (like lorazepam or intramuscular neuroleptics (like levomepromazine). Depot injections (which release medication over weeks) are particularly useful if compliance is a problem – and compliance is not to be expected if insight is poor. Inpatient and day hospital stays might be from a few weeks to a year.

MEDIUM-TERM SERVICE OPTIONS

Patients in remission can be managed in the community with the help of community teams, clinics and day hospitals. Patients may attend a variety of voluntary and state support services designed to rehabilitate them. Such facilities include social service drop-in centres, MIND day centres, and clinics. CPN support and computer follow-up to monitor and give treatment is essential to prevent patients 'falling through the net'. Where compliance has been a problem some people are referred to an assertive outreach team who try to ensure compliance by the patient and family. Depot medications may be vital in ensuring the constant delivery of antipsychotics to patients with poor insight who will not comply. Use of community treatment orders may also be considered to enforce treatment, although there are important ethical issues to do with autonomy to consider.

Some patients will inevitably relapse even though compliance may be achieved, perhaps due to overwhelming life events, drug misuse, or intrinsic factors.

LONG-TERM SERVICE OPTIONS

If relapse occurs, rapid treatment responses by crisis teams may prevent a further inpatient stay. Further episodes may require readmission to inpatient facilities. Once the episode is under control, return to the community can be renegotiated. Persistent psychosis may require altered treatment strategies, e.g. with clozapine, or admission to dedicated rehabilitation wards. There will always be a need for long-term hospitalisation in a minority of cases. Such hospitalisation may be in open, low secure or medium secure facilities, often now provided by the independent sector.

Some dedicated sheltered housing is sometimes available through the voluntary and independent sector, social services and other agencies.

Most cases can be managed in the community, usually in their own homes by liaison between community mental health teams, GPs, psychiatrists and social services.

The NHS has moved away from inpatient units to community teams. The move has been conducted without substantial research evidence to back it up and is in the nature of a well-intentioned intuitive policy initiative. Many teams lack experienced staff and revenue savings mean that newly employed staff may not even have a mental health background. There is therefore a question as to how skilled NHS community teams actually are. We lack clear epidemiological studies to monitor the current burden of unnoticed mental illness in the community on patients and their families. Historically there has always been a need for 'asylum' in the best sense of the word for the treatment-resistant mentally ill and it is likely that the rush towards community teams in the early 2000s will be seen by history as being overly enthusiastic.

SCHIZOAFFECTIVE DISORDER

The early psychopathologists debated whether psychosis is a single entity or not. Kraepelin proposed that **affective** psychoses and psychoses affecting **thought** were separate. This led to a separation of affective psychoses from the illness which is currently known as schizophrenia. However, there are people whose illnesses do not conveniently fit into either category and share features of schizophrenia and affective disorders. Their illness is sometimes termed schizoaffective disorder. This has strong features of affective disorder and schizophrenia at varying times during the same illness episode. People with this may have psychotic features such as delusions or hallucinations in the absence of affective symptoms and also severe symptoms of mania or depression at other times in the same illness episode. Treatment may involve an antipsychotic and often a mood stabiliser or antidepressant as well.

SELF-ASSESSMENT
MCQs

1 Features associated with a good prognosis in a first episode of schizophrenia include:
  A astereognosis
  B poor psychosexual functioning
  C sudden onset of symptoms
  D emotional blunting
  E social withdrawal

2 Antipsychotic drugs include:
  A haloperidol
  B sulpiride
  C risperidone
  D flupenthixol
  E dexamphetamine

3 Positive features of schizophrenia include:
  A anhedonia
  B avolition
  C thought disorder
  D visual hallucinations
  E delusions of reference

SHORT ANSWER QUESTIONS

1 List the first rank features of schizophrenia.
2 What are neurological soft signs?
3 What agencies contribute to the care of patients with schizophrenia in the community?
4 What investigations would you use to assess a patient presenting with auditory hallucinations, and why?

MCQ answers

1 A=F, B=F, C=T, D=F, E=F.
2 A=T, B=T, C=T, D=T, E=F.
3 A=F, B=F, C=T, D=T, E=T.

EXPLORATIONS

LINKS WITH NEUROLOGY AND NEUROANATOMY

➤ What tests can be done in neurological examination to detect 'soft signs' such as dysgraphaesthesia?

➤ What is the neuroanatomical basis of such soft signs?

➤ What is 'cerebral localisation'?

➤ What links can you establish between symptoms in schizophrenia and the possible site of brain pathology? For instance, where might problems such as thought disorder be located in the brain?

LINKS WITH PHARMACOLOGY

➤ How are antipsychotic drugs metabolised?

➤ What different neurotransmitter systems do the drugs chlorpromazine and clozapine act upon?

LINKS WITH OBSTETRICS AND GYNAECOLOGY

➤ What evidence is there to link birth trauma, perinatal brain damage and schizophrenia?

➤ How good is that evidence?

FURTHER READING AND REFERENCES

TEXTS

Gelder M, Harrison P, Cowen P. *Shorter Oxford Textbook of Psychiatry*. Oxford: Oxford University Press; 2006. (Chapter 9: Schizophrenia, p. 267.)

Johnstone E, Freeman CPL, Zealley A (2004) *Companion to Psychiatric Studies*. 7th ed. Edinburgh: Churchill Livingstone; 2004. (Chapter 19: Schizophrenia and related disorders, pp. 390–420.)

Shorter E. *A History of Psychiatry*. New York: John Wiley & Sons; 1997.

Sims A. *Symptoms in the Mind*. 3rd ed. London: WB Saunders; 1995.

PAPERS

Andreasen N. Magnetic resonance imaging of the brain in schizophrenia. *Arch Gen Psychiatry*. 1990; **47**: 35–44.

Arseneault L, Cannon M, Witton J, Murray RM. Causal association between cannabis and psychosis: examination of the evidence. *British Journal of Psychiatry*. 2004; **184**: 110–17.

Geddes J. Prenatal and perinatal risk factors for early onset schizophrenia, affective psychosis, and reactive psychosis. *BMJ*. 1999; **318**: 426.

Geddes J. Suicide and homicide by people with mental illness. *BMJ*. 1999; **318**: 1225–6.

McNeil TF, Harty B, Bennow G, *et al*. Neuromotor deviation in offspring of psychotic mothers: a selective developmental deficiency in two groups of children at heightened psychiatric risk. *J Psychiatric Research*. 1993; **27**(21): 39–54.

Murray RM, Jones P, O'Callaghan E, *et al*. Genes, viruses and neurodevelopmental schizophrenia. *J Psychiatric Research*. 1992; **26**(4): 225–35.

Shepherd M, Watt D, Falloon I, *et al*. The natural history of schizophrenia: a five-year follow-up study of outcome and prediction in a representative sample of schizophrenics. *Psychological Medicine*. 1989; Suppl 15: 46.

Tsuang MT, Woolson RF, Fleming JA. Long-term outcome of major psychoses. *Arch Gen Psychiatry*. 1979; **36**: 1295.

Vaughn CE, Leff JP. Influence of family and social factors on the course of psychiatric illness. *British Journal of Psychiatry*. 1976; **129**: 125.

SCHIZOPHRENIA IN FILM

➤ *A Beautiful Mind* (2002) was directed by Ron Howard. It centres around Nobel Prize-winning mathematician John Nash who was a student in 1947 reading mathematics at Princeton University. He delivered a paper on game theory (the mathematics of competition) that overthrew the accepted ideas about economics, only for his mind to later succumb to what was then diagnosed as paranoid schizophrenia.

➤ Scott Hicks' film *Shine* (1996) depicts the psychosocial decline of a talented pianist, David Helfgott, with what appears to be schizophrenia. The film spends a considerable time detailing how work and social relationships are eroded as the illness takes hold.

➤ Roman Polanski directed *Repulsion* in 1964, a London-based film that starred

Catherine Deneuve as a beautiful but sexually avoidant young woman, Carol. From the outset Carol appears preoccupied and early on appears to be suffering with visual hallucinations brushing imaginary objects from her face and shoulders. Carol is tortured by hallucinatory experiences where walls crack, hands project from walls to feel her, and in bed phantom lovers come to sexually assault her. The film portrays the psychotic process fairly authentically, and Carol's perplexity, self-neglect, asocial speech and disordered thought processes are really well done.

RESOURCES

Rethink
National Schizophrenia Fellowship
28 Castle Street, Kingston-upon-Thames KT1
1SS
Tel: 0845 456 0455
www.rethink.org

Richmond Fellowship
80 Holloway Road, London N7 8JG
Tel: 020 7697 3300
www.richmondfellowship.org.uk

SANE – schizophrenia: a national emergency
1st Floor Cityside House, 40 Adler Street,
London E1 1EE
Tel: 0845 767 8000
www.sane.org.uk

MIND
National Association for Mental Health
15–19 Broadway, London E15 4BQ
Tel: 020 8519 2122
www.mind.org.uk

Making Space
Tel: 01925 571680
www.makingspace.co.uk

National Institute of Mental health (USA)
www.nimh.nih.gov

OTHER WEB RESOURCES

Royal College of Psychiatrists information page
www.rcpsych.ac.uk/mentalhealthinformation/mentalhealthproblems/schizophrenia.aspx –

Clinical guidelines – information from National Institute for Clinical Excellence (NICE)
www.nice.org.uk/page.aspx?o=42424

Psychiatry On-Line – review on schizophrenia
www.priory.com/schizo.htm

Psychiatry Research Trust
www.iop.kcl.ac.uk/iop/prt/schizophrenia.htm

CHAPTER 6

Eating disorders

Eating disorders involve abnormal patterns of behaviour where people consistently eat too much or too little, and other behaviours such as bingeing and vomiting. Eating disorders are surprisingly common. There is a spectrum of eating disorders ranging from mildly abnormal attitudes about eating to severe anorexia nervosa. Examples of eating disorders are anorexia nervosa, bulimia nervosa and arguably obesity.

CONTENTS

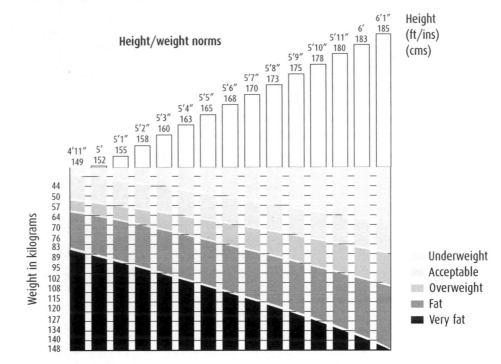

Figure 6.1 Mean weights for height

ANOREXIA NERVOSA

The principal psychological problem is a morbid fear of fatness. In order to keep his or her body mass down, the anorexic patient will diet excessively, combining this technique with strenuous exercise, the abuse of laxatives and diuretics and self-induced vomiting. Although the sufferer may be almost cachexic he or she may see themselves as overweight. Sometimes such skeletal patients may draw self-portraits which are really caricatures of themselves showing themselves as obese.

One of the criteria used for the diagnosis of anorexia nervosa is a body mass 15% or more below the expected mass for a person of that age, sex and height. Another criterion is amenorrhoea in women and loss of libido in men (secondary to reduced gonadotrophin levels because of self-starvation).

Young children and old people can be anorexia nervosa sufferers, but the preponderance of sufferers are teenagers. Ninety per cent or more of patients are women.

CASE HISTORY 1

Anna, 16, was brought to her family doctor by her worried mother. Her mother explained that her daughter was losing weight and looking increasingly frail and ill. With some difficulty she mentioned her fear that her daughter might have leukaemia or cancer. When the doctor asked about her daughter's appetite her mother said that Anna had 'gone off her food because she was too ill'.

From across the room the doctor could see how painfully thin Anna was, despite her having dressed in thick, baggy, woollen clothes. Although the weather outside was sunny, Anna's hands looked bluish and were cold to the touch. The doctor noted that there were abrasions on the knuckles of Anna's right hand.

Table 6.1 The differential diagnosis of anorexia nervosa

Physical	• thyrotoxicosis
	• malabsorption syndromes, e.g. coeliac disease
	• malignant disease, e.g. leukaemia, oat cell carcinoma
	• diabetes mellitus
	• hypothalamo-pituitary
	• tumours
	• Crohn's disease
Psychological	• depression (with appetite loss)
	• schizophrenia (with delusions involving food, e.g. that it is poisoned)
	• bulimia nervosa
	• abnormal eating attitudes

How would you proceed with the interview?

There is a choice between continuing a conversation with the mother about Anna, or interviewing Anna separately, possibly followed by the mother in turn on her own. Interviewing Anna on her own would allow you to assess her concerns and build a rapport with her. She is 16 and capable of answering for herself. Her cooperation will be essential whatever the diagnosis turns out to be.

Any medical illness must be excluded, so the mother's fears will need to be explored. Questions to Anna might include 'What other symptoms you have noticed, Anna?' or 'What do you feel is the matter?'

If there is little history to suggest physical illness, questions should be asked about dieting behaviour, feelings about her figure and appearance. More probing questions about her maximum ever weight and what her present weight is may encounter resistance, but should be asked.

What weight does Anna see as ideal? Does she see herself as very thin? Have her periods stopped? How much food does she eat in a day? How often does she make herself sick? (The abrasions on the dorsum of her hand suggest she makes herself sick by sticking her fingers down her throat. The abrasions arise because the skin rubs against the teeth.)

Does she use laxatives or diuretics to reduce her weight? How much does she exercise? Can she concentrate on her schoolwork or is she constantly thinking about her weight?

This barrage of questions may generate vital information, but the experience is likely to feel unpleasant to Anna if she does have anorexia nervosa. Proceeding to an immediate physical examination may well humiliate her further, although such an examination does need to be done at some time. The doctor might make a mental note to do this at a subsequent visit, choosing to concentrate on gaining Anna's confidence on the first visit.

What physical features of anorexia nervosa might be found on physical examination?

Table 6.2 Features on physical examination

Weight 15% or more below mean body mass for height/age
Retarded growth
Delay of onset of secondary sexual characteristics

(continued)

Dental enamel erosion and caries
Peripheral cyanosis
Hypothermia
Hypotension
Bradycardia
Cardiac arrhythmias
Constipation
Oedema (if heart failing)
Lanugo hair (fine downy hair on arms and lower back)
Carotenaemia (orange skin pigmentation due to reliance on carrot diet. Diets mainly of oranges can also lead to skin pigmentation.)

What physical investigations might assist Anna's management?

Investigations would be used to seek the effects of long-term malnutrition and the severity of risk faced by the patient. A full blood count will identify any anaemia, and help exclude any white cell dyscrasia. Urea and electrolyte screening will give a guide as to renal function and the possibility of hypokalaemia due to excessive vomiting. Thyroid function tests will exclude the differential diagnosis of thyrotoxicosis, but will also give a guide as to any secondary hypothyroidism associated with anorexia nervosa. A random glucose screen might help exclude diabetes mellitus. More specialised investigations such as growth hormone assays and an ECG might await any hospital referral.

Table 6.3 Abnormal physical investigations in anorexia nervosa

Hypokalaemia
Alkalosis
Leucopaenia
Anaemia

(continued)

Growth hormone levels raised
Plasma cortisol raised
Reduced gonadotrophins
Triiodothyronine (T3) reduced
ECG abnormalities
Hypoglycaemia
Raised urea
Reduced GFR
Reduced bone density
Hypercholesterolaemia

CASE HISTORY 2

Mandy had been in hospital with anorexia nervosa for two weeks. Although she was 14 she looked much younger, and weighed only four and a half stone (28.5 kg). She had been admitted after fainting at boarding school. Since admission she had been put on to bed rest, and kept in a private room. Visits by her family and phone calls to them were strictly regulated. Visits and phone calls were used as rewards by the nursing staff for eating her high-calorie diet (3000 kcal/day). Every Monday and Thursday Mandy was weighed to see if her weight was improving. If there was improvement then she was rewarded by greater freedom. In her first few days in hospital the nurses had noted that even though Mandy was eating her food, she was vomiting it down the sink unit in her room as soon as the nurse left the room with her empty tray. Nurses had also noticed that on the days she was weighed Mandy would try to drink as much water as she could just before she was weighed. Since noticing these things the nurses had watched Mandy very closely, which she did not like at all.

In her third week she had confided in a female occupational therapist that for a long time she had been receiving the unwanted sexual attentions of her form teacher. Staff acted to protect Mandy and to resolve family issues, as well as encouraging Mandy to gain weight. Three months after her weight returned to the average for her age, Mandy's periods restarted.

What made Mandy faint at school?

The metabolism of anorexic patients is mainly catabolic, and they are prone to hypoglycaemia. Cardiac arrhythmias and hypotension also predispose to syncope. School is also the place where her abusing teacher was, and the stress of this situation may also have been a contributing factor.

What are the aims of her hospital admission?

In severe anorexia nervosa the physical state of the patient may warrant admission for re-feeding and to correct any metabolic abnormalities. There is a substantial mortality associated with anorexia nervosa. Long-term follow-up studies show a mortality rate of 15–20% over 10–20 years (causes of death include frank starvation and oesophageal rupture). For this reason re-feeding is not the only aim of admission. Although some psychological factors can be caused or worsened by starvation (e.g. cognitive impairment, social withdrawal, irritability, depression and preoccupation with food), anorexic tendencies persist after re-feeding. After discharge from hospital relapse is unfortunately common. To prevent relapse other work needs to be done: educating the patient about the illness, about nutrition and the body's needs, and psychotherapeutic work with the patient and the family. Occasionally, chlorpromazine or amitriptyline may be prescribed (both stimulate appetite and weight gain). Some new antidepressants like fluoxetine help with the preoccupation with food.

What role did the sexual abuse play in the genesis of Mandy's illness?

It has been estimated that up to 50% of anorexics have been sexually abused (set against a community prevalence of 20–30%). Some people see anorexia nervosa as the pubertal teenager's way of rejecting adult sexuality. Put together with a previous history of abuse, you can see why the sufferer might starve themselves to delay the onset of puberty, and avoid the complications of adopting an adult shape.

BOX 6.1 RE-FEEDING SYNDROME

Re-feeding syndrome may occur when intervening and feeding patients with body mass index less than 18 or when patients have eaten little for >10 days. It involves potentially fatal shifts in electrolytes and fluids, e.g. hypophosphataemia, sodium imbalances, thiamine deficiency, etc. Adapted NICE guidelines for management follow:

Step 1: Check serum potassium, calcium, phosphate and magnesium.

Step 2: **Before** feeding give oral thiamine 200–300 mg, high dose vitamin B, and multivitamins and trace elements and continue throughout treatment. (Consider carefully whether to use adjusted intravenous doses.)

Step 3: Start feeding 0.2–0.5 MJ/kg/day and slowly increase over 4–7 days

Step 4: Rehydrate carefully: correcting potassium, phosphate, calcium and magnesium as necessary. Use extreme care when checking dosages, especially with potassium supplementation.

Step 5: Monitor electrolyte levels for first two weeks and amend treatment as necessary.

Other people see anorexia nervosa as a 'battle for control' over the patient's body. In a world where the sufferer perceives him or herself to be relatively helpless, it is sometimes a relief to at least be able to control their eating habits (although ultimately to their own detriment). The control itself is of paramount importance. This is why helping some anorexic patients sometimes feels like a battle for control for their families and their doctors. The 'battle for control' model can fit in with the sexual abuse theory too, because in sexual abuse the victim often feels helplessly out of control and seeks any means of establishing some control over the outside world.

Although sexual abuse is an important factor in some cases it must be remembered that abuse may not be present in others.

LEARNING POINTS: ANOREXIA NERVOSA

➤ Anorexia nervosa involves overvalued ideas about weight and shape – a 'morbid fear of fatness', and a preoccupation with food and its calorific value.
➤ Weight loss 15% or more below norm for age/sex/height.
➤ 90% of sufferers female.
➤ Amenorrhoea in teenage women, low sex drive in boys.
➤ Anorexia nervosa is associated with multiple physical signs and metabolic complications.
➤ Physical causes of emaciation should be excluded (e.g. Crohn's or malabsorption syndromes).
➤ Patients may use a variety of covert means to keep their weight low (e.g. secret vomiting).
➤ Long-term mortality is high (15–20%).
➤ Gaining the patient's trust helps long-term compliance.
➤ High-calorie diets may be needed to reverse starvation.
➤ Inpatient units may use behavioural management regimes (preventing vomiting and other means of reducing weight and

drawing up a programme of weight goals and associated rewards).
➤ Individual and family therapy help prevent relapse.
➤ There is an association with child sexual abuse.
➤ More common in higher socioeconomic classes (community prevalence 1% of women) and in higher educational settings (2–3% of women).

BULIMIA NERVOSA

Bulimia nervosa differs from anorexia nervosa in three key respects:
➤ the body weight may be normal or excessive and periods may be present (although sometimes irregular)
➤ frequent binge eating
➤ more common than anorexia nervosa (2–3% of all women).

The sufferer is usually female and older than those with anorexia nervosa (presenting in their twenties). Although anorexics display a profound control over their eating behaviour bulimics are characterised by their lack of control. Although concerned about their weight for most of the time, uncontrollable impulses may lead sufferers to binge on high-calorie foods. A typical binge might involve a tub of ice-cream and a packet of chocolate biscuits followed by half-a-loaf's worth of buttered toast. After such a binge the bulimic patient commonly feels extreme remorse and is thrown into despair. Self-induced vomiting may re-establish some self-esteem, but generally the self-esteem of bulimic patients is very low.

CLINICAL FEATURES

Table 6.4 Clinical features of bulimia nervosa

Past history of anorexia nervosa common (in about a third)
Frequent binge eating
Concern about weight and shape

(continued)

Guilt and low self-esteem

Vomiting, laxative abuse and diuretic abuse, moderate exercise all used to try to reassert control

Irregular or absent menses

Dental decay (due to gastric acid)

Parotid gland enlargement

Calluses on the dorsum of the hand

Normal, high or low weight

Alkalosis, hypokalaemia

Electrolyte imbalance

CASE HISTORY 3

Shortly after her wedding to Michael, Andrea attended her family doctor. She looked quite fit and well, but began by talking about how tired she was feeling and how unsympathetic her husband was. Picking up on her cues, her doctor asked about the experience of being a newlywed. He went on to ask about the quality of their sexual relationship and it was at this point in the consultation that Andrea felt able to unburden herself.

Now aged 24, Andrea had been sexually active with several boyfriends in the past. This her family doctor already knew, but he was surprised to hear that every relationship had had the same pattern to it. At first Andrea had been head over heels in love with each new boyfriend and their sexual relationship had been marked by its intensity and freedom. Soon after the beginning of each relationship Andrea would feel an overwhelming guilt and an irresistible urge to stop seeing the boyfriend. This had led to a large number of very short but very intense relationships, some of them little more than 'one night stands'.

Andrea had met her husband only two months before. Theirs was a whirlwind romance and the honeymoon had been graced by a closeness that Andrea had at first enjoyed, but now found oppressive.

To make matters worse she had begun doing something she had not done for many years. She had started raiding the fridge in the middle of the night to gorge herself on food, which she had stocked there over the past few days. She would eat a family-size trifle in a matter of seconds and follow it by a plate of salami and mayonnaise, then chocolate biscuits on which she had sprayed whipped cream. A few minutes after gorging herself she would go to the bathroom and stick her fingers down her throat to make herself sick. Full of guilt and despair she would return to her marital bed and lie awake thinking about what a bad and fat person she had become.

She had found that a hefty measure of sherry sometimes sent her off to sleep straight away and was enough to prevent her going downstairs to the fridge. Unfortunately, Andrea had begun to see this as an occasional way of keeping bad feelings about herself at bay during the day. Every few days she bought a bottle of sherry and drank it steadily through the day, finishing it last thing at night.

What can the family doctor do to help?

The diagnosis of bulimia nervosa is a fairly clear one. There are repeated binges on highly calorific food, low self-esteem, feelings of fatness, and the patient has a 'normal' appearance, like many bulimic patients (which is why the behaviour often goes undetected for many years).

The family doctor, though, notices that there are echoes of this 'bingeing' behaviour in the rest of her life – there is a repeating 'bingeing' on men and alcohol. Like the food after a binge, the men are discarded once Andrea is racked by guilt. The family doctor might worry here about how Andrea's bulimic behaviour patterns could jeopardise her marriage.

The family doctor needs to collect more data about the extent of the bingeing behaviour and help the patient see a link between her feelings and behaviour and the events in her life. One way of raising these issues is to use self-treatment manuals. Sometimes doctors treating eating disorders ask their patients to complete a food diary for each day. The diary logs food eaten, vomiting behaviour, events and feelings at various times through the day. Reading through the diary with the patient can help both doctor and patient see the pattern of behaviour – what things trigger bulimic behaviour?

Such diaries can be used in cognitive behavioural therapy. Other forms of psychotherapy used to help can be individual dynamic psychotherapy and group therapy.

Some psychiatrists see such behaviour as resulting from disturbances in hypothalamic function. Since serotonin has been found to be important in the regulation of the hypothalamic appetite centre, the regular use of selective serotonin re-uptake inhibitors (SSRIs) has been found useful in reducing the

Time	Food Eaten and Drinks Consumed	Place	Binge	Vomiting	Events around eating	Feelings
8:15 am	1 grapefruit 1 orange black tea	Lounge			Watching breakfast TV	Anxious about day
10:15 am	16 choc biscuits sweet tea	Cafe at Supermarket	Binge		Tempted whilst shopping	Felt hungry
10:30 am		Toilets at Supermarket		Vomit		Guilty. Feel fat
Noon	Ate nothing Black coffee					Making up after binge
4:00 pm	Two Mars bars	Way home from shops	Binge			
4:10 pm		Home		Vomit		Felt sick
7:00 pm	Spaghetti bolognese Glass of wine	Dining room			Listening to Radio	Feel lonely, fat and unwanted
10:00 pm	half litre of choc ice cream half a loaf 2 bowls of cornflakes 4 defrosted cream cakes half bottle of wine	Bedroom floor	Binge			Feeling bloated and guilty
11:00 pm		Bathroom toilet		Vomit		Feel dreadful, can't sleep, Take sleeping tablet.

Figure 6.2 Example of a food diary kept by a bulimic patient

frequency and severity of bulimic binges. An example would be fluoxetine 40–60 mg daily.

LEARNING POINTS: BULIMIA NERVOSA

➤ Prevalence about 2% – presentations are mainly women in their twenties.
➤ Weight may be normal, high or low.
➤ There is a loss of control over eating and sometimes other behaviours such as alcohol or sex.
➤ Frequent binges of high calorie food.
➤ Associated with low self-esteem.
➤ Relatively few physical signs on examination.
➤ Patients may have a past history of anorexia nervosa or obesity.
➤ Psychological treatments include cognitive behavioural therapy, individual dynamic therapy and family therapy.
➤ Drug treatments include SSRIs and other antidepressants.

OBESITY

Obesity is the commonest form of malnutrition in the developed world. Possibly as many as 30% of adults are more than 20% overweight. Extreme obesity is associated with excess mortality from a variety of causes including cardiovascular disease, diabetes mellitus, respiratory dysfunction and gallstones. Obesity is also associated with social, psychological and occupational difficulties. Obesity is seven to 12 times more common in low socioeconomic groups. Genetic factors seem to play a large part too, accounting for a significant proportion of the variance of the body mass index.

Overweight people consistently underestimate their food intake and overestimate their energy expenditure by as much as 50%.

Obese people are often subject to low self-esteem and prejudice. Such prejudice and loneliness leads to further 'comfort eating' and a resultant worsening of the obesity. Intervention can interrupt this cycle, but up to now obesity problems form an insignificant part of the psychiatrist's workload and the problem is not traditionally seen as psychiatric.

Health benefits can accrue from only a 10% reduction in weight. Diets have their problems too, though. There is some evidence to show that weight instability (through alternating periods of dieting and overeating) may be more damaging than weight stability, even at an overweight level.

Table 6.5 Differential diagnosis of obesity

Common causes	Excess calorie intake
	Low physical activity
Rare causes	Endocrine causes (hypothyroidism, Cushing's disease)
	Hypothalamic lesions
	Insulinomas
	Rare genetic causes (e.g. Prader-Willi syndrome)

Table 6.6 Treatment initiatives

First-line	Calorie restriction
	Exercise
	Weight Watchers® or similar group
Second-line	Psychotherapy/cognitive behavioural therapy
	Total fasting (only with close medical supervision)
	Fluoxetine
	Amphetamines
Last resort	Gastric reduction surgery
	Jejunoileal bypass

LEARNING POINTS: OBESITY

➤ Excess weight increases morbidity and mortality from cardiovascular disease.
➤ Weight instability increases the relative risk of death over and above weight stability.
➤ Social, economic and genetic factors play their part in the aetiology of obesity.

➤ Overweight people underestimate their calorie intake and overestimate their energy expenditure.

➤ Health benefits may begin to accrue from modest weight loss (10%).

➤ Treatment options include low-calorie diets, moderate exercise programmes, self-help and commercial programmes, cognitive therapy, pharmacotherapy (e.g. fluoxetine, orlistat or rimonabant) for those more than 30% overweight, and possible surgery for people 100% or more overweight.

SELF-ASSESSMENT
MCQs

1 Clinical features of anorexia nervosa include:
   A loss of secondary sexual characteristics
   B a morbid desire for food
   C reduced growth hormone serum levels
   D leucopenia
   E raised serum levels of triiodothyronine

2 Anorexia nervosa:
   A involves intrusive delusional ideas about food
   B is best treated by psychoanalysis
   C can be diagnosed only when 25% of body mass is lost
   D affects less than 1/1000 teenage women
   E involves a dread of fatness which is an overvalued idea

3 Generally available treatments for bulimia nervosa include:
   A intensive psychoanalysis
   B family therapy
   C fluoxetine
   D cognitive behavioural therapy
   E risperidone

SHORT ANSWER QUESTIONS

1 List 10 physical complications of anorexia nervosa.
2 Explain the similarities and differences between anorexia nervosa and bulimia nervosa.

ESSAY
Describe the principles of the management of severe anorexia nervosa.

MCQ answers
1 A=F, B=F, C=F, D=T, E=F.
2 A=F, B=F, C=F, D=F, E=T.
3 A=F, B=T, C=T, D=T, E=F.

EXPLORATIONS
LINKS WITH PHYSIOLOGY AND BIOCHEMISTRY

➤ What biochemical changes in metabolism are associated with starvation?
➤ What calorific intakes are required for differing lifestyles?
➤ What psychological changes are associated with biochemical changes in starvation?

LINKS WITH EPIDEMIOLOGY RESEARCH

➤ How would you design research to establish the prevalence of anorexia nervosa in a community?
➤ How would you design research to establish the outcome of a treatment for anorexia nervosa?

LINKS WITH COMMUNITY MEDICINE/ GENERAL PRACTICE

➤ What self-help groups and voluntary organisations exist for anorexia nervosa and bulimia nervosa sufferers in your local area?
➤ How can you assess the quality of the service they offer?
➤ What would the benefits and disadvantages be to clients of these services?

FURTHER READING AND REFERENCES

Bruch H. *The Golden Cage: the enigma of anorexia nervosa*. London: Open Books; 1978.

Crisp AH. *Anorexia Nervosa: let me be*. London: Academic Press; 1980.

Fairburn C. *Cognitive Behaviour Therapy and Eating Disorders*. London: Guilford Press; 2008.

Hsu LKG. *Eating Disorders*. New York: Guilford Press; 1990.

King MB. Eating disorders in a general practice population: prevalence, characteristics and follow-up at 12–18 months. *Psychological Medicine*. 1989; **s14**.

Mann AH, Wakeling A, Wood K, Monck E, Dobbs R, Szmukler G. Screening for abnormal eating attitudes and psychiatric morbidity in an unselected population of 15 year old schoolgirls. *Psychological Medicine*. 1983; **13**, 573–80.

Mazzola A. Skin signs in eating disorders. *Psychiatry On-Line*; 2007. www.priory.com/psychiatry/Skin_signs_anorexia.htm

Mehenna M, Mooledina J, Travis J. Refeeding syndrome: what it is, and how to prevent and treat it. *BMJ*. 2008; **336**: 1495–8.

National Institute for Health and Clinical Excellence. *Nutrition Support in Adults. Clinical Guideline CG32*. London: NIHCE; 2006. www.nice.org.uk/CG32

Palmer RL. *Helping People with Eating Disorders: a clinical guide to assessment and treatment*, London: John Wiley & Sons; 2008.

Rathner G, Messner K. Detection of eating disorders in a small rural town: an epidemiological study. *Psychological Medicine*. 1993; **23**: 175–84.

Russell GFM. Bulimia nervosa: an ominous variant of anorexia nervosa. *Psychological Medicine*. 1979; **9**: 429.

Russell GFM, Szmukler GI, Dare C, Eisler I. An evaluation of family therapy in anorexia nervosa and bulimia nervosa. *Arch Gen Psychiatry*. 1987; **44(12)**: 1047–56.

Sharp CW, Freeman CPL. The medical complications of anorexia nervosa. *British Journal of Psychiatry*. 1993; **162**: 452–62.

Treasure J, van Furth E, Schmidt U. *Handbook of Eating Disorders*. 2nd ed. London: John Wiley & Sons; 2003.

ANOREXIA NERVOSA IN LITERATURE

Life-size by Jenefer Shute. Mandarin paperbacks; 1997.

The Art of Starvation by Sheila MacLeod. Virago Paperbacks; 1989.

Anorexic by Anna Patterson. Westworld International; 2000.

RESOURCES

Beating Eating Disorders
103 Prince of Wales Road, Norwich NR1 1DW
0870 770 3256
www.b-eat.co.uk/

Section of Eating Disorders
Division of Psychological Medicine and Psychiatry, PO59
Institute of Psychiatry
De Crespigny Park, London SE5 8AF
Tel: 020 7848 0160
Fax: 020 7848 0182
www.iop.kcl.ac.uk/

Academy for Eating Disorders
111 Deer Lake Road, Suite 100, Deerfield, IL 60015 USA
www.aedweb.org/

NIMH eating disorders web pages
www.nimh.nih.gov/health/publications/eating-disorders/what-are-eating-disorders.shtml

CHAPTER 7
Addiction

A wide variety of exogenous substances have addictive properties. Naturally occurring substances such as tobacco, cannabis and alcohol have been used by humankind for thousands of years. Synthetic compounds such as heroin, cocaine and benzodiazepines have become available in the last few centuries. For a substance to be addictive it must usually provide some psychological reward, e.g. relief of anxiety, and be capable of inducing physical dependence. Substance addicts often crave the substance when it is not available because of psychological and physical withdrawal effects.

CONTENTS

ADDICTION, TOLERANCE, DEPENDENCE AND WITHDRAWAL

Addiction is defined differently by different people. In this book addiction refers to a state of craving for a particular external substance which, for various reasons, the addict feels he or she needs and cannot do without. Addicts often act in ways that damage themselves or others in order to get and use the desired substance. Repeated exposure to the same dose may result in a diminishing response. This is known as *tolerance*, where the addict feels that they need to up the dose to achieve the same effect as before. *Dependence* can be physical or psychological. Abusers of alcohol may drink in order to cope with stressful situations. Without alcohol they may feel unable to cope. Physical dependence implies that there are physical symptoms when the drug is withdrawn, i.e. a *withdrawal syndrome*. An example of a *dependency cycle* is given in Figure 7.1.

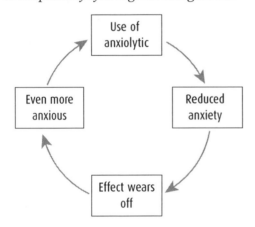

Figure 7.1 Addiction cycle for anxiolytics

In this cycle the use of an anxiolytic, e.g. a benzodiazepine, is prompted by anxiety, but once the benzodiazepine is metabolised the anxiety returns, prompting reuse. Since benzodiazepines are associated with tolerance and withdrawal effects, there is a drive to take higher and higher doses more often to reduce anxiety. The faster the cycle spins, the greater the risk of addiction. Short half-life drugs spin the cycle quicker than long half-life drugs,

so that benzodiazepines with short half-lives are more addictive than those with long half-lives. Table 7.1 gives the half-lives of various benzodiazepines. Long-term benzodiazepine use is associated with a notorious withdrawal syndrome, which includes rebound anxiety, rebound insomnia and convulsions. Some of the symptoms are given in Table 7.2.

CLINICAL FEATURES OF ADDICTION

These include:

- tolerance
- persistent desire for the substance
- unsuccessful attempts to cut down or stop using
- a great deal of time, effort or risk expended in obtaining the substance
- difficulty fulfilling social obligations at work, college or home
- persistent use despite awareness of adverse effects of drug on health or well-being of self or others
- withdrawal symptoms
- substance taken specifically to avoid going into withdrawal.

THE EPIDEMIOLOGY OF ADDICTION

It is difficult to get accurate figures for the prevalence and incidence of substance misuse. An approximate top 10 list of misused substances is given in Table 7.3 (p. 110). To estimate alcohol consumption in the country epidemiologists look at government revenue statistics of alcohol sales, population surveys, and sometimes use indirect but correlated data, such as deaths from liver cirrhosis. Certain occupational groups are at higher risk of alcoholism: publicans, bartenders, businessmen, service personnel, doctors and lawyers. In General Hospitals 20 to 30% of all male admissions and 5 to 10% of all female admissions are probably related to heavy alcohol use. At least 5% of all men and about 2% of all women in the UK have a drinking problem.

Statistics for illicit drug consumption are more difficult to obtain since there is no legal duty on illicit drugs. Information only arises

Table 7.1 The half-lives for four benzodiazepines

Drug	T ½ (hours)	Volume of distribution (L/kg)	% bound to plasma proteins
Chlordiazepoxide	6–28	0.3–0.6	95
Diazepam	20–40	1–2	98
Temazepam	8–16	1.3–1.6	97
Nitrazepam	18–31	1.5–2.8	87

Table 7.2 Some withdrawal symptoms associated with long-term benzodiazepine use

Rebound insomnia	Dysarthria
Rebound anxiety	Frequency
Panic	Metallic taste
Convulsions	Polyuria
Excitability	Diarrhoea
Depersonalisation	Nausea and vomiting
Poor concentration	Palpitations
Illusions	Hyperventilation
Depression	Thirst
Craving	Loss of libido
Vivid dreams	Skin rash
Stiffness	Stuffy nose
Paresthesiae	Hyperacusis
Hallucinations	Temporal lobe fits
Pain	Obsessions
Weakness	Menorrhagia
Tremor	Mammary pain
Formication	Flushing and sweating
Muscle twitches / fasciculation	Ataxia
Blurred vision	Tinnitus

therefore when addicts come into contact with official departments such as the Home Office. Doctors in the UK are supposed to notify the Home Office of addicts of certain controlled substances. Most notifications concern opiate abuse. Substance abuse is generally more common in men than in women. Other information comes from criminal statistics, drug seizures, offences against drug laws and self-report surveys. Regular drug use in inner city schools may be as high as 20% of 16 year olds and is rising. In 1991 in the United States at least 40% of males arrested for burglary and assault tested positive for some drug. Between 9 and 64% of these drug users were using cocaine. Addicts indulge in a variety of crimes to get the money they need to fuel their addiction. Some of these activities, for instance prostitution, may put them at particular risk of HIV infection.

PSYCHIATRIC CONSEQUENCES OF ALCOHOL ABUSE

There are consequences for the individual, his or her family and society.

CONSEQUENCES FOR THE INDIVIDUAL

The features of the dependence syndrome mean that the individual underperforms at work, functions poorly socially and in the family. Sexual relationships may be threatened by loss of employment, disinhibition, violence and impotence. Cravings for alcohol dominating the individual's waking hours may mean that other activities are excluded, and so the alcoholic's life begins to revolve only around alcohol. Substance addicts may be so focused on getting their next drink or fix that they will steal or deceive in order to fund their habit.

Table 7.3 Most popular non-prescribed addictive drugs in the UK

Rank	Drug	Regular users
1	Alcohol	Majority of adults
2	Tobacco	12.5 million
3	Ecstasy	800 000
4	Cocaine	800 000
5	Amphetamines	650 000
6	Alkyl nitrites	550 000
7	Benzodiazepines	160 000
8	LSD	70 000
9	Heroin	40 000
10	Khat	40 000
11	Anabolic steroids	38 000
12	Solvents	37 000

Table 7.4 UK street costs of illicit drugs

Drug	UK street cost
Heroin	£45 per gram
Cannabis	1 ounce herbal £87–£134 depending on quality, resin £55 per ounce
Cocaine	£43 per gram
Ecstasy	£2.40 per pill
Amphetamine	£10 per gram
Ketamine	£25 per gram
Methadone	£2 a dose
Anabolic steroids	£8 a tablet
GHB	£15 a bottle
LSD	£4 a tablet

Source: The Independent and Drugscope (www.drugscope.org.uk)

In persistent heavy drinkers cessation of drinking may lead to a withdrawal syndrome. This typically begins 8 to 24 hours after stopping drinking. Typical withdrawal symptoms include anxiety, withdrawal fits, tremor, sweating, insomnia and loss of appetite. Withdrawal signs include pupillary dilatation, tachycardia and raised blood pressure.

Delirium tremens
Delirium tremens is an acute confusional state. This may occur 24 to 96 hours after stopping drinking. Symptoms include pronounced tremor, restlessness, disorientation, illusions and hallucinations (visual, auditory or tactile), fever, sweating and tachycardia. There is a mortality of 10%, requiring medical management on a medical ward.

Alcoholic hallucinosis
Alcoholic hallucinosis is a rare condition where hallucinations, usually auditory, occur in clear consciousness.

Morbid jealousy
Morbid jealousy, or the *Othello syndrome*, involves firmly held delusions of the partner's infidelity. The alcoholic researches partner's belongings for signs of infidelity or interrogates them about their daily activities to try to catch them out. Under continual pressure of this kind unwise partners may confess to an infidelity that they haven't committed. Such an admission may provoke a violent assault or even murder. Even in partners who maintain their innocence geographical separation may be necessary to save their lives.

Depression and suicide
Depression and suicide are more common among alcoholics. Suicide is made more likely because of all the social consequences of alcohol abuse, for instance job loss and divorce, and also because of the disinhibiting effect of alcohol. Depression may resolve without the use of antidepressants once the alcoholic has stopped drinking for some time.

Cognitive effects
Cognitive effects may occur secondary to alcohol toxicity, brain trauma while inebriated and thiamine deficiency. Among heavy users

of alcohol, short-term memory problems, narrowness of thinking and impairment of visio-spatial awareness are common findings. A high proportion of alcoholics develop cortical atrophy and ventricular enlargement on brain imaging. Severe thiamine deficiency may produce an acute brain syndrome called Wernicke's encephalopathy, which is characterised by delirium, confabulation, memory impairment, ataxia, nystagmus, and a peripheral neuropathy. A chronic form of Wernicke's encephalopathy is the Korsakoff state. This is a chronic form of memory impairment, without the delirium. Often the two syndromes are classified together as the Wernicke-Korsakoff syndrome. High dose thiamine replacement may help reverse some of the cognitive deficits. Such thiamine replacement may need to be introduced as an emergency via intramuscular or intravenous routes.

FAMILY CONSEQUENCES

The use of alcohol may impact on the family in terms of childhood physical or sexual abuse. Those who are children of alcoholics themselves have an increased vulnerability to developing substance misuse problems, and this may be a genetic or environmental effect. Other members of the family may suffer reactive depression or adjustment disorders as a consequence of the alcoholic individual's effect on the family. Mothers who misuse alcohol during pregnancy may have children with foetal alcohol syndrome. This is sometimes recognised in infants due to problems such as growth retardation, small head circumference, small eyes, a flattened bridge of the nose, elfin features and learning disability. Sometimes foetal alcohol syndrome may be missed in infants, and may present in adolescence with behavioural problems.

CONSEQUENCES TO SOCIETY

Sixty per cent of convicted criminals report alcohol problems. One-third of all drivers killed on the roads have excess alcohol in their bloodstream. As a consequence of offending behaviour such as sexual assault or drink driving, unrelated third parties may be psychologically damaged and suffer post-traumatic stress disorder or bereavement reactions.

Alcoholism and cirrhosis

National hepatic cirrhosis rates are directly linked to per capita alcohol consumption. Cirrhosis mortality rates are rising sharply in Britain. Between 1987–91 and 1997–2001 cirrhosis mortality in men in Scotland rose by 112% and in England and Wales by 67%. Mortality for cirrhosis in women rose 63% in Scotland and 35% in England and Wales. Cirrhosis rates in Scotland are the highest in Western Europe: about 30/100 000 in men and 13/100 000 in women.

ADVERSE EFFECTS OF STREET DRUGS

Drug users will often deny to themselves and to others that drugs have any adverse consequences, but unfortunately they do, especially if they are derived from an impure source or a rogue batch. Some of the common side-effects of street drugs are given in Table 7.5 (p. 112). Paradoxically, addicts may be at risk from unusually pure supplies of street drugs. Street heroin is often adulterated with other substances. When a pure supply enters the dealing system this may mean that the addict consequently uses too much and overdoses themself unwittingly.

TREATMENT OPTIONS FOR ALCOHOLICS

The main attribute necessary for a recovery is the will of the patient to conquer their own alcohol problem. It may seem obvious to say that before the problem can be conquered it must be recognised, but alcohol problems often persist for a long time before the individual accepts that he or she even has a problem. The alcoholic's psychological defence mechanisms are used to deny the problem, and to project the responsibility for the problem onto other people. External agencies such as hospitals can assist with detoxification, and specialist hostels

Table 7.5 Key facts about street drugs

Heroin	Derived from poppies grown, e.g. in Afghanistan and Pakistan. Sedative and highly addictive. Can be smoked or injected. Associated with 'cold turkey' withdrawal syndrome. Addicts may 'mature out' of using heroin after several years. Adverse effects include respiratory depression, constipation, pupillary constriction, coma.
Amphetamines	Synthetic stimulant: can be in tablets, snorted, mixed in drinks, injected. Increased heart rate and alertness. Associated with paranoia and depression. Methamphetamine particularly addictive. Made in labs in UK, Netherlands, Scandinavia and US.
Cannabis	Easily cultivated – plant leaves can be smoked or eaten. More potent forms can cause hallucinations and panic attacks. The major biologically active chemical compound in cannabis is delta-9-tetrahydrocannabinol, commonly referred to as THC. Adverse effects include fatigue, apathy, impaired memory and concentration, bronchitis, also carcinogenic.
Psilocybin	Drunk in teas made from magic mushrooms. Adverse effects include: tachycardia, hypertension, papillary dilatation, illusions and hallucinations, nausea and stomach pains.
LSD	Highly potent synthetic hallucinogen. Affects perception of time. Associated with later flashbacks.
Anabolic steroids	Synthetic hormones used by bodybuilders. May be associated with irritability, paranoia and mood disturbance. Other adverse effects include liver and kidney damage.
GHB	Gammahydroxybutyrate – sold as 'liquid ecstasy' – relaxant, disinhibiting, associated with fits and rape. Sudden withdrawal in addicts is associated with agitated psychosis, delirium, and autonomic instability.
Organic solvents	From paints, glues, lighter fluid – euphoriant, disinhibiting and may cause arrhythmias and death. Other risks include: suffocation, fires, ataxia, slurred speech, nausea, hallucinations, and coma.
Ecstasy	3,4-Methylenedioxymethamphetamine. Used in dance scene, causes feelings of well-being and amiability, anxiety and paranoia in some. Pyrexia may cause dehydration and muscle cell death. Other adverse effects include pupillary dilatation, fits, and rarely death. MDMA causes impaired cognitive function in attention/concentration, verbal and nonverbal learning and memory, psychomotor speed and executive system functioning.
Ketamine	Developed as intravenous anaesthetic. In tablet form may be hallucinogenic, probably through affecting glutamate receptor neurotransmission, and by causing secondary increases in glutamate release.
Cocaine	Derived from coca shrubs in Colombia and Bolivia. Cocaine powder, freebase and crack are all forms of cocaine. Can be snorted, smoked and injected. Stimulant and increases confidence. Raises heart rate and blood pressure. Associated with pyrexia, fits and heart failure. May cause panic attacks and precipitate psychosis. Cocaine addiction has sometimes been treated with disulfiram, topiramate, tiagabine and propranolol.

can provide support in terms of shelter and encouragement, but the fundamental change in behaviour required is ultimately the responsibility of the addict him- or herself. Family members can be co-opted as co-therapists, and this is often useful, and ongoing support from self-help and other groups may be vital.

MEDICAL HELP FOR ALCOHOLICS

Detoxification and withdrawal regimes may rely heavily on benzodiazepines. These can be useful in allaying withdrawal symptoms such as rebound anxiety and also useful because they raise the threshold and reduce the likelihood of alcohol withdrawal fits. Detoxification regimes therefore require the addict to switch over to a regular high dose of benzodiazepines. These detoxification programmes can be done in hospital, or in the community. The advantage of a hospital withdrawal programme means that closer monitoring is possible, and trained staff are theoretically immediately on hand to act if there is a withdrawal fit which may have fatal consequences if not properly treated. The object of the use of benzodiazepines is to avoid full-blown alcohol withdrawal symptoms with all the dangers this entails. Additional components of medical withdrawal from alcohol would include thiamine and multivitamin supplements to prevent Wernicke-Korsakoff syndrome. Attention to hydration, electrolyte balance and glucose levels is important. Specific advice on the physical consequences of alcoholism can be given if liver function tests are analysed on admission. Psychological problems may warrant onward referral, particularly if there is coexisting post-traumatic stress disorder, for instance. Psychological cravings for alcohol can sometimes be treated in the medium term with acamprosate. Disulfiram (Antabuse) can be used as a psychological and physical support to an abstinence programme. Those people who take Antabuse regularly are aware that should they lapse and begin to drink alcohol they will suffer a severe and unpleasant reaction because of the disulfiram in their bloodstream. The reaction involves flushing, nausea, headache, tachycardia, difficulty in breathing and effects on blood pressure.

For patients in whom there is evidence of abnormal liver function, abstinence is the most desirable way forward. Abstinence may be promoted and maintained by the use of either NHS Support Groups for Recovering Alcoholics, or voluntary sector support groups such as Alcoholics Anonymous. Regular attendance at such groups yields the best chance of sustained abstinence and better outcomes long term.

MEDICAL TREATMENT OPTIONS FOR DRUG ADDICTS

Withdrawal programmes for heroin addicts often use the opiate substitute methadone. The choice of either methadone or heroin in withdrawal/maintenance programmes is controversial. Maintenance programmes seek to replace the street supply of heroin/methadone with a Health Service derived alternative, which is obviously pure, without adulteration with other substances, and if given with sterile needles, less likely to produce HIV and hepatitis than shared 'works'. In a withdrawal course, methadone may be supplied in a reducing course over several weeks or months. In maintenance programmes the Health Service prescribed drugs are prescribed almost indefinitely with a view being that addicts sometimes 'mature out' of using the drug after several years. Advocates of maintenance programmes point to the advantages of clean needle supplies in reducing infections in the general population, and a reduced local crime rate. Problems with maintenance programmes include the increased death rate in methadone users long term, the selling on of the methadone/heroin, or the topping up of prescribed sources with other street drugs by the addict. Naltrexone is an oral long-acting antagonist which the detoxified addict can take. Further drug use is not associated with any effect because of the antagonism, thereby eliminating any reward effect.

Drug rehabilitation units in hostels are available, but rare. They may follow various principles including rehabilitation techniques in a drug- and alcohol- free environment. The 'therapeutic community' approach is key in some hostels where group therapy work with peers is seen as important with peers often being particularly able to point out where an individual is using psychological defence mechanisms such as denial or projection. Some hostels are run along the '12 step' model for alcohol / drug addiction.

In some areas of the NHS community drug teams focus specifically on opiates. In other areas help can be given for users of other drugs, such as cocaine and cannabis.

Withdrawal from amphetamines and other stimulants can sometimes be aided by the use of antidepressants.

Benzodiazepine addiction can be managed by switching the addict on to a longer half-life benzodiazepine, and gradually withdrawing this over weeks or months.

CASE HISTORY 1

A 34-year-old married man called Nicholas was brought to hospital by ambulance. His colleagues at the college where he worked as a librarian had found him slumped over a desk in the library archives. He had drunk an entire bottle of vodka. He had been sick everywhere, but was also nearly unconscious. He was admitted to the medical ward, and seen the next day by a duty psychiatrist who noted that Nicholas had a clammy handshake, was shaking all over and looked very sweaty. While he was talking Nicholas kept wringing his hands and seemed very anxious. He cried twice during the interview.

He gave a history of heavy drinking for the past six months ever since his supervisor at work had set certain targets for his department. The drinking had caused many arguments with his wife, whom he had hit twice. He said that this was 'out of character' and 'because of the drink'. He describes his wife as an 'unforgiving and hard woman'.

He was particularly annoyed that she had left him, taking their two children with her. He had tried to phone her at her mother's house, but the family had had the telephone number changed, and she had changed her mobile since leaving him. Feeling very sorry for himself, Nicholas had bought a bottle of vodka, intending to drink it all at work and kill himself through alcoholic self-poisoning. The psychiatrist enquired about various other symptoms, and learnt that Nicholas had initial insomnia, early morning wakening, loss of appetite and had been having memory problems which he called 'blackouts'. He kept forgetting what had happened the day before.

How do you assess this man further?

He needs to have full history taken, a mental state examination, particularly an assessment of his cognitive function. He requires a physical examination, some physical investigations and a corroborative history.

What cognitive tests would you be most interested in?

Orientation, and providing that his attention and concentration are adequate, tests of short-term memory such as three objects (apple, table, penny) and a new name and address. It might be worth investigating whether he repeatedly gets lost on the ward, because visio-spatial memory is often impaired. It may also be important to check out his recall of the ward routine and corroborate this with the nurses. For instance, it may be worth asking him about his visitors, what he has been doing that morning, and what he has had to eat. Sometimes patients may *confabulate* where they will fill in gaps in their memory with plausible sounding information. Checking this information against a corroborative history can be revealing, and may point to the presence of a Wernicke-Korsakoff syndrome.

The importance of checking orientation would be to exclude a delirium. When people tend to forget the previous day's events, this is sometimes called palimpsest.

What would the immediate management of this patient be?

It appears that he is in alcohol withdrawal (he is anxious and sweating, has a tremor and may well also have pupillary dilatation and tachycardia on examination). Not only is the withdrawal unpleasant for the patient to experience, but there is also a risk of epileptic fits, as the alcohol withdrawal reduces the epileptic threshold. A detoxification regime using benzodiazepines such as chlordiazepoxide should be employed. It would also be important to exclude metabolite disturbances, coexisting infection and too much use of high dose vitamins, particularly thiamine.

CASE HISTORY 2

Kevin was 21 when he arrived as a new patient at the health centre. He claimed he had just moved into the area and needed to register with a new family doctor that day. He seemed very keen to see the doctor immediately, but wouldn't explain why to the receptionist and was rude to her when she probed further. When he did see his new doctor he told the doctor that he had been using drugs since the age of 13 when he had started sniffing glue out of plastic bags. When one of his friends had died from sniffing butane from aerosols Kevin had moved on to 'safer drugs'. He gave a history of using cannabis for a few years, but said that he had latterly been injecting heroin. He said that his mother had thrown him out of her house and he was living in a squat nearby. He told the doctor that he used money from burglaries and from car thefts to fund his habit. He told the doctor that he was now very keen to come off heroin and was seeking a supply of methadone. When the doctor explained that he wasn't an approved prescriber of methadone and that he referred all his patients to the regional drug clinic, Kevin became very abusive, much to the doctor's alarm. Kevin then became very tearful and asked the doctor to 'give me a break and just prescribe something'. The doctor was beginning to type out a prescription on the computer when the receptionist rang him. Over the telephone the receptionist said that she had checked Kevin's details, and his name, date of birth and address were incorrect. When the doctor looked up from the computer screen he saw that the consulting room door was ajar and Kevin was gone.

What feelings are aroused in health professionals by such patients?

Although carers may start out with good intentions and high ideals with such patients, they run the risk of becoming cynical when faced with numerous patients like Kevin who cheat and thieve to fulfil their cravings. The negative feelings evoked by such patients need to be acknowledged. If carers deny their own feelings about the patient they may deceive themselves and they may be fooled by their responses which they initially may think are justifiable, but are in fact motivated by cynicism and dislike. Negative feelings may lead carers to ignore vital information. For instance, a doctor may fail to examine an unconscious patient properly in casualty due to the mistaken belief that they are merely drunk as they are smelling of alcohol, when in fact they may be drunk but also have a skull fracture. Furthermore it is important to realise that some addicts do mean what they say, and can carry out their promises to reform themselves. Studies tend to show that addicts are best helped by care and encouragement from staff with a high motivation.

CASE HISTORY 3

Private Henson was a 20-year-old soldier admitted as an emergency under a Section of the Mental Health Act. He had been assessed in accident and emergency after being airlifted from a NATO base in Germany. He was psychotic and paranoid and had attacked his Military Police guards, rendering one unconscious, and then assaulted a nurse. He was rapidly tranquillised with intramuscular haloperidol and lorazepam and transferred into a locked psychiatric intensive care unit (PICU). As he got onto the ward he became frightened of the staff grade doctor, saying he was 'a spy' and tried to attack him. Private Henson was restrained and placed in seclusion. Blood and urine samples were taken from him when he settled under further sedation. Such history as could be obtained said he had been in action in Iraq and had become anxious and depressed. He had been managed at an army medical facility in Germany with a view to repatriation, when he became even more disturbed after a brief period of leave into the nearby German town. He had returned drunk and profoundly scared. There was no history of past psychiatric illness prior to service in Iraq.

What is the most likely diagnosis?

There is a suggestion of past mood disturbance severe enough to warrant his leaving the front line. The illness has become more severe still with fearfulness and violence, possibly based on misidentification.

Noticeably the deterioration occurred after a period of leave, and this might point towards a drug-induced psychosis.

What might be the cause of his depression?

Active service might suggest that he has been exposed to some combat-related trauma. Post-traumatic stress disorder could manifest as depression.

What drugs might cause such a drug-induced psychosis?

Amphetamines or cocaine could be potential candidates. These drugs could have exacerbated an underlying depression or PTSD to induce a psychotic reaction.

What's the link between PTSD and drug use?

Drug misuse and alcohol misuse are commonly associated with PTSD, probably as a self-administered means of coping with PTSD symptoms. Alcohol may be used to cope with initial insomnia and other drugs used to cope with dysphoria.

LEARNING POINTS: ADDICTION

➤ Tolerance implies that the repeated use of the drug of abuse produces less effect for the same dose.

➤ Dependence may be physical or psychological, and implies that without the drug the addict may suffer withdrawal syndrome characterised by physical or psychological symptoms of withdrawal.

➤ Substance abuse is more common in men than in women.

➤ The main attribute necessary for long-term recovery is the will of a patient to conquer his or her addiction.

➤ Alcoholism is linked to a 15% lifetime risk of suicide.

➤ Ten per cent of alcoholics have had withdrawal fits.

➤ Delirium tremens is an acute confusional state which may occur 24 to 96 hours after stopping drinking. Symptoms include marked tremor, restlessness, disorientation, illusions and hallucinations, fever, sweating and tachycardia. There is a mortality of 10%.

➤ In General Hospitals 20 to 30% of all male admissions, and 5 to 10% of female admissions are probably heavy drinkers.

➤ Addiction is not confined to any single portion of society, and is endemic throughout the world.

➤ Street drug use is rising, and drug users are getting younger. It is difficult to control access to addictive substances such as solvents which are widely available. Small laboratories are easily set up to create supplies of crack cocaine, LSD, amphetamines and ecstasy. In view of the drugs' ready availability, combating drug abuse requires health education which will modify people's attitudes towards drugs and alcohol.

➤ Although alcohol and drug abuse does not tend to bring people directly into contact with psychiatry, people who misuse drugs are at increased risk of affective disorders, psychotic disorders and suicide.

BOX 7.1

The CAGE MAST Questionnaires are examples of questionnaires used to screen for alcohol problems. The CAGE questions were derived from work by Mayfield and others in 1974. They represent a validated screening instrument. Two positive answers on the CAGE are strongly suggestive of alcoholism. The shortened Michigan Alcoholism Screening Test (MAST) is a series of 10 alternative questions. To score the MAST an individual would get 2 for a negative answer to the first and second questions, and for positive answers to the remainder of the questions you score either 5 or 2. For question 3, a yes would give you 5; for question 4 a yes would give you 2; for questions 5, 6, 7, 8, 9 and 10, score 2, 2, 2, 5, 5 and 2 respectively for positive answers. A score above 18 indicates severe problems. Most-non alcoholics score less than 5 on the MAST.

THE CAGE QUESTIONNAIRE

C Have you ever felt that you should CUT down on your drinking?

A Have people ANNOYED you by criticising your drinking?

G Have you ever felt bad or GUILTY about your drinking?

E Have you ever had a drink first thing in the morning to steady your nerves or get rid of a hangover (EYE OPENER)?

THE MAST QUESTIONNAIRE

1 Do you feel you are a normal drinker?

2 Do friends or relatives think you are a normal drinker?

3 Have you ever attended a meeting of Alcoholics Anonymous (AA)?

4 Have you ever lost friends or girl/boyfriends because of drinking?

5 Have you ever got into trouble at work because of drinking?

6 Have you ever neglected your obligations, your family, your work for more than two days in a row because you were drinking?

7 Have you ever had delirium tremens, severe shaking, heard voices or seen things that weren't there after heavy drinking?

8 Have you ever gone to anyone for help about your drinking?

9 Have you ever been in a hospital because of your drinking?

10 Have you ever been arrested for drunken driving or driving after drinking?

SELF-ASSESSMENT
MCQs

1 Features of the chronic Korsakoff's syndrome include:
   A delirium
   B anterograde amnesia
   C confabulation
   D psychotic symptoms
   E vertical nystagmus

2 Benzodiazepine withdrawal may produce:
   A tremor
   B insomnia
   C anxiety
   D convulsions
   E muscle fasciculation

3 Methadone:
   A is a benzodiazepine
   B can be prescribed intravenously
   C has a shorter half-life than heroin
   D may induce vomiting
   E is not excreted in breast milk

4 Clinical feature of chronic opiate dependence include:
   A dilated pupils
   B tremors
   C tiredness
   D constipation
   E impotence

MCQ answers

1 A=F, B=T, C=T D=F, E=F.
2 All true.
3 A=F, B=T, C=F D=T, E=F.
4 A=F, B=T, C=T D=T, E=T.

EXPLORATIONS
LINKS WITH PUBLIC HEALTH

Look at the data in Table 7.5 (p. 112) about alcohol consumption and cirrhosis of the liver. What conclusions can you draw?

LINKS WITH MEDICINE

➤ What are the long-term physical consequences of alcohol dependence?

➤ How might these consequences fit in with psychological problems such as jealousy, memory problems and delirium?

➤ What physical investigations could be used to identify alcohol abusers in general medical practice?

LINKS WITH PRIMARY CARE

What evidence is there that screening questionnaires, such as those in Box 7.1 (p 117), are useful in identifying alcoholics in general practice?

FURTHER READING AND REFERENCES

Abadinsky H. *Drug Use and Abuse: a comprehensive introduction.* London: Wadsworth; 2007.

Brecht M-L, Anglin MD. Conditional factors of maturing out of narcotics addiction: long term relationships. *Proceedings of the Social Statistics Section, American Statistical Association.* 1993. pp. 209–14.

Edwards G, Lader M, editors. *The Nature of Drug Dependence*, Oxford: Oxford University Press; 1991.

Kalechstein AD, De La Garza R II, Mahoney JJ III, Fantegrossi WE, Newton TF. MDMA use and neurocognition: a meta-analytic review. *Psychopharmacology.* 2007; **189**(4): 531–7.

Kamal A, Cheung R. Positive CAGE screen correlates with cirrhosis in veterans with chronic hepatitis C. *Digestive Diseases & Sciences.* 2007; **52**(10): 2564–9.

Landabasoa M, Iraurgib I, Jiménez-Lermac J, Callea R, Sanza J, Gutiérrez-Frailed M. Ecstasy-induced psychotic disorder: six-month follow-up study. *Eur Addict Res.* 2002; **8**: 133–40.

Leon DA, McCambridge J. Liver cirrhosis mortality rates in Britain from 1950 to 2002: an analysis of routine data. *Lancet.* 2006; **367**: 52–6.

Ponicki WR, Gruenewald PJ. The impact of alcohol taxation on liver cirrhosis mortality. *Journal of Studies on Alcohol.* 2006; **67**(6): 934–8.

Sofuoglu M, Kosten TR. Emerging pharmacological strategies in the fight against cocaine addiction. *Expert Opinion on Emerging Drugs.* 2006; **11**(1): 91–8.

ADDICTION IN LITERATURE

Amis KW (1969) *The Green Man.*
Baudelaire C (1860) *Artificial Paradises.*

Dick P (1977) *A Scanner Darkly.*
De Quincey T (1821) *Confessions of an English Opium Eater.*
Welsh I (1993) *Trainspotting.*

RESOURCES

Action on Addiction
East Knoyle, Wiltshire SP3 6BE
www.actiononaddiction.org.uk

Alcoholics Anonymous
PO Box 1, 10 Toft Green, York YO1 7NJ
www.alcoholics-anonymous.org.uk

Al-Anon
(Family Groups)
61 Great Dover Street, London SE1 4YF
Tel: 020 7403 0888 (Helpline 10 am to 10 pm, 365 days a year)
www.al-anonuk.org.uk

Alcohol Concern
64 Leman Street, London E1 8EU
Tel: 020 7264 0510
Email: contact@alcoholconcern.org.uk
www.alcoholconcern.org.uk

Drugscope
40 Bermondsey Street, London SE1 3UD
Tel: 020 7940 7500
Email: info@drugscope.org.uk
www.drugscope.org.uk

Release
Tel: 020 7729 9904
www.release.org.uk

Talk to Frank
Tel: 0800 77 66 00
www.talktofrank.com

Turning Point
Standon House, 21 Mansell Street, London E1 8AA
Tel: 020 7481 7600
Email: info@turning-point.co.uk
www.turning-point.co.uk

CHAPTER 8

Post-traumatic stress disorder

Post-traumatic stress disorder (PTSD) is a severe psychological reaction to a life-threatening trauma. It can also be provoked by threats to a person's physical integrity, prolonged stress such as torture or being a prisoner of war, or witnessing the death of a loved one. It involves anxiety, depression and specific features such as nightmares, flashbacks, hyper-arousal and avoidance behaviours.

CONTENTS

CLASSIFICATION OF PSYCHIATRIC REACTIONS TO TRAUMA

Psychiatric reactions can be provoked by various traumas including assault, rape, severe road traffic accidents, surviving a fire, surviving a terrorist incident, being mugged, or witnessing someone being badly injured or killed. **Acute stress reactions** involve feelings of intense anxiety, dizziness and feeling faint, numbness and detachment, and poor sleep. These occur in the first few hours after a trauma, may be self-limiting and may last just a few days.

An initial stress reaction may evolve into an **acute stress disorder (ASD)**. This may occur in the first month after a trauma and may last a few days or weeks. It may occur in 10 to 20% of people involved in assaults and road accidents. Symptoms resemble those of **post-traumatic stress disorder (PTSD)**, which is conventionally only diagnosed when over a month has elapsed since the trauma. PTSD is a more chronic disorder than ASD and may last a year or even several years. A diagnosis of ASD often predicts a later diagnosis of PTSD.

Where the predominant feature of a psychiatric reaction is low mood following some loss or trauma (and where some PTSD features are missing) doctors may sometimes diagnose an **adjustment disorder**.

EPIDEMIOLOGY

The estimated lifetime prevalence of PTSD among adults in the general population is about 7–10%, with women twice as likely as men to have PTSD at some point in their lives. This is a small proportion of those who actually have had major traumas. About 50–60% of people will experience at least one major traumatic event in their lives. The main risk factors for developing PTSD include: being female, and a past history of trauma, PTSD, or psychiatric disorder. Childhood exposure to abuse (sexual or physical) or bullying may also predispose people.

Specific populations may have a higher prevalence of PTSD, e.g. military veterans and police officers.

CASE HISTORY 1

A 41-year-old woman was seen in clinic for her problem of repeated self-harm. Her GP was most concerned about the self-harm. She would cut and burn her skin most days and had done so from the age of 30 when she said she was raped by two men. She said she always felt calmer when she saw her own blood. She said she had thoughts about suicide but would not kill herself because she has two young children. She admitted to drinking three litres of cider a day and to having withdrawal symptoms in the morning unless she had alcohol. She said she had had some fits when she had tried to stop drinking once before. She was irritable and her neighbours had been seeking an 'antisocial behaviour order (ASBO)' against her. She avoided talking about the rape and avoided the place where it had happened as reminders of the incident made her panicky. She described nightmares about the rape most weeks and said that she sometimes felt it was as if she could hear the voices of the men in her head. She felt low in mood and her concentration was always poor.

The GP referred the patient for deliberate self-harm (DSH) – how does this link with PTSD?

PTSD is often missed as a diagnosis because other associated behaviours seem to claim the attention of services – excessive alcohol use, self-harming and anger towards her neighbours may all seem to be more pressing problems to agencies than the underlying problem.

The self-harm is a maladaptive way of coping with inner tension and possible guilt. Patients often describe no pain during the act of self-harm because they are 'dissociated'. They often experience a release of tension when they see the injury or the blood caused by the injury. This is the psychological reward that makes future DSH more likely.

Table 8.1 Symptom frequencies in cases of PTSD

Symptom	Percentage of patients
Insomnia	95
Anxiety at reminder cues	93
Intrusive thoughts, images, sounds and sensations (flashbacks)	91
Poor concentration	91
Irritability	91
Diminished interests	85
Recurrent dreams of the trauma	83
Avoidance of people or places associated with trauma	83
Foreshortened expectations of life	78
Detachment from others	76
Avoidance of thinking or talking about the trauma	73
Low mood	71
Absent or diminished libido	69
Poor appetite	67
Hypervigilance	53
Mood lability (e.g. being easily moved to tears)	50
Startle reactions	45
Acting as if the event was recurring	36
Alcohol and substance use increase	36
Restricted affect	18

What is it about the case that justifies the diagnosis of PTSD?

Rape is followed by PTSD in a large proportion of cases. It does not tend to be seen by services, however, until secondary problems – such as the use of alcohol ('to blot things out') brings the issue to light. Rape involves a loss of the person's sense of integrity and victims often feel they are about to be killed – more than

sufficient for the diagnostic requirements for the condition.

In this case the patent describes nightmares, flashbacks (the men's voices) and avoidance behaviour. These are key features of PTSD that often distinguish it from other conditions.

Irritability and disinhibition from alcohol often bring PTSD sufferers into contact with the law. It is difficult for rape and trauma survivors to trust others and they often feel detached from friends and family.

About 30% of people with PTSD abuse alcohol and about 30% of people with alcohol problems have PTSD. It is very important to consider the issue of PTSD with alcohol patients.

How could the patient be managed?

Initial management would be to engage the patient and offer detoxification. As she has had withdrawal symptoms, management of her detoxification would best be on an inpatient unit. A dual approach with long half-life SSRI antidepressants and psychotherapy would be indicated. The antidepressant would treat the depressive component and the psychotherapy – probably cognitive behavioural therapy would address features of PTSD including avoidance behaviour. Some sensitivity would need to be given to whether a female psychiatrist/psychotherapist would be needed.

CASE HISTORY 2

A 42-year-old police officer noticed a young man sitting alone on a wall in the city centre on a cold February morning. He sat with his knees up touching his head. He was wearing only shorts and a vest. Concerned for his welfare, the police officer went over to him. As he did so, the young man produced an automatic weapon and pointed it at the police officer's head. As he stood up he distinctly said, 'Today I'm going to kill a policeman and you are that policeman.'

The muzzle of the gun was held to the policeman's head. The policeman was aware that the young man was muttering to himself unintelligibly and shouting at unseen people. The officer was convinced he was about to be killed. Eventually, after a protracted dialogue with unseen people the young man took the gun from the officer's head and wandered off. An armed response team was summoned. The officer suffered with frequent nightmares for 10 months, which gradually tailed off over the next year. He had flashbacks where he could see the gun and hear the man saying, 'Today I'm going to kill a policeman and you are that policeman.' His alcohol consumption increased to 20 units a day and he started smoking again. Irritability and detachment combined with reduced libido led to a relationship breakdown with his partner of 10 years.

What can be done to preserve patients' social networks?

It's all too easy to see that being the partner of someone who has become unaccountably and unpredictably angry is unpleasant. When this is coupled with a lack of motivation, alcohol misuse and a lack of libido a relationship can easily founder. This is extremely unfortunate. Often explaining the diagnosis to the patient and, with their permission, to the partner – not to excuse behaviours but to provide a rationale, that it isn't the victim's partner who is to blame and that the condition may improve with treatment – can be enough to help the couple through.

Similarly, detached and irritable parents can be frightening and worrying for their children to deal with. Family therapy may be indicated to help the parents see their responsibilities and modify the impact that their behaviours are having.

A HISTORICAL CASE OF PTSD: CHARLES DICKENS

Charles Dickens (1812–70), the most successful author of his day – an international traveller – then aged 53, was returning from a trip to Paris on 9 June 1865. In the train coach with him on their way to London were his partner Ellen Ternan and her mother.

The train track was being repaired near Staplehurst in Kent. Part of the track over the bridge had been dismantled and a mistake had been made about when the express was due. The oncoming train was unaware that there was a gap of 42 feet long in the tracks over the bridge. At the last minute the engineer saw the situation, but it was far too late to stop. The engine and the first part of the train sped across the gap in the tracks, but the coaches in the centre and the rear of the train fell into the river bed below. Dickens' coach dangled from the bridge.

Dickens and Mrs Ternan were physically uninjured. Ellen had only minor injuries. Others weren't as lucky. Ten people were killed and about 50 were injured.

Dickens scrambled from his coach, and using brandy from a flask and water carried from the river in his top hat did what he could to aid and comfort the injured. He described the scene as 'unimaginable'.

He saw a dying man, still pinned under the train. At one point Dickens gave an injured lady who was resting under a tree a sip of brandy. The next time he passed her she was dead. Over the next three hours Dickens did what he could to alleviate people's suffering.

He described the incident in a letter to his friend Mitton:

My dear Mitton

I should have written to you yesterday or the day before, if I had been quite up to writing. I am a little shaken, not by the beating and dragging of the carriage in which I was, but by the hard work afterwards in getting out the dying and dead, which was most horrible.

I was in the only carriage that did not go over into the stream. It was caught upon the turn by some of the ruin of the bridge, and hung suspended and balanced in an apparently impossible manner. Two ladies were my fellow passengers; an old one, and a young one. [Author's Note – Dickens conceals the identity of his mistress and her mother.] This is exactly what passed:- you may judge from it the precise length of the suspense. Suddenly we were off the rail and beating the ground as the car of a half emptied balloon might. The old lady cried out 'My God!' and the young one screamed.

I caught hold of them both (the old lady sat opposite, and the young one on my left) and said: 'We can't help ourselves, but we can be quiet and composed. Pray don't cry out.' The old lady immediately answered, 'Thank you. Rely upon me. Upon my soul, I will be quiet.' The young lady said in a frantic way, 'Let us join hands and die friends.' We were then all tilted down together in a corner of the carriage, and stopped. I said to them thereupon: 'You may be sure nothing worse can happen. Our danger must be over. Will you remain here without stirring, while I get out of the window?' They both answered quite collectedly, 'Yes,' and I got out without the least notion of what had happened.

Fortunately, I got out with great caution and stood upon the step. Looking down, I saw the bridge gone and nothing below me but the line of the rail. Some people in the two other compartments were madly trying to plunge out of the window, and had no idea there was an open swampy field 15 feet down below them and nothing else! The two guards (one with his face cut) were running up and down on the down side of the bridge (which was not torn up) quite wildly. I called out to them 'Look at me. Do stop an instant and look at me, and tell me whether you don't know me.' One of them answered, 'We know you very well, Mr Dickens.' 'Then,' I said, 'my good fellow for God's sake give me your key, and send one of those labourers here, and I'll empty this carriage.'

We did it quite safely, by means of a plank or two and when it was done I saw all the rest of the train except the two baggage cars down in the stream. I got into the carriage again for my brandy flask, took off my travelling hat for a basin, climbed down the brickwork, and filled my hat with water. Suddenly I came upon a staggering man covered with blood (I think he must have been flung clean out of his carriage) with such a frightful cut across the skull that I couldn't bear to look at him. I poured some water over his face, and gave him some to drink, and gave him some brandy, and laid him down on the grass, and he said, 'I am gone', and died afterwards.

Then I stumbled over a lady lying on her back against a little pollard tree, with the blood streaming over her face (which was lead colour) in a number of distinct little streams from the head. I asked her if she could swallow a little brandy, and she just nodded, and I gave her some and left her for somebody else. The next time I passed her, she was dead.

Then a man examined at the Inquest yesterday (who evidently had not the least remembrance of what really passed) came running up to me and implored me to help him find his wife, who was afterwards found dead. No imagination can conceive the ruin of the carriages, or the extraordinary weights under which the people were lying, or the complications into which they were twisted up among iron and wood, and mud and water.

I don't want to be examined at the Inquests and I don't want to write about it. It could do no good either way, and I could only seem to speak about myself, which, of course, I would rather not do. I am keeping very quiet here. I have a – I

don't know what to call it – constitutional (I suppose) presence of mind, and was not in the least flustered at the time. I instantly remembered that I had the MS of a Novel with me, [Author's Note – *Our Mutual Friend*] and clambered back into the carriage for it. But in writing these scanty words of recollection, I feel the shake and am obliged to stop.

Ever faithfully
Charles Dickens

This letter begins to demonstrate the features of PTSD for us – some evidence of anxiety on being reminded of the accident and the start of some avoidance behaviour.

Dickens returned to Gad's Hill Place the day after the accident, and told the landlord of the Falstaff Inn that 'I never thought I should be here again', which emphasises that he felt his life had been at risk – a partial diagnostic requirement for PTSD.

His eldest son found that soon after the accident his father was 'greatly shaken, though making as light of it as possible – how greatly shaken I was able to perceive from his continually repeated injunctions to me by and by, as I was driving him in the basket-carriage, to "go slower, Charley" until we came to foot-pace, and it was still "go slower, Charley."' This is suggestive of an initial 'acute stress reaction'. Further evidence for this acute stress reaction is that even days after the accident he was still overwhelmed by 'the shake'. He felt weak, experiencing 'faint and sick' sensations in his head and he felt nervous.

He wrote letters, in which he mentioned the horrors of the accident and attributes his shakiness not to his work among 'the dying and dead'. In the longest letter (to Thomas Mitton), he made it clear that he wanted to avoid being examined at the inquest into the disaster. Sufferers of PTSD often make every effort to avoid thinking or talking about the trauma.

Later when travelling by train (which he again tried to avoid) he suffered from the illusion that his carriage was 'down' on the left side. This sounds altogether like a 'flashback' or reliving a phenomenon, as seen in PTSD.

Further avoidance behaviour is evidenced by the fact that travelling became for him a most distressing activity – and this was in a man who previously used to relish walking and travelling the length and breadth of the country and lecturing abroad. His international travels ceased.

He tried to overcome his fear of trains by going back in them almost at once (exposure therapy). He had to travel on a slow train rather than the express, however, and even the traffic noise of a London carriage distressed him.

Patients with PTSD often lose interest in their usual activities and become withdrawn. After the crash Dickens withdrew from all scheduled public engagements, and 'the shake' affected his writing: the rest of that number of *Our Mutual Friend*, snatched from the crash, was too short.

PTSD can last for years and two years after the crash Dickens wrote that the effect of the Staplehurst accident 'tells more and more'. A year later he confessed: 'I have sudden vague rushes of terror, even when riding in a hansom cab, which are perfectly unreasonable but quite insurmountable.'

Dickens's son, Henry, stated that 'I have seen him sometimes in a railway carriage when there was a slight jolt. When this happened he was almost in a state of panic and gripped the seat with both hands.' And his daughter Mamie recalled that 'my father's nerves never really were the same again . . . we have often seen him, when travelling home from London, suddenly fall into a paroxysm of fear, tremble all over, clutch the arms of the railway carriage, large beads of perspiration standing on his face, and suffer agonies of terror. We never spoke to him, but would touch his hand gently now and then. He had, however, apparently no idea of our presence; he saw nothing for a time but that most awful scene.' Dickens often had to leave his train at an early station, and walk the rest of the way home.

His son later said that Dickens 'may be said never to have altogether recovered'. Dickens even died on the fifth anniversary of the Staplehurst disaster.

SELF-ASSESSMENT
MCQs

1 Key diagnostic features of PTSD include:
   A loss of appetite
   B avoidance behaviours
   C ritualised behaviours
   D pseudohallucinations
   E depersonalisation
   F nightmares about the traumatic event

2 Evidence-based treatments for PTSD include:
   A antidepressants
   B cognitive behavioural therapy (CBT)
   C counselling
   D psychological debriefing
   E antipsychotics

3 With regard to the epidemiology of PTSD:
   A the prevalence in the general UK population is less than 1%
   B the prevalence in military combat veterans is more than 20%
   C the course of the acute illness is usually less than six months
   D about 10% of motor vehicle accident survivors suffer PTSD
   E about 10% of rape survivors develop PTSD

MCQ answers

1 A=F, B=T, C=F, D=F, E=F, F=T.
Although PTSD can present with varying symptoms only a few are relatively specific to the disorder.

2 A=T, B=T, C=F, D=F, E=F.
There is an evidence base for antidepressants and CBT. There is less of an evidence base for some therapies people intuitively think might be useful, such as counselling. Indeed, there is some evidence that some counselling may worsen the prognosis for people after trauma. Antipsychotic drugs are sometimes used for intractable cases of PTSD, but there is no substantial evidence base.

3 A=F, B=T, C=T, D=T, E=F.
The lifetime prevalence of PTSD is about 5% in men and 10% in women. The prevalence of PTSD in rape survivors exceeds 30%.

EXPLORATIONS
LINKS TO MEDICINE

If PTSD can arise as a sequel to life-threatening traumas such as a plane crash, how many medical patients suffer PTSD as a result of life-threatening medical crises such as a heart attack? Search the research literature to find incidence and prevalence data.

LINKS TO HISTORY AND ETHICS

➤ PTSD is a modern term for a phenomenon which has been present in earlier times. What terms were used in the past to describe the psychiatric casualties of war?

➤ How were such casualties dealt with historically?

➤ There are tensions in military psychiatry where the primary aim of the military is to guarantee a return to the 'front' as soon as possible. What ethical problems can you envisage for military psychiatrists?

FURTHER READING AND REFERENCES

Brewin CR, Andrews B, Rose S, Kirk M. Acute stress disorder and posttraumatic stress disorder in victims of violent crime. *American Journal of Psychiatry.* 1999; **156**: 360–6.

Bryant RA, Harvey AG. *Acute Stress Disorder: a handbook of theory, assessment, and treatment.* Washington, DC: American Psychological Association; 2000.

Green BH. Post-traumatic stress disorder: symptom profiles in men and women. *Current Medical Research and Opinion.* 2003; **19**: 3.

PTSD IN FILM

Jacob's Ladder (1990), directed by Adrian Lyne and written by Bruce Joel Rubin, could be summarised in psychiatric terms as '*PTSD or not PTSD*'. The hero, Jacob Singer (played by Tim Robbins), appears to be a survivor of the Vietnam War. There are graphic scenes depicting his war traumas in which his platoon is destroyed and he is bayoneted in the stomach.

The next portion of the film describes his new life as a divorced postal worker, living with a new woman, Jezebel. He suffers with recurrent nightmares derived from his experiences, seems hypervigilant, has flashbacks during the day, is irritable and distant from others and in many ways is a classic case of post-traumatic stress disorder (PTSD). The memory of his dead son (acted by a very young Macaulay Culkin) also haunts him, and these include horrid images of his son being run over.

RESOURCES

The Centre for Anxiety Disorders and Trauma
99 Denmark Hill, London SE5 8AF
Tel: 0203 228 2101 and 0203 228 3286
Email: anxietydisordersunit@slam.nhs.uk
Web: http://psychology.iop.kcl.ac.uk/cadat/default.aspx

Combat Stress
Ex-Services Mental Welfare Society
Tyrwhitt House, Oaklawn Road, Leatherhead, Surrey KT22 0BX
Tel: 01372 841600
www.combatstress.org.uk/

International Society for Traumatic Stress Studies (US)
www.istss.org/

National Center for PTSD (US)
www.ncptsd.va.gov/

National Institute for Clinical Excellence (NICE) Guidance on PTSD
www.nice.org.uk/guidance/CG26

CHAPTER 9

Suicide and deliberate self-harm

The annual UK suicide rate for men runs at 15–20 per 100 000 and 4–5 per 100 000 for women. Most completed suicides are associated with prior psychiatric illness. Depression, schizophrenia, alcoholism and most other mental disorders greatly increase the risk of suicide. About 10% of people with severe mood disorders and 5% of people with schizophrenia eventually kill themselves. Careful assessment and management of psychiatric patients may help prevent some of these deaths. Repetitive deliberate self-harm such as self-cutting or self-burning behaviour is becoming more common in Europe with up to 4% of adolescents self-harming in this way.

CONTENTS

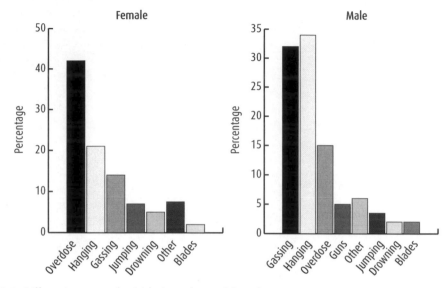

Figure 9.1 Different means of suicide in males and females

WHAT IS SUICIDE?

Suicide is the deliberate taking of a person's own life. Attempted suicides can be by a variety of means: self-poisoning (drug overdoses and the like), self-strangulation, failed attempts at hanging and so on. *Deliberate self-harm* is abnormal behaviour aimed at causing physical harm to the body, but without clear intent to take life, such as repeated minor cutting of the wrists or forearms.

HOW COMMON IS SUICIDE?

There are about 4500 recorded suicides in the United Kingdom every year. This works out as a recorded suicide every two hours. Suicide is about four times as common in men as in women, although there are more suicide *attempts* by women. Women are far more likely to choose drug overdoses as a method. In drug overdose there is a greater chance of intervention than in traditionally male means of attempting suicide such as hanging, gassing or firearms.

RISK FACTORS FOR SUICIDE

➤ Unemployed men are two to three times more likely to kill themselves.
➤ Certain occupations such as vets, doctors,

dentists, pharmacists and farmers are at high risk.
➤ Single, widowed and divorced people are more likely to kill themselves than married or co-habiting people.
➤ About 5% of people with schizophrenia, 10% of alcoholics and 10% of people with mood disorders go on to kill themselves.
➤ Young people with conflicts about their sexuality.
➤ Drug misuse and homelessness.
➤ Terminal or disabling illness and chronic pain.
➤ Family history of suicidal behaviour.
➤ Loneliness and social isolation.
➤ Command hallucinations – telling the patient to kill themselves.
➤ Certain occupations are at high risk: dental practitioners, medical practitioners (particularly female), farmers, vets, waitresses, construction workers and nurses.

CASE HISTORY 1

Steph was a 17 year old, brought to casualty by her sister. Steph had told her sister that she had taken a handful of her mother's antidepressant tablets to kill herself. The overdose had followed a row with her 18-year-old boyfriend, Kyle.

She had locked herself in her bedroom, drunk half a bottle of vodka and swallowed the contents of a bottle containing her mother's amitriptyline tablets (amitriptyline is a tricyclic antidepressant). She had written an angry letter to Kyle, blaming him for ruining her life and causing her suicide. When she began to feel drowsy Steph felt scared and called down to her elder sister in the kitchen. The sister drove her to casualty with the empty bottle and the suicide note.

On admission Steph smelt of alcohol and was lapsing into unconsciousness.

What are the dangers associated with a toxic dose of tricyclic antidepressants?

Tricyclic antidepressant overdoses are difficult to manage. Drowsiness, coma, epileptic fits and cardiac problems may result. In addition to coma, anticholinergic activity may produce mydriasis, tachycardia and hallucinosis. Conduction abnormalities and myocardial depression are common. Doses above 2 or 3 g have a 20% mortality (because of hypotension and heart failure).

Initial management may include gastric lavage and repeated doses of activated charcoal. Correction of acidosis may prevent cardiac problems. Heart monitoring is essential in the initial stages and for some time afterwards. Ventricular arrhythmias and epileptic fits will require active intervention, say, with lignocaine or diazepam respectively.

On the day after the overdose what questions would a psychiatrist want to ask Steph?

The psychiatrist will be trying to assess whether Steph has a mental disorder and whether it is treatable. The psychiatrist will also want to try to assess whether there is an immediate risk of a further suicide attempt (and whether there is a risk of harm to others).

The psychiatrist will try to assess whether there is a treatable depressive illness by asking about depressive symptoms in the weeks leading up to the overdose (tearfulness, insomnia, anorexia, reduced libido and weight loss for instance). Because alcohol was used in the overdose it would be important to assess whether Steph had an alcohol problem and questions about daily intake and symptoms of dependence would be warranted. In the mental state examination, questions used to elicit psychotic symptoms might determine whether there was a schizophrenic illness.

The psychiatrist will also try to assess how determined a suicide attempt this was – the type and number of pills taken is not a good guide to motivation, but things like precautions taken by the patient to avoid discovery suggest a certain determination to kill him- or herself.

A large number of overdoses have an 'impulsive' quality to them. They sometimes follow a major family row, difficulties at school or work, or – as in Steph's case – a breakdown in a romance. Impulsive overdoses are made more likely by drinking alcohol, because alcohol disinhibits the individual, making unwise decisions more likely. Overdoses can be the means of expressing anger or revenge (e.g. 'They'll miss me when I'm gone – they'll be sorry then') or of manipulating people – for instance forcing someone to their point of view (e.g. 'If you don't rehouse me today I'll kill myself'). Despite this unpleasant flavour, impulsive overdoses can be as fatal as any other kind. Paracetamol overdoses are notorious for their medium-term effects on liver function. Days after the patient has regretted their paracetamol overdose, they may still succumb to hepatic failure. Overdoses are a common suicide method in women. Men opt for more violent means such as hanging, shooting or gassing. These more violent means are often more fatal and an 'impulsive' suicide attempt may be as fatal as a suicide attempt within the setting of long-standing mental illness.

> ### CASE HISTORY 2
>
> Adam was a farmer who lived by himself on a hill farm. He was aged 47 and had never married. He had no close relatives and apart from a few drinking companions in the local pub he had no friends. The village doctor had treated him for two depressive episodes, when Adam was 30 and 35. In the past year he had had several setbacks. His herd of cows had had to be destroyed after a foot-and-mouth outbreak. The bank had threatened to foreclose on his business loan. An EU grant had failed to materialise and his hired help was suing him for negligence after a farming accident. The village doctor had diagnosed a depressive illness after Adam had come to the surgery complaining of sleeplessness. He had prescribed a course of antidepressants for Adam and arranged for a psychiatrist to visit him at home.
>
> The next week the doctor was called to the farm by the village postman who had called round to deliver a parcel. The doctor found Adam dead in the kitchen. He had shot himself in the head with his shotgun.

What factors suggested a high risk of suicide for Adam?

Adam lived alone, was single, male, had multiple financial and legal problems, had no support network and had a past psychiatric history. This case highlights the problem of working in remote areas where perhaps resources are few. In this case the village doctor may have done everything he reasonably could. He correctly diagnosed the depressive illness. He correctly prescribed treatment and he arranged follow-up. Even so, the people who 'survive' suicide, i.e. the people who are left behind, such as relatives or carers, after someone else has killed themselves are often left with a mixture of sadness, guilt and anger.

LEARNING POINTS: SUICIDE

> ➤ Males are particularly likely to choose violent and 'non-reversible' means of killing themselves.
> ➤ Loneliness, certain key occupations and psychiatric illness are all important risk factors for completed suicide.
> ➤ Always include questions about suicidal ideas and plans in your psychiatric assessment.
> ➤ Those left behind after a suicide need special attention for their own feelings of betrayal and sadness.
> ➤ Suicide is exceedingly rare in children, but becomes much more likely after adolescence and in young adulthood.

> ### CASE HISTORY 3
>
> Dawn was a regular attender at the accident and emergency department. She had been cutting her wrists and forearms regularly since the age of 13. She was now 18 and her arms were covered in scar tissue. One night she attended after a violent row with a young man at the hostel where she lived. She had been drinking and was verbally abusive towards the doctor who saw her to stitch up a couple of lacerations on her wrist. She winced as he put the local anaesthetic injection into her skin. He asked her, 'Why do you cut yourself if you're afraid of the pain?'
>
> 'It doesn't hurt at the time,' she said. 'At the time nothing seems to matter. You just have to do it. Then you feel better. You feel better when you see the blood coming out.'
>
> She denied any wish to kill herself, but did complain of poor sleep in the past week so the accident and emergency doctor was careful to ask a psychiatrist to see Dawn before she was discharged from casualty.

Why didn't Dawn feel any pain when she cut herself, but did feel pain when the anaesthetic injection was given?

Alcohol may have had some role in limiting the pain she felt at the time of the cutting, but in deliberate self-harm the patient is often dissociated into a state a bit like a trance. The awareness of the cutting and the awareness of the pain derived from it are split. Often the cutting provides a kind of relief after building tension over the previous hours or days. Dawn experiences the relief as she sees her own blood flow.

The relief from tension is a psychological reward for the cutting behaviour. Since the behaviour is associated with a reward, the behaviour is more likely to be repeated in the future. This explains why acts of deliberate self-harm are often repeated.

Deliberate self-harm is particularly common in younger patients, who are female and who have abnormal personality traits. Sexual abuse and poor relationship functioning are particularly associated.

CASE HISTORY 4

Ruby was a 24-year-old woman who attended A&E on a Saturday night asking for help. She had drunk a bottle of wine and said she had taken an overdose. The triage nurse was sceptical as Ruby was a regular attender and often claimed to have taken an overdose or had cut herself. Her paracetamol levels were found to be zero, she was conscious and deemed 'medically fit' by overworked staff who thought she was 'crying for attention again' and the duty liaison psychiatry nurse was pressurised into seeing her. The notes were later scrutinised by the coroner and found to be brief. The Mental Health Trust's risk assessment sheet was filled in, and so was a 'suicide prediction screening instrument'. This yielded a 'mild risk' score. The records showed that Ruby was discharged to the 'crisis team' for a home visit in a week's time. Later that night Ruby scaled the hospital stairs and threw herself from the hospital roof.

What pointers, if any, are there to a diagnosis in the above scenario?

Most completed suicides are associated with psychiatric illness prior to the act. There are suggestions of numerous episodes of past self-harm and self-poisoning. Repeated acts of self-harm and attempted suicide are associated with the diagnosis of **borderline personality disorder**.

Borderline personality disorder is a complex and controversial condition. There is dispute as to what it is and how it can best be treated. People with the condition place high demands on healthcare systems – repeated overdoses can be viewed judgementally by medical and nursing staff in A&E who are hard-pressed to cope with medical and surgical emergencies.

The term *personality disorder* is an unpleasant one and seems to place much of the onus for unwanted behaviour on the sufferer. This can be difficult as the healthcare system may sometimes turn into a persecutor by both judging the individual and refusing them various help they seek. Whatever the condition is, it affects behaviour from the early teens on and is associated with unpleasant moods that distress the individual. The association between the condition and depression is close. There is also an association between the condition and completed suicide. This makes it important to challenge any assumptions or attitudes that frontline staff may have about the condition. These attitudes may be that all suicide attempts are merely 'cries for help', 'not serious' or 'attention seeking'. Other attitudes that mental health staff have and may require challenging are that 'personality disorders are not genuine psychiatric illnesses', 'personality disorders cannot be treated' and 'personality disorders should not receive any psychiatric drugs'.

A psychiatric post-mortem report for a clinical negligence case brought on behalf of Ruby's two-year-old son elicited the following facts about her history: that she had a history of alcohol binges, bulimic eating patterns and numerous short-lived but intense relationships with boyfriends. Her overdoses often followed a breakdown in such relationships. Boyfriends, rather than being sympathetic to such overdoses, were often repelled and overwhelmed by the intensity of her reaction to an argument or a break in the relationship. Ruby had begun self-cutting when she was 13 after she claimed her uncle abused her. The family did not believe her. When she started taking overdoses aged 15 the family severed links with her and she went into care for a while. From 18 she had several admissions with severe depressions where she stopped eating and received ECT. At this time she also claimed to hear the voice of her abuser taunting her. A psychiatrist then started a mood stabiliser and gave her antidepressants. She improved and started studying hotel management and managed to hold down a job as a junior manager at a health spa. She became pregnant, and her medications were stopped. The baby was born but her relationship with the father broke down and she had a relapse of depression. A psychiatrist restarted her medication and arranged for her to join a 'therapeutic community'. The 'community' disapproved of her medication and sought to get Ruby to accept responsibility for her moods and behaviour. She was discharged after getting drunk once too often. Six months later she attended A&E for the last time.

The psychiatric report also focused on the fact that for the purposes of economy Ruby's frontline care was devolved to relatively junior nurses using 'screening tools'. No in-depth account was taken of her past history or lack of social support. Risk assessments of a 'tick box' variety yielded a 'mild risk' score. However, analysis of the actual research papers about the Trust's scales used to rate suicide risk revealed that they were designed for use only as research tools and that subsequent research has shown they were of no value whatsoever in predicting whether patients actually completed suicide.

What lessons can be drawn from the above scenario?

The extended history obtained by an analysis of all the materials about Ruby available to the Trust indicated she was at high risk of suicide, not low risk. The failure of the Trust to provide a psychiatrist to take a full history and mental state examination and its over-reliance on screening tools (of no proven value) led to a decision that the Trust was indeed negligent.

The underlying lesson is about stigmatisation and how labels and attitudes can seriously affect how people with mental health problems are treated. Ruby had met with repeated rejections in her life – her family after her abuse, various boyfriends and individuals within the health system – her treatment on her final night may have felt like a further rejection and an unstable mood state, or maybe even a frank depressive episode alongside her personality problems became too much to bear.

BOX 9.1 DELIBERATE SELF-HARM

Richey Edwards, co-lyricist and rhythm guitarist of the band Manic Street Preachers self-harmed. His deliberate self-harm (DSH) led to a slogan: '4 Real' – a grim reference to an incident dating back to a gig in 1991 where, challenged by a journalist to prove the weight of his convictions, he carved the term '4 Real' into the flesh of his arm with a razor.

He spoke about his own self-harm: 'When I cut myself I feel so much better, all the little things that might have been annoying me suddenly seem so trivial because I'm concentrating on the pain. I'm not a person who can scream and shout, so this is my only outlet. It's all done very logically.'

In February 1995, at the age of 27, Richey Edwards went missing. Police found his car at a service station near the Severn Bridge, a notorious suicide spot. It was assumed that he had killed himself. His body was never found and he was declared legally dead in March 2009.

Nevertheless, even where Trusts do not rely on spurious screening tests and assessments by inexperienced and minimally trained staff, and provide first rate support and care, suicides among recognised patients will sporadically occur.

Deliberate self-harm may involve behaviours such as self-cutting, self-burning, self-strangulation or punching a wall. DSH often starts in adolescence and may be associated with sexual abuse, domestic violence, school bullying, parental separation, psychological conflicts to do with emerging sexuality or other stressors. DSH may be occasional or repetitive.

DSH as a behaviour may be becoming more frequent. Old textbooks of psychiatry make little mention of the behaviour, which could reflect that DSH was rare or that it was a hidden behaviour, even from psychiatrists. Even today most DSH does not begin to reach the attention of professionals, and may be hidden from parents and siblings. Teenagers who self-harm may instead engage with subcultures that promote DSH on the Internet or other peer groups. Research in Germany has indicated that maybe 4% of adolescents at school may 'repeatedly' self-harm and 10% may 'occasionally' self-harm. DSH has been estimated to occur in 6.2% of Australian schoolchildren. Part of the problem in estimating the size of the problem is to do with the covert nature of the behaviour and how DSH is defined. For instance, should self-poisoning be classified as DSH or as attempted suicide?

DSH is not an entirely human phenomenon. There are animal correlates which are recognised in veterinary medicine as 'self-injurious behaviour' where animals that are stressed in terms of living conditions or who are experimented upon may exhibit behaviours such as self-biting or pulling out their fur or feathers.

LEARNING POINTS: DELIBERATE SELF-HARM

- Repetitive DSH may occur in about 5% of adolescents at school.
- Patients who self-harm often repeat the behaviour if it is associated with a psychological reward.
- Deliberate self-harm adolescents are more than 15 times more likely to go on to kill themselves than those who do not self-harm.
- DSH used to be most common in females, but is approaching parity between the sexes in some communities.
- Abnormal personalities are associated with deliberate self harm behaviour, but like anybody else abnormal personalities can suffer with treatable mental illness and so they must receive a careful assessment.
- Severity of inflicted harm is not a reliable guide as to the likelihood of completed suicide in the future.
- Suicide prediction scales show little ability to predict eventual suicide in DSH patients.

EXPLORATIONS

1 There are about 4500 recorded suicides in the United Kingdom every year. Why is this likely to be an underestimate of the true number of suicides?

2 The 10 occupations in Table 9.1 (p. 136) have the highest suicide rates in England and

---

BOX 9.2 ANIMAL SELF-HARM

Laboratory monkeys separated from their mothers during the first year of life become excessively fearful and aroused and may engage in self-mutilation; biting themselves, head banging, slapping their own faces, and sometimes attempting to chew off a limb. After self-injuring, the monkeys would become calm.

Table 9.1 Male suicides by occupation: the top 10

Occupation	PMR	Deaths
Vet	364	35
Pharmacist	217	51
Dental practitioner	204	38
Farmer	187	526
Medical practitioner	184	52
Therapist	181	10
Librarian	180	30
Typist, secretary	171	16
Social scientist	179	11
Chemist	169	70

Wales. (It uses the Proportional Mortality Ratio or PMR – the extent by which suicide is more or less frequent compared with the general population. So a PMR of 100 would be the same as for the general public.) What factors about these occupations make them more at risk?

3 The range of self-harming behaviours among humans could be extended depending on the definition. What would you make of behaviours such as self-harm as political protest, as part of religion, or self-harm in art? Should obesity or anorexia nervosa be classified as self-harming behaviours?

4 The following graphs show the number of deaths from suicide and self-inflicted injury in young men and young women (15–44) in the United Kingdom over the period 1991–2006. What trends can you see? What would you predict from this trend? How could you investigate what actually happened in the years after 1991? What real explanations might there be for the trend? Check out changes in government policy, car exhaust system manufacture, alterations in OTC painkiller packaging as possible explanations.

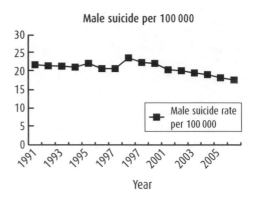

Male suicide per 100 000

Figure 9.2 UK: Age standardised male suicide rate in 15–44 year olds, 1991–2006 (Source: National Statistics)

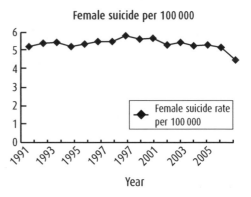

Female suicide per 100 000

Figure 9.3 UK: Age standardised female suicide rate in 15–44 year olds, 1991–2006 (Source: National Statistics)

FURTHER READING AND REFERENCES

Biddle L, Brock A, Brookes ST, Gunnell D. Suicide rates in young men in England and Wales in the 21st century: time trend study. *BMJ.* 2008; **336**: 539–42.

Brunner R, Parzer P, Haffner J, Steen R, Roos J, Klett M, Resch F. Prevalence and psychological correlates of occasional and repetitive deliberate self-harm in adolescents. *Arch Pediatr Adolesc Med.* 2007; **161**: 641–9.

Charlton J, Kelly S, Dunnell K, Evans B, Jenkins R. Suicide deaths in England and Wales. *Population Trends.* 1993; **71**: 34–42.

Hawton K, Catalan J. *Attempted Suicide: a practical guide to its nature and management.* 2nd ed. Oxford: Oxford Medical Publications; 1987.

Hawton, K, Harris L. Zahl D. Deaths from all causes in a long-term follow-up study of 11,583 deliberate self-harm patients. *Psychological Medicine.* 2006; **36**(3): 397–405.

Kaltreider NB. The impact of a medical student's suicide. *Suicide Life Threat Behav.* 1990; **20**: 195–205.

Kessel N. Self-poisoning. *BMJ.* 1965; **ii**: 1265–70, 1336–40.

London Gay Teenage Project. *Something to Tell You.* London: LGTP; 1984.

Marzok P, Tierney H, Tardiff K, Gross EM, Morgan EB, Hsu MA, Mann JJ. Increased risk of suicide in people with AIDS. *JAMA.* 1988; **259**: 1333–7.

Meltzer H, Griffiths C, Brock A, Rooney C, Jenkins R. Patterns of suicide by occupation in England and Wales: 2001–2005. *British Journal of Psychiatry.* 2008; **193**: 73–6.

Murphy GE, Wetzel R. The lifetime risk of suicide in alcoholics. *Archives of General Psychiatry.* 1990; **47**: 383–92.

Paykel ES, Prusoff BA. Suicide attempts and recent life events: a controlled comparison. *Archives of General Psychiatry.* 1975; **32**: 327–33.

Roy A. Suicide in chronic schizophrenia. *British Journal of Psychiatry.* 1982; **141**: 171–7.

Runeson B, Beskow J. Reactions of suicide victims to interviews. *Acta Psychiatrica Scandinavica.* 1991; **83**: 169–73.

Van Dongen CJ. Experiences of family members after a suicide. *J Fam Pract.* 1991; **33**, 375–80.

Varah C. *The Samaritans.* London: Constable; 1965.

SUICIDE ATTEMPTS AND SUICIDE IN LITERATURE AND FILM

You've Had Your Time (1990) by Anthony Burgess (autobiography – author's wife repeatedly attempts suicide).

Girl, Interrupted (2000), film directed by James Mangold, with Angelina Jolie and Winona Ryder, depicts borderline personality disorder.

Madame Bovary (1856), by Gustave Flaubert, suicide following reactive depression.

Sorrows of Young Werther (1774), by Johann W Goethe.

Romeo and Juliet (1597), by William Shakespeare.

The Virgin Suicides (2000), film directed by Sophia Coppola.

RESOURCES
The Samaritans
The Upper Mill, Kingston Road, Ewell, Surrey KT17 2AF
Tel: 0845 790 9090
Email: jo@samaritans.org
www.samaritans.org/

Official Suicide Statistics
www.statistics.gov.uk/

CHAPTER 10

Psychiatry in old age

Although elderly people generally enjoy relatively good health, the ageing brain is more susceptible to physical insults than the brain of a younger adult. Various pathological processes such as cerebrovascular disease and amyloid plaque formation may cause a global deterioration in brain function called dementia. The elderly with normal cognitive functions are susceptible to a range of mental disorders that affect younger adults too. Affected by bereavements, loneliness and failing health, some elderly people may begin to suffer with depressive illness.

CONTENTS

THE AGEING BRAIN

The brain of a 75 year old has been subjected to a lifetime of brain insults which may have included events such as birth injuries, head trauma, viral infections, episodes of hypoxia, exposure to environmental toxins such as lead and transient ischaemic attacks among others. This catalogue of events, together with normal ageing processes in the brain, means that the functional reserves of the aged brain are diminished compared with those of a healthy 25 year old. This fall in the 'cerebral reserve' is diagrammatically represented in Figure 10.1. Memory function in elderly persons is less good, partially because of the reduced ability to learn new information. Although memories of long ago may still be as bright, the ageing brain is functionally less plastic and new memories are less easily required. This is usually a relatively benign memory impairment.

Because the cerebral reserve has been diminished, further brain insults such as an episode of chest infection may not be coped with. A similar infection in a 25 year old with higher cerebral reserves may pass without any observable deterioration in brain function. In a 75 year old, however, the infection may so use up the reserve capacity that confusion or an acute brain syndrome supervenes. In other words, the ageing brain is increasingly vulnerable to new insults and, if burdened, easily descends into a transient confusional state.

THE PREVALENCE OF MENTAL DISORDERS IN THE ELDERLY

Dementia from all causes may be present in about 5% of the population over the age of 65. Over the age of 85 the prevalence rises to about 30%. Depression requiring treatment may be present in about 10% of the population over 65. However, unfortunately, most cases of depression in the elderly go unrecognised and are consequently untreated.

DEMENTIA

Dementia is a chronic and progressive global deterioration of brain function. The causes

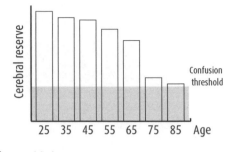

Figure 10.1

of dementia are varied, although Alzheimer-type dementia is one of the commonest with 60–75% of diagnosed dementias being of this kind. Ten to 15 per cent of dementias are of the Lewy body dementia type. Some of the causes of dementia are partially or wholly reversible with treatment. These include conditions such as hypothyroidism, Wilson's disease, and normal pressure hydrocephalus. Accurate diagnosis is therefore very important.

Table 10.1 Causes of dementia

Alzheimer's disease
Lewy body disease
Multi-infarct dementia (arteriosclerotic dementia)
Alcoholic dementia
Binswanger's disease
Creutzfeldt-Jakob disease (CJD)
Huntington's chorea
AIDS-related dementia
Parkinson's disease
Normal pressure hydrocephalus
Wilson's disease (disorder of copper metabolism)
Metabolic diseases such as hypothyroidism
Malnutrition, e.g. vitamin deficiencies
Traumatic or toxic injury, e.g. carbon monoxide poisoning or traumatic brain damage
Malignant disease: primary or metastatic
Infections, e.g. neurosyphilis

Table 10.2 Some clinical features in cortical dementia syndromes

Short-term memory impairment – forgetting appointments – losing personal possessions – self-neglect, forgetting to wash, forgetting meals

Long-term memory impairment – late feature.

Agnosias – visual agnosia, topical agnosia (getting lost), hemisomato agnosia (failure to recognise half of the body)

Dyspraxias, e.g. constructional or dressing

Dysphasias, e.g. expressive, receptive, nominal

Dyscalculia

Difficulty remembering names or recognising others (or even self in the mirror – mirror sign)

Disinhibition and poor judgement, risk of being exploited (vulnerability)

Perseveration, echolalia, palilalia, echopraxia

Disorientation in time, place and person

Incontinence

Return of primitive reflexes

Emotional lability – tearfulness or anger

Depression

Mistaken beliefs, e.g. that parents are still alive or that grown up children are still at school

Unlike an acute organic brain syndrome (delirium) the onset of a dementia is often gradual. Its progress is often slow. In senile dementia of the Alzheimer type (SDAT) the median survival from first symptoms to death is about five years or so, but may be as long as 10 years.

The symptoms and signs of dementia reflect the parts of the brain which are damaged by the disease process so that difficulties with the task of dressing or the order of tasks in dressing may reflect cortical damage in the parietal lobe. Some dementias affect corti-cal *and* sub-cortical structures. Others, like Binswanger's disease, tend to affect just the sub-cortical structures and therefore have different symptom profiles. A key early clinical feature of most dementias, however, is short-term memory loss, which is really an inability to form new memories (anterograde amnesia). Long-term memories may be intact, although later in the illness these too may be lost so that patients may fail to remember their marriages or fail to recognise their spouses.

Carers may have to cope with changes in the patient's personality. From earlier chapters you will have learnt how lesions in the frontal lobe can affect personality by removing inhibitions. For example, dementia patients with lesions in their frontal lobe may swear (where they haven't done before), insult others or make inappropriate sexual advances to strangers. Frontal lesions are also associated with a loss of continence. Dementia patients may occasionally be violent where this has never been a feature of their personality before. Psychotic symptoms such as vision hallucinations may also occur. Not every patient with a dementia has exactly the same symptoms or follows the same course.

CASE HISTORY 1

Mary had been married for 42 years when her husband, Fred, died of lung cancer. She found coping with the arrangements after his death very difficult and leaned heavily on her friends and relatives. This they could understand, but weeks after the funeral Mary seemed very disorganised. Friends would call round to the house and find it in a mess, with half-empty milk bottles and partly finished meals in odd places about the house. When they made arrangements to see her, Mary would not keep these appointments. When they mentioned these missed appointments to Mary she would become upset.

Her brother-in-law first noticed there was something seriously wrong when Mary phoned him and asked where he was claiming that he had forgotten to come and

> pick her up to take her to work. For one thing Mary had retired some years ago and for another thing it was 2 o'clock in the morning. Two days later she turned up at their house in a taxi at 5 am. Her brother-in-law was so concerned that he took her in to see her doctor.

What probably are the main problems identified by the friends and relatives?

These centre around Mary's disorganisation. She forgets appointments and seems to have lost her sense of time doing daytime things when she should be asleep. Her mistake about whether or not she is working suggests a serious disorientation in time.

Why has this problem presented now?

The answer to this question depends upon the diagnosis. Mary is presenting after her husband's death. It is possible that her bereavement reaction is so bad that she has become severely depressed. In older people depression can seem to change their cognitive abilities so much that they appear demented. This is called a pseudo dementia, and it tends to resolve after the depression is appropriately treated. This could explain the time relationship between the death and her confused presentation.

On the other hand, the problems related above do not highlight low mood as a prime feature and there may be an alternative explanation for the presentation after Fred's death. Mary may have been becoming more disorientated and more disorganised for some time before his death and he *may have been compensating for her.* He may have been tidying away after her, and making sure she didn't miss her appointments, for instance. Sometimes a couple can be so symbiotic that the outside observer may not pick up the dementia symptoms in one of the partners at all. For instance, people with dementia sometimes have difficulty in remembering names or small details. If their partner is with them, he or she may prompt the other in such a naturalistic way that any observer may think nothing of it. It is only when the partner is not present that the symptoms and signs of the dementia begin to be apparent.

How would you establish the diagnosis?

A full history from the patient and informant may yield important information such as a family history of early deaths from dementia or a cerebrovascular disease. A past medical history of hypothyroidism, anaemia or stroke may be equally important. Look at the differential diagnoses of dementia (*see* Table 10.3) and work out what features might be present in the history for each. Classically, senile dementia of the Alzheimer's type (SDAT) follows a gradually deteriorating course whereas a cerebrovascular dementia follows a stepwise deteriorating cause with each sudden deterioration following a cerebrovascular event. This is information that can be gained from the history. Informants may be able to tell you how much the patient can do for him- or herself. Dressing dyspraxia can be detected in this way.

A physical examination is absolutely essential to pick up signs of Parkinsonism, say, or hypertension. Treatable causes of dementia such as hypothyroidism must be found and a physical examination could turn up features such as dry skin, hair loss, slow reflexes, or bradycardia.

Physical investigations also need to be done: a full blood count (why?), serum B12 and folate, urea and electrolytes, thyroid functioning tests, liver function tests and syphilis screening would all be very relevant. If you find features in the history or physical examination which make you think of a specific disorder, more specialised tests may also be warranted. If you found features of Wilson's disease, for instance, what blood tests would you order? Radiological examinations such as chest X-rays and increasingly brain scans are routine initial assessments for dementia. An ECG is very important to exclude rhythm disturbances. Atrial fibrillation may, for example,

Table 10.3 Distinguishing features of some dementias

Dementia	Onset	Brain pathology	Transmission	Key clinical features
SDAT	Early from 50+	Cortical thinning and ventricular dilation	Early onset form possibly autosomal dominant	Anteretrograde amnesia and cortical dementia features
	Late from 65+	Senile plaques and neurofibrillary tangles	Late onset form four times more likely in first degree relatives	
Multi-infarct	65+	Focal infarcts in white matter showing as areas of low attenuation on CT/MRI scans		Stepwise, deterioration Onset sometimes sudden Focal neurological signs
Huntington's	30–40 years	Abnormal GABA and dopamine systems in basal ganglia Reduced volume of caudate and putamen on CT/MRI	Autosomal dominant gene on chromosome 4	Involuntary movements, gait abnormalities
Parkinson's	65+	Subcortical dementia in 20% of Parkinson's		Associated with Parkinsonian features
Normal pressure hydrocephalus	Usually 60+	Dilation of ventricles without cortical thinning on CT/MRI scans		Unexplained incontinence and gait abnormalities
Prion dementia (Creutzfeldt-Jakob disease)	Adulthood	Accumulated prion protein Astrocytosis Spongiform appearance No cerebral atrophy	Horizontal rather than vertical	Rapidly progressive dementia, most dead within 2 years Abnormal movements and EEG
AIDS	<65	Brain atrophy Thickened meninges Demyelinaton Astrocytosis	Horizontal and vertical	Slow onset Tremor, ataxia, hyperreflexia, dysarthria Frontal release signs
Wilson's	<65	Copper deposition in basal ganglia	Autosomal recessive	Kayser-Fleischer rings around iris Abnormal movements

(continued)

Dementia	Onset	Brain pathology	Transmission	Key clinical features
Pick's	55–60	Frontal and temporal lobe atrophy Pick's bodies and balloon cells	Incomplete penetrance of autosomal dominant gene	Personality change and euphoric mood
Neurosyphilis (general paralysis of the insane)	5–25 years after the infection	Neuronal cell loss Astrocytosis Treponema pallidum in cortex	Horizontal and vertical	Small, unequal, unreactive pupils Disinhibition

predispose to embolus formation.

A mental state examination would help elicit whether depressive symptoms are present. Specialised cognitive screening tests can be done at the assessment clinic, for instance looking for parietal lobe signs like dyscalculia or constructional dyspraxia which, if positive, would increase the likelihood of a dementing illness.

WHAT CAN BE DONE FOR DEMENTIA?

Dementias with treatable causes such as hypothyroidism and Wilson's disease may wholly or partially remit with treatment. Other dementias such as Huntington's are not yet treatable although research is ongoing. Alzheimer's disease in recent years has been found to be slowed or inhibited in its course by agents such as the cholinesterase inhibitors. These include donepezil (Aricept), galantamine (Reminyl), and rivastigmine (Exelon). There are no major differences between these drugs and they all help to alleviate certain symptoms such as memory loss, apathy and anxiety. They may help patients remember new information and recall old information, improve alertness and motivation. Side-effects include nausea, loss of appetite, tiredness, diarrhoea, and sometimes sleep problems. They work by improving acetyl choline activity. Acetyl choline is used in the memory centres. Cholinesterase inhibitors reduce the destruction of acetyl choline and increase levels in the brain. Fifty to 60 per cent of people who take these drugs show a slight improvement or stabilisation of their condition. They are expensive drugs.

The treatment of such patients usually emphasises care rather than cure, however. Care is tailored, in ideal cases, to prolong people's independence as much as possible and reduce the burden on their carers to the use of day hospitals, day centres, and respite care.

CASE HISTORY 2

Edna, 78, did not go out of the house very often. It was a huge effort for her because she was plagued by osteoarthritis of the hips and was waiting for a hip replacement. Her home help did all her cleaning and cooking. She got her groceries delivered. Edna's closest friend had died in the summer and now in October she felt 'blue' as she described it. She struggled down to the family doctor one day to ask for sleeping tablets as her joints were hurting more than usual. She said, 'It was either that or a slug of whisky' although she had always been teetotal.

During the five minute conversation she had with her, the family doctor noted how much weight Edna had lost. Although she knew that this would be good from the point of view of Edna's joints, she suspected that Edna had lost her appetite. When asked Edna confirmed that the food did not taste as good as it used to and that her appetite was poor.

The family doctor acquiesced and gave Edna a short course of sleeping tablets, but arranged for the community practice nurse (CPN) to call round to see her. He was able to spend much more time speaking to Edna about her loneliness and the loss of her lifelong friend. He also spoke to Edna's home help who said that lately Edna would sit silently in her chair for hours on end. The home help made her hot drinks, wrapped blankets about her and made sure the heating was on but was worried in case the old lady developed hypothermia. When the home help knew Edna was not listening she told the CPN that Edna often 'shed a tear' nowadays.

What are the main problems here?

They include:

➤ painful arthritic joints
➤ loneliness following bereavement
➤ risk of hypothermia
➤ insomnia
➤ low mood with tearfulness and psychomotor retardation
➤ poor appetite and weight loss.

The last three problems suggest that the patient has a depressive illness. It will be important to clarify the exact type of insomnia. Is the insomnia due to depression or physical causes? Is early morning wakening present? Is waking purely due to arthritic pain? If waking were the only problem and was purely due to pain, suitable analgesics might be more appropriate than an antidepressant. However, there are other features of depression and depressive illness often interacts with pain to make pain seem much worse. The weight loss as a symptom is perhaps more diagnostic of depression than in younger adults. It is also important to realise that weight loss in older people can indicate other illnesses such as heart failure, respiratory failure and malignant disease. Is it

worth treating depression if the cause is mainly either physical or out of the doctor's control? One of the reasons that older people may not receive the treatment that they need for depression is the mistaken belief that if a depression is 'understandable', it does not merit treatment. A doctor might say to himself, 'Well Edna is 78; she hasn't got much to look forward to. She is crippled with arthritis and her best friend died recently, I'd be depressed if I were her.' The important thing to remember is that depression is not normal in old age and that treatment is extremely worthwhile. Successful treatment for Edna would mean a better quality of life, might reduce her pain levels, increase her mobility and give her the confidence to go out and make new friends.

What treatments could be available?

Most treatments available for younger adults are also suitable for the elderly with some alterations.

SSRI antidepressants are relatively safe and may be used in slightly lower doses than in younger adults. Tricyclic antidepressants are cardio-toxic and should also be avoided in older people as they may also produce confusion due to cholinergic effects, and because they also can cause urinary retention in males.

Cognitive behavioural therapy may be a helpful adjunct.

In severe cases ECT is possible, although there may be reservations about using anaesthetics and an anaesthetist may need to advise regarding this. In psychotic cases of depression it is important to realise that antipsychotics may produce postural hypotension and this is a complication which must be guarded against since it may lead to falls and fractures.

Bereavement counselling may also be useful in the elderly.

Day centres and day hospitals can be useful to combat loneliness and monitor recovery.

CASE HISTORY 3

A woman, 51 years of age, presented with a striking symptom: ideas of jealousy concerning her husband. Soon after, mental deterioration was noticed; she would lose her way about in her own home, throw things around and hide herself for fear of being killed. In hospital she seemed perplexed, was disoriented in time and place, and occasionally complained that she understood nothing and that she found it difficult to express her thoughts. She frequently greeted her psychiatrist as she might a social caller, making excuses that her housework was still unfinished. At other times she would cry because she thought that her doctor would cut her or interfere with her. At times she called out for her husband and daughter and appeared to be hallucinated. Sometimes she shouted out for hours at a time.

Whenever she was unable to grasp a situation she would cry. Retention of information was markedly impaired. When shown objects she named them for the most part correctly, but immediately forgot them. In reading she went from line to line spelling out the words or read without inflection. In writing she repeated many syllables, left out others, but executed the tests rapidly. In speaking she misplaced words – an occasional paraphasia – and perseveration was frequent. Many questions asked of her were simply not understood. Her gait was normal and hand coordination was equally good. Patellar reflexes were present; the radial arteries firm; no increase in the area of cardiac dullness; no albumin in the urine. The patient was eventually completely demented; confined to bed with contractures of the lower extremities; and passed urine and faeces involuntarily. In spite of greatest care decubitus developed. Death occurred after four and a half years of the illness.

What features of dementia are described?

The case history describes disorientation in time, place and person. There is mention of a global cognitive decline and an inability to retain information. There is misidentification and gradual decline of language function with receptive aphasia. There is progression over 4.5 years from first symptoms to a state of being bed-ridden with double incontinence.

The description is a case history written by Alois Alzheimer himself (1864–1915). His case records also describe his analysis of brain pathology in this case with global cortical atrophy, arteriosclerosis, glial proliferation and neurofibrillary tangles.

OTHER PSYCHIATRIC DISORDERS IN THE AGED

First time presentations of hypomania and neurotic disorders are rare in the elderly and may signify some treatable organic illness. Once treatable organic causes have been ruled out, symptomatic relief with conventional treatments in altered doses are useful. Schizophrenia does not tend to present in the elderly, but a variant sometimes termed paraphrenia exists and is characterised by persecutory delusions and hallucinations. This disorder is more common in those elderly people who have sensory deficits such as deafness. The emergence of paraphrenia may herald a dementing process.

LEARNING POINTS: PSYCHIATRY IN OLD AGE

➣ Ten per cent of the population over 65 has depressive illness. Despite this, most cases of depression in the elderly go unrecognised and untreated.

➣ Depression in the elderly is not normal and can be effectively treated.

➣ Depression can mimic dementia when attention and concentration are badly affected. This pseudo-dementia usually resolves with antidepressant therapy.

➤ Dementia affects about 5% of the elderly population.

➤ Some dementias are long illnesses (e.g. Alzheimer's which lasts about six years from onset to death) while others are short (e.g. Creutzfeldt-Jakob which lasts about two years).

➤ Symptoms and signs of dementia can help you localise lesions to specific areas in the grey and white matter.

➤ Most people with dementia are cared for at home by spouses or other relatives. These carers need practical and emotional support but this support is usually underprovided.

SELF-ASSESSMENT
MCQs

1 Reversible causes of dementia include:
   A Pick's disease
   B Huntington's chorea
   C hypothyroidism
   D Creutzfeldt-Jakob disease
   E Wilson's disease

2 In a community of 2000 people over the age of 65:
   A about 200 will have dementia
   B about 200 might have depression
   C 300 would have obsessive-compulsive disorder
   D about 10 would have Huntington's chorea
   E at least 100 would have cerebrovascular dementia.

3 Features of sub-cortical dementias include:
   A memory loss
   B dyscalculia
   C receptive aphasia
   D disorientation
   E tactile agnosia

MCQ answers
1 A=F, B=F, C=T, D=F, E=T.
2 A=F, B=T, C=F, D=F, E=F.
3 A=T, B=F, C=F, D=T, E=F.

EXPLORATIONS
Sources listed in the resources and further reading sections will help you with the following.

LINKS WITH ANATOMY, PHYSIOLOGY, PATHOLOGY, NEUROLOGY

➤ Using the anatomy of the cerebral vasculature, find out which areas of the brain are mainly supplied by which arteries.

➤ Which of these arterial systems is the most likely to become occluded?

➤ What therefore are the most likely brain areas to be damaged by strokes?

➤ How would these present to the doctor?

➤ What clinical signs may be elicited by the examining doctor initially and after several days?

LINKS WITH SOCIOLOGY AND PSYCHOLOGY

➤ What changes in their roles do older people face?

➤ How do they and their families adapt to this changing role?

➤ How might the doctor or the healthcare team be called upon to help in this adjustment by the individual family?

LINKS WITH PUBLIC HEALTH MEDICINE

➤ What proportion of your local population is over 65?

➤ How are their mental health needs addressed in terms of *finding* morbidity, and treatment once morbidity has been detected?

➤ Using prevalent and instance statistics for depression and dementia in the elderly, estimate the actual number of cases in your local population.

➤ What services (local and central government run, voluntary and private) are available in your area?

➤ What changes are expected in the numbers of people in various age bands in your local population?

➤ What service changes are currently being planned to coincide with this change?

LINKS WITH HISTOPATHOLOGY

➤ What are the histological changes present in the normal ageing brain?

➤ How do these changes differ from those seen in various types of dementia?

FURTHER READING AND REFERENCES

Aarsland D, Kurz M, Beyer M, Bronnick K, Piepenstock Nore S, Ballard C. Early discriminatory diagnosis of dementia with Lewy bodies. The emerging role of CSF and imaging biomarkers. *Dementia & Geriatric Cognitive Disorders*. 2008; **25**(3): 195–205.

Atkinson JH, Grant I. Natural history of neuropsychiatric manifestations of HIV Disease. *Clinics of North America*. 1994; **17**(1): 17–33.

Benbow SM. The role of electroconvulsive therapy in the treatment of depressive illness in old age. *British Journal of Psychiatry*. 1989; **155**: 147–52.

Bennett DA, Schneider JA, Arvanitakis Z, Kelly JF, Aggarwal NT, Shah RC, Wilson RS. Neuropathology of older persons without cognitive impairment from two community-based studies. *Neurology*. 2006; **66**(12): 1837–44.

Bertram L, Tanzi RE. The genetic epidemiology of neurodegenerative disease. *Journal of Clinical Investigation*. 2005; **115**(6): 1449–57.

Blennow K, de Leon MJ, Zetterberg H. Alzheimer's disease. *Lancet*. 2006; **368**: 387–403.

Devito EE, Pickard JD, Salmond CH, Iddon JL, Loveday C, Sahakian BJ. The neuropsychology of normal pressure hydrocephalus (NPH). *British Journal of Neurosurgery*. 2005; **19**(3): 217–24.

Green BH, Copeland JRM, Dewey ME, *et al.* Risk factors for depression in old age. *Acta Psychiatrica Scandinavica*. 1992; **86**(3): 213–17.

Green BH, Dewey ME, Copeland JRM, *et al.* Risk factors for recovery and recurrence of depression in the elderly. *Int J Geriatric Psychiatry*. 1994; **9**: 789–95.

Green RC, Cupples LA, Go R, Benke KS, Edeki T, Griffith PA, Williams M, Hipps Y, Graff-Radford N, Bachman D, Farrer LA. MIRAGE Study Group (2002). Risk of dementia among white and African American relatives of patients with Alzheimer disease. *JAMA*. 2002; **287**(3): 329–6.

Hesdorffer DC, Hauser WA, Annegers JF, Kokmen E, Rocca WA. Dementia and adult-onset unprovoked seizures. *Neurology*. 1996; **46**(3): 727–30.

Lennox G. Lewy body dementia. *Bailliere's Clinical Neurology*. 1992; **1**(3): 653–76.

McCusker J, Cole M, Abrahamowicz M, Primeau F, Belzile E. Delirium predicts 12-month mortality. *Archives of Internal Medicine*. 2002; **162**(4): 457–63.

Mitchell AJ, Subramaniam H. Prognosis of depression in old age compared to middle age: a systematic review of comparative studies. *American Journal of Psychiatry*. 2005; **162**(9): 1588–601.

National Institute for Health and Clinical Excellence. *Donepezil, Rivastigmine and Galantamine for the Treatment of Alzheimer's Disease*. London: NIHCE; 2001.

Neary D, Snowden JS, Gustafson L, Passant U, Stuss D, Black S, Freedman M, Kertesz A, Robert PH, Albert M, Boone K, Miller BL, Cummings J, Benson DF. Frontotemporal lobar degeneration: a consensus on clinical diagnostic criteria. *Neurology*. 1998; **51**(6): 1546–54.

O'Brien JT. Role of imaging techniques in the diagnosis of dementia. *British Journal of Radiology*. 2007; **80**(Spec No 2): S71–7.

Parkes M. The effects of bereavement on physical and mental health: a study of the case records of widows. *BMJ*. 1964; **ii**: 274–9.

Pinquart M, Duberstein PR, Lyness JM. Effects of psychotherapy and other behavioral interventions on clinically depressed older adults: a meta-analysis. *Aging & Mental Health*. 2007; **11**(6): 645–57.

Vicioso BA. Dementia: when is it not Alzheimer disease? *American Journal of the Medical Sciences*. 2002; **324**(2): 84–95.

Wilson K, Mottram P, Sivanranthan A, Nightingale A. Antidepressants versus placebo for the depressed elderly. *Cochrane Database of Systematic Reviews*. 2001; (**4**).

Wilson KC, Mottram PG, Vassilas CA. Psychotherapeutic treatments for older depressed people. *Cochrane Database of Systematic Reviews*. 2008; (**1**): CD004853.

Xie J, Brayne C, Matthews FE and the MRC Cognitive Function and Ageing Study collaborators. Survival times in people with dementia: analysis from population based cohort study with 14-year follow up. *BMJ*. 2008; **336**: 258–62.

RESOURCES

Age Concern
Astral House, 1268 London Road, London
SW16 4ER
Helpline: 0800 009 966
www.ageconcern.org.uk/

Alzheimer's Association
www.alz.org/index.asp

Alcoholics Anonymous
PO Box 1, 10 Toft Green, York YO1 7ND
Tel: 0845 769 7555 (National Helpline) or
01904 644 026 (York)
www.alcoholics-anonymous.org.uk

Alcohol Concern
1st Floor, 8 Shelton Street, London WC2H 9JR
Tel: 020 7395 4000
www.alcoholconcern.org.uk

Alzheimer's Society
Devon House, 58 St Katharine's Way, London
E1W 1JX
Tel: 0845 300 0336
www.alzheimers.org.uk/site/index.php

Counsel and Care
Twyman House, 16 Bonny Street, London NW1
9PG
Tel: 0845 300 7585
www.counselandcare.org.uk/

Crossroads – caring for carers
10 Regent Place, Rugby, Warwickshire, CV21
2PN
www.crossroads.org.uk/

Cruse Bereavement Care
PO Box 800, Richmond, Surrey TW9 1RG
Day by Day Helpline 0844 477 9400
Email: info@cruse.org.uk
www.crusebereavementcare.org.uk/

Help the Aged
207–21 Pentonville Road, London N1 9UZ
Tel: 020 7278 1114
Fax: 020 7278 1116
Email: info@helptheaged.org.uk
www.helptheaged.org.uk/en-gb/

LEWYNET
www.nottingham.ac.uk/pathology/lewy/
lewyinfo.html

National Association of Widows
3rd floor, 48 Queens Road, Coventry CV1 3EH
Tel: 0845 838 2261 (local rate)
Email: info@nawidows.org.uk
www.nawidows.org.uk/

The Princess Royal Trust for Carers
www.carers.org/

CHAPTER 11

Child and adolescent psychiatry

Children with psychological problems are dependent on others, such as parents or teachers, to recognise their distress and arrange help for them. It is likely that much of this psychological distress is overlooked. Child psychiatrists differ in their practice from adult psychiatrists in three ways. Firstly, they must take into account the developmental stage that the child has reached. Secondly, the family and their stage in the family life cycle must be considered. Finally, child psychiatrists tend to rely on psychological methods of treatment rather than physical methods.

CONTENTS

PSYCHIATRIC DISORDERS IN CHILDREN

Some disorders may occur in children in forms that are similar to those in adults, e.g. phobias and obsessive-compulsive disorder, but generally diagnoses in child psychiatry are less precise and are often formulated in terms of family or other problems. Some diagnostic terms are more specific to childhood.

Mental health problems in children are known somehow to be linked to socioeconomic factors. Psychiatric problems are more prevalent among children in families where neither parent works (20%) compared with those in which both parents work (8%), and one parent works (9%).

Hyperkinetic disorders involve overactivity, poor attention, poor concentration on tasks, and disorganisation in most situations. Hyperkinetic disorders generally arise in the first five years of life. Hyperkinetic children are often impulsive, accident prone, and may be seen as cheeky by adults, and are unpopular with other children. Motor and language skills may be delayed. Hyperkinesis may be associated with a *conduct disorder*. Hyperkinetic disorder is sometimes termed attention deficit hyperactivity disorder (ADHD). The term ADHD is probably better understood by the public who are more familiar with this through its use in the lay media.

Conduct disorders involve antisocial and aggressive or defiant acts on a repeated basis, and are more severe than simple mischief or high spirits. Conduct disorders are more common in boys than in girls. Recognised features include aggression towards people or animals, e.g. bullying and cruelty; destruction of property, e.g. by fire setting, deceitfulness or theft and rule breaking. They are linked to the diagnosis of antisocial personality disorder, which is reserved for people over the age of 18. There is some dispute as to whether such antisocial childhood behaviours should receive a medical diagnosis. Prevalence rates vary: in the UK 6% of 5–10-year-old boys and 8% of 11–16-year-old boys. Only 3% of 5–10-year-old girls and 5% of 11–16-year-old girls have the diagnosis.

Emotional disorders are slightly more common in girls than in boys. Six per cent of 11–16-year-old girls compared with 4% of 11–16-year-old boys have emotional disorders. The category of emotional disorders contains such problems as low mood, separation anxiety, phobic anxiety, social anxiety, PTSD, OCD and sibling rivalry. Separation anxiety disorder of childhood occurs when children undergo real or imagined separation from attachment figures.

In the 12 months leading up to March 2007, 4241 children under 14 were admitted to hospitals in England after attempting to kill themselves. Deliberate self-harm may be found in 5–7% of 15–16-year-old adolescents. The number of prescriptions for depression in children under 16 for depression has quadrupled in a decade.

Other problems associated with childhood may include tics (involuntary, rapid, recurrent non-rhythmic motor movements) like eye blinking and grimacing, non-organic enuresis (bedwetting) and non-organic encopresis (passage of faeces in inappropriate places). Tics are relatively common (10–20%) and usually resolve themselves. Rarely tics may form part of Gilles de la Tourette syndrome and may respond to small doses of haloperidol. Non-organic enuresis occurs in 10% of five year olds, 4% of eight year olds and 1% of 14 year olds. Management involves excluding organic problems (such as urinary tract infection), family assessment and behavioural therapies such as 'star charts' and 'bell and pad' alarms.

ASSESSING CHILDREN

Assessment starts with consideration of the referral and who has made it. The child does not usually trigger referrals – referrals originate from concerned parents, teachers, social workers, GPs or paediatricians. Sometimes childhood psychiatric problems can be essentially normal reactions to family disorders occasioned by bereavements or divorce. The actual assessment may involve interview of the child with – and ideally without – parents. Older children can usually spend longer in individual interviews without their parents. Sometimes extra techniques can be used to help communication – working alongside the child doing artwork, or playing with Lego or dolls' houses. Family interviews may assist either as a whole family group or split into siblings or parental subgroups.

Some areas feature more prominently in child assessments: the pregnancy and any prematurity or problems with delivery affecting bonding, school and peer group relationships; early developmental milestones; and family history and membership. Physical and mental state examinations are essential. Investigations such as blood counts and biochemistry may be routine. Less common investigations may include electroencephalography (EEG) to exclude temporal lobe epilepsy for instance, or chromosomal testing, or brain imaging.

GENERAL TREATMENT OPTIONS

General practitioners and health visitors are important primary care resources and can help with advice and assessment. Child psychiatrists are a relatively scarce resource, but they often work through child guidance clinics or special community mental health teams. Most of their work is done on an outpatient basis. Inpatient facilities are rare. Child psychiatrists may use behavioural regimes, and family and group therapy. Rarely, they may use physical treatments. Community mental health teams may also include community psychiatric nurses, child psychologists and special child social workers who often have family therapy skills.

NICE recommends group-based parent-training/education programmes in the management of younger children with conduct disorders. Such programmes last 8–12 sessions and should be based on principles of social learning theory and attempt to improve family relationships. Parents should be helped to identify their own parenting goals. There is role play within sessions and homework given for between sessions, so that parents can try out newly acquired parenting techniques.

Educational psychologists are available within the school system and can help not only in identifying specific educational problems, e.g. dyslexia, but also managing school-related anxieties and may be vital in managing school refusal. Educational welfare officers also assist in managing school refusal and truancy.

ATTENTION DEFICIT HYPERACTIVITY DISORDER (ADHD)

Abnormalities of frontostriatal circuits, modulated by dopamine, have been found in brain patients with ADHD – with the focus being on the dopamine transporter (DAT), which has a key function in dopamine metabolism. Methylphenidate lowers DAT availability and this may explain some of its efficacy in ADHD.

Although the disorder may aggregate in some families, there is no evidence of a specific gene being involved and there may be an implication that several genes each of relatively small effect plus environmental factors combine to produce the disorder.

Prescriptions for methylphenidate and similar medications have soared in this decade with estimates now of over 420 000 youngsters aged between five and 19 being prescribed such agents in the UK. Prescriptions for such medicines increased by 20.1% in Scotland between 2005/06 and 2006/07. The cost of ADHD prescriptions to the NHS in England was £7 million in 2002 and predictions are that this will rise to somewhere between £49 and £101 million per year by 2012.

Benefits of treating ADHD with agents like methylphenidate may include less school absenteeism and increased reading ability.

Methylphenidate's most common side-effects include loss of appetite and insomnia. Methylphenidate has been linked with stunted growth (through growth hormone suppression) and doubts have been cast on its long-term efficacy.

THE FAMILY LIFE CYCLE

The family is like an organism which is born, lives, gives birth, ages and dies. A man and woman from different families meet and form a permanent relationship, the nucleus of a new family. Their relationship together changes forever when a new child is born and develops as more children are added. This growth phase of the family is followed by a plateau phase during which children are nurtured, trained and educated. One by one the children are ready to assume their own autonomous existence and leave the closeness of the family to begin their own separate lives. Contact may be maintained but the nuclear family is ageing now and contracting as a result. Parents may react in a variety of ways to their offspring leaving them. Some parents may see themselves as desolated and others feel rewarded by the successful completion of their parental roles. Some children may never feel able to leave. Some do, however, and often seek out their own partners often to renew the family life cycle. Of course the above cycle concerns a stereotypical view of a family. Not all families conform to this traditional pattern. Some families may exist together in an extended form and other families consist of a single parent and child.

CASE HISTORY 1

Tony, 12, was brought to the accident and emergency department by his father, who had just stopped him trying to climb out of his bedroom window. The paediatrician on call noted that Tony was unsteady on his feet and that his speech was slurred. Tony did not seem to know where he was. His father told him off for giggling at the doctor and for pulling a rude face. His father said that when he had pulled Tony away from the window his son had talked about seeing a 'stairway to heaven'. There had been no previous contact with psychiatrists and Tony's general health had always been good.

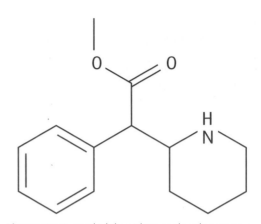

Figure 11.1 Methylphenidate molecular structure

What are the main problems?

Tony appears to be disorientated and disinhibited. He sounds as if he was misperceiving his environment at home because he was trying to climb out of the window in response to what sounds like a visual hallucination.

What could have caused these problems?

The key feature is the sudden onset of all these symptoms. The symptoms themselves have a strongly organic character: ataxia, slurred speech, visual hallucinations and disorientation. The sudden onset in a child may reflect pyrexial illness or some epileptic phenomenon, but perhaps more likely in this case some drug-induced phenomenon. The doctor would need to know if Tony has been prescribed anything recently or whether he could have had access to any prescribed medications in the house. An overdose of a parents' tricyclic antidepressant could cause a sudden acute organic reaction. Street drugs may be to blame and the parents may or may not know if these were available in Tony's school or neighbourhood. Similarly, they may or may not know whether Tony has in fact been experimenting with solvents or aerosol gas. Street drugs or solvent abuse can cause similar presentations. Trying to establish the cause of the reaction is important because of the physical consequences of some substances, e.g. arrhythmias with solvents. If a psychotic reaction is caused by a substance misuse, it should subside fairly quickly, although some recreational drugs like LSD and ecstasy may have long-term psychological effects.

CASE HISTORY 2

Sue came to the doctor explaining about her two-year-old son Mark. He would not sleep at night, she said, and now he is hyperactive and 'into everything' during the day. 'You will probably think I'm just neurotic,' she said to the doctor. 'My husband does.' And, indeed, as if to confirm, Mark sat quietly on his mother's lap throughout the entire interview.

The doctor eventually moved the interview then to talking about Sue's relationship with her husband since Mark's birth and also to discussing Sue's own sleeping pattern.

The doctor learnt that since the birth Sue and her husband, Richard, had drifted apart a bit and that she focused her attention on Mark. She was very careful about what he ate, how he dressed and his 'untidiness' during play. Sue was not sleeping well and had early morning wakening, instead of sleeping at 5 am she went into Mark's room and busied herself getting his clothes ready for the morning. Mark, hearing his mother moving about in his room, woke and began to play. During the day Sue felt irritable, frustrated, lonely and cried easily. When her husband came home from work she usually had a row with him because he took 'no interest' in his son.

What is the main problem according to Sue?

Mark is overactive and will not sleep at night.

How does the husband perceive the problem?

It is difficult to say because his opinion is only reported by his wife, but it does sound as if there is some conflict between the parents. Sue says that her husband thinks she is neurotic and

it seems as if the arrival of Mark is related to an increase in distance between Sue and her husband.

How might the doctor perceive the problem?

If the doctor listens purely to what Sue says about Mark he might think that some simple remedy to help Mark sleep at night would solve the problem. This 'linear' thinking might lead some doctors to prescribe night sedation as a solution with all the inherent problems with dependence that are associated with this.

There is a mismatch between what Sue reports and how Mark behaves in the surgery and this might direct the doctor towards other solutions. In particular it does sound as if Sue may be unwell herself. Perhaps she has had an untreated post-natal depressive illness which is worsening her problems. Is her nocturnal insomnia leading her to seek out contact with Mark and stopping him from sleeping at night? Treatment for Sue's depression might be considered, although Sue has already signalled that she doesn't accept her husband's suggestion that the problem lies with her. She feels the solution is somewhere outside herself. If the doctor focused purely on this he might conflict with Sue who might assume that he was blaming her for the family's problems.

So the problem cannot be represented by a simple linear cause and effect model. In other words, it is not Mark's overactivity or Sue's depression that is the single origin of all their problems. There is a *circular* process here, partly because the whole family is involved. Figure 11.2 (p. 156) shows diagrams of how the family must have originally looked and how the arrival of Mark may have changed things. First, there was a couple and then a third person moved into the house and changed forever the relationship between husband and wife, leading to alternate distance and conflict. Sue's relationship with Mark may appear to be so strong to her husband that he feels excluded and is left apart occasionally on the periphery of the family. The family doctor might ask

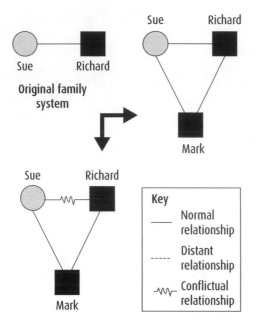

Figure 11.2 Diagram showing the changing relationships in Case History 2.

to see the whole family or ask a community psychiatric nurse to visit the family home to work with the family. Some simple suggestions to support the original family subsystem (the couple) could be made; for instance, to leave Mark to sleep through the night and encourage the couple to maintain their joint interests and activities. If there are serious problems, marital therapy might be necessary. If Sue does have a depressive illness, treatment could be valuable and there may be corresponding benefits in her relationship with her husband and child, but it is helpful to recognise the changes within the family and assist the family to move forward together.

CASE HISTORY 3

Mrs Han brought her 11-year-old son, Jordan, into the practice. The doctor knew from his records that Jordan was an only child and that his parents had divorced a few years ago. In the surgery Jordan sat solemnly in a chair with his arms folded, avoiding eye contact. 'There must be something wrong with him, Doctor. He is never well enough to go to school.' Jordan had not been into school for a year despite the best efforts of Mrs Han and an educational welfare officer. 'I sometimes get him as far as the school gates and he turns white and says that he feels shaky and unwell so he comes home and I ask him whether he will try again the next day but he never goes past those gates. During the day he just lies in bed at home or plays computer games on his Nintendo.'

Is Jordan a truant?

No, because he does not absent himself from school to go off with friends or to go off on his own to places that others do not know about. He stays at home with his mother. His problem is one of *school refusal*, not truancy.

Should doctors be concerned about school refusal?

On the surface the problem may appear to be more a province of an educational welfare officer or educational psychologist, but the doctor can have a useful role to play. The family doctor could, for instance, help exclude physical illness (Jordan often says he feels unwell before coming home) and also explore whether there might be other health factors at play. A family doctor might want to exclude solvent or substance abuse.

The psychological factors in the case are also unclear. Perhaps Jordan is being bullied at school. Bullying causes a great deal of emotional distress and has been linked with completed suicide. Being bullied at school is also a vulnerability factor for developing PTSD later in life. Bullying may lead to a childhood emotional disorder.

The doctor may also want to explore the psychological rewards that *reinforce* and maintain Jordan's behaviour. Staying at home may reduce his anxiety and be the *primary gain*, but there may be *secondary gains* such as his mother's attention and kindness, special food and computer games. A more unconscious reward may be his mother's approval. He might notice that when she describes how she tries to get him into school she says that she *asks* him whether or not he will go in the next day. It is clear that she yields her authority in this matter to him, but that it may suit her own needs for her to have his company during the day.

Mrs Han says she wants Jordan to go to school so how might she also want Jordan at home?

Deep down Mrs Han may prefer Jordan at home. He might provide her with someone to talk to and she may be afraid that he may ultimately grow away from her and leave her as her husband did. Although she acknowledges his need to be educated, she may also like him at home and may be only half hearted in her attempts to get him into school. She may be content just to have been seen to try and fail. Although she has brought her son to the doctor, this may have been at the insistence of her other agencies such as the educational welfare officer. It may also be that she may not wholly want the doctor to succeed. She and her son may have a relationship which is over-close or *enmeshed*.

What can be done?

The situation is unfortunate because Jordan is losing contact with his peer group and not gaining the skills that will help him develop satisfying relationships later in life. He is losing out on his education and may never fulfil his potential in terms of any career. The stakes are quite high but any helping agency would have to acknowledge that they may be working against the family system. If both Mrs Han and Jordan want him to stay at home, there is going to be little motivation for either of them to change. Explaining the situation may help, although the arguments are probably very familiar to everybody concerned. Some work might be aimed at reducing Jordan's anxieties about school. The educational psychologist and his teachers could work together so that

he could become gradually reintroduced into the school a bit at a time as in a *systematic desensitisation* programme. Jordan might be encouraged to air his feelings about his absent father as an individual or even in family therapy. Any depressive condition present in Jordan or his mother could be treated. Family work may encourage Mrs Han to change the language she uses with Jordan. For instance, instead of asking Jordan she might start *telling* him to go into school. Even so, if mother and son lack sufficient motivation to make any changes it could be necessary for local authorities to invoke legal proceedings that require her to send her child to school. A legal dimension may show Mrs Han how serious the problem is and enable her to summon enough courage and authority herself to send Jordan to school.

CASE HISTORY 4

The concerned parents of William, eight years old, brought him along to see the child psychiatrist. William was less than 60% of the normal body mass for his height. When he could exercise he would exercise as hard as he could, although recently he had become too tired to run cross country, a sport for which he had several junior medals.

His breakfast consisted of only hot water, for lunch he would drink juice, eat an orange and eat a few portions of rye bread. For supper he would eat an egg and an orange. His family doctor suggested putting him on a weight chart but William had cheated by drinking extra water on the days he was to be weighed.

When the psychiatrist interviewed William on his own William cried. He seemed preoccupied with the death of his grandfather the previous year and was also worried that his father was spending weeks away from home. His father worked for a petroleum company in Dubai. He said that he was worried about his father dying in an aeroplane crash on his way to and from his work.

At the family interview it transpired that his father was in conflict with his wife about his absences and that his wife resented his time away from home.

William's mother revealed that she had had anorexia nervosa when she was a teenager. Although she was no longer anorexic she confessed to being a 'fitness freak'.

What are the main problems outlined above?

William has made, and is still making, strenuous efforts to lose weight and has succeeded in reducing his weight to levels that would go towards fulfilling the criteria for anorexia nervosa. About 10% of anorexia nervosa sufferers are male.

His mood appears to be low following the loss of his grandfather and he appears to be concerned about his parents' marriage.

Besides anorexia nervosa what other diagnoses might be made?

William may have a depressive illness, i.e. an emotional disorder of childhood. His concerns about his grandfather's death and his parents' marriage sound as if they consume him. The doctor would be interested in assessing the depth of his depression and its associated symptoms and signs. Although suicide is thankfully rare in children, particularly so young, it could be that William feels that life is not worth living and this might be an indicator of how severe his depression is. This would be one of the factors that would be weighed in the decision as to whether William needed to be admitted to hospital or whether he could be treated in the community. His doctor could arrange some grief counselling or individual psychotherapy such as cognitive behavioural therapy to help improve his mood, reduce his grief, and tackle eating issues.

Antidepressants could be another option especially if it is felt that part of William's refusal to maintain his body weight is due to depressive appetite loss.

Family issues sound particularly important in this case. William's mother seems to have had anorexia and may have some dysfunctional attitudes to food and fitness, which may have influenced William as he has been growing up.

Family therapy might be helpful to try to defuse any direct or indirect criticism that exists within the family between members and also to explore the family's ideas about eating, living together or apart and the role of grandparents. In some ways it may be useful to reassure William that, to some extent, the relationships of his parents (*the parental subsystem*) are not his to try to control and conversely the family therapy may endeavour to communicate to his parents that they should maintain the boundaries of that subsystem, i.e. not allow worry to spill over unnecessarily into their offspring (*the children's subsystem*).

LEARNING POINTS: CHILD AND ADOLESCENT PSYCHIATRY

➤ Boys are more prone to conduct disorders; girls are more prone to emotional disorders.
➤ The prevalence of childhood mental health problems appears to be increasing.
➤ Suicidal attempts and DSH in childhood appear to be becoming more frequent.
➤ Family and marital problems often manifest as childhood psychiatric problems so family dynamics should be assessed before assuming the pathology rests with the child alone.
➤ Childhood schizophrenia is very rare.
➤ Solvent abuse and substance abuse are relatively common in the young and may precipitate brief psychotic episodes.

SELF-ASSESSMENT
MCQs

1 First line treatments for childhood depression include:
   A tricyclic antidepressants

B electroconvulsive therapy
C individual psychotherapy
D family therapy
E group therapy

2 Which of the following statements are true, and which are false?
  A Girls (aged less than 11) whose mothers die are at risk of becoming depressed as adults.
  B Children aged 5–10 years with emotional disorders are at greatly increased risk of psychiatric disorders as adults.
  C Many adults with schizophrenia showed signs of neuro-developmental immaturity as children.
  D Adults with bipolar affective disorder frequently had emotional disorders as a child.
  E Children with conduct disorders usually become adults with dissocial personality.

3 Methylphenidate:
  A may impair growth
  B is prescribed in childhood depression
  C is sometimes prescribed in narcolepsy
  D may induce hallucinations
  E is a dopamine re-uptake inhibitor

SHORT ANSWER QUESTIONS

Write short notes on:
1 The emotional reactions of children to change in family structures.
2 The differences between conduct and emotional disorders.
3 Cognitive behavioural therapy in childhood psychological disorders.

MCQ answers
1 A=F, B=F, C=T, D=T, E=T.
2 A–T, B–F, C=T, D=F, E=F.
3 A=T, B=F, C=T, D=T, E=T.

EXPLORATIONS

Sources listed in the resources and further reading sections will help you with the following.

LINKS WITH PUBLIC HEALTH

➢ What are the most common childhood mental disorders?
➢ What are the most common adolescent mental disorders?
➢ What is the ratio between boys and girls in these disorders?
➢ How can prevalence figures be obtained about childhood mental disorders?

LINKS WITH PRIMARY CARE

➢ What proportion of children presenting to family doctors with abdominal pain have *no* physical diagnoses that account for the pain?
➢ How can GPs know when a child's abdominal pain is physical and when the pain is more to do with psychological or social factors?
➢ What might these non-physical factors be?
➢ How can the family doctor manage such a case?

FURTHER READING AND REFERENCES

Barbaresi WJ, Katusic SK, Colligan RC, Weaver AL, Jacobsen SJ. Modifiers of long-term school outcomes for children with attention-deficit/hyperactivity disorder: does treatment with stimulant medication make a difference? Results from a population-based study. *Journal of Developmental & Behavioral Pediatrics.* 2007; **28**(4): 274–87.

Barker P. *Basic Family Therapy.* 5th ed. London: Wiley; 2007.

Carr A, editor. *What Works with Children and Adolescents? A critical review of psychological interventions with children, adolescents and their families.* London: Brunner-Routledge; 2007.

Gopfert M, Webster J, Seeman MV. *Parental Psychiatric Disorder: distressed parents and their families.* Cambridge: Cambridge University Press; 2004.

Graham J, Coghill D. Adverse effects of pharmacotherapies for attention-deficit hyperactivity disorder: epidemiology, prevention and management. *CNS Drugs.* 2008; **22**(3): 213–37.

Green C. *New Toddler Taming: a parent's guide to the first four years.* London: Vermilion; 2003.

Krause J. SPECT and PET of the dopamine transporter in attention-deficit hyperactivity disorder. *Expert Review of Neurotherapeutics.* 2008; **8**(4): 611–25.

Mick E, Faraone SV. Genetics of attention deficit hyperactivity disorder. *Child & Adolescent Psychiatric Clinics of North America.* 2008; **17**(2): vii–viii, 261–84.

Minuchin S, Lee W, Simon G. *Mastering Family Therapy.* London, Wiley; 2006.

Office for National Statistics. *Mental Health of Children and Young People in Great Britain, 2004.* London: HMSO; 2005.

Rutter M, Taylor E, editors. *Child and Adolescent Psychiatry.* 4th ed. London: Blackwell; 2002.

Scott A, Shaw M, Joughin C. *Finding the Evidence: a gateway to the literature in child and adolescent mental health.* 2nd ed. London: Gaskell; 2001.

RESOURCES

Conduct disorder
http://en.wikipedia.org/wiki/Conduct_disorder

Conduct disorder – parent training programmes
www.nice.org.uk/guidance/TA102

The National Attention Deficit Disorder Information and Support Service
www.addiss.co.uk/

Methylphenidate (prescribed for ADHD)
http://en.wikipedia.org/wiki/Methylphenidate

American Academy of Child and Adolescent Psychiatry
http://aacap.org/

Child abuse and conduct disorder
www.priory.com/psych/abuse.htm

NICE Guidance on prescribing for ADHD
www.nice.org.uk/nicemedia/pdf/TA098guidance.pdf

Young Minds
www.youngminds.org.uk/

CHAPTER 12
Personality

Every individual's personality is unique. One definition of personality is that it is an individual's characteristic way of thinking, feeling or acting. Personality is a combination of biological temperament, willingness to explore and socialise, intelligence, education and accumulated experience in reaction to life events. Personality may dictate how people react to physical and mental illness. Some personalities are so different from others that they are sometimes called personality disorders. The behaviour or people with such extreme personalities may lead to them harming themselves or harming others.

CONTENTS

PERSONALITY DEVELOPMENT
PERSONALITY IN THE NEONATE AND INFANT

If you listen to mothers describing their children they will often tell you how each pregnancy had its own characteristics and how even at birth each child differed in some way from its siblings. Some babies seem to be very active in the womb and to react to their mother's behaviour and others seem relatively inactive. At birth some babies are relatively alert and excitable and others are more stolid and slow to react. Obviously, some of these stories are altered by circumstance over the years to explain the temperament or character of a child: 'He was always outgoing – how he made his voice heard when he was born!' and suffer from the problems of retrospective recall. Some events cloud observations of neonate character; for instance, if pain relief is given to the mother in labour the neonate may have depressed levels of consciousness. However, there is work to suggest biological differences in excitability and even learning ability (in terms of habituation to stimuli) in embryos and neonates. These biological differences probably form some core of personality.

Temperament is the name given to this genetically directed core of personality. Features of temperament that have been focused on are: **activity** – related to the energy levels of the child – are they constantly on the move or sedate?; **regularity** in areas such as sleep, eating and bowel; **approach or withdrawal to new stimuli** – are they bold or do they shy away?; **adaptability** – how long and how well does the child adjust to change?; **intensity** refers to the level of response to a new situation – intensely or calmly, for instance?; **mood** – a general tendency towards happiness or unhappiness; **distractibility** – how easily they are sidetracked; **persistence and attention span** refers to a similar ability to stay focused on a task; **sensitivity** refers to how easily a child is disturbed by changes in the environment, similar to irritability.

Mother and child

The newborn baby and his or her mother react and adapt to each other. The components and effect of this dyadic relationship are difficult to unravel because there are symbiotic needs and behaviours involved. People often think that the needs in such a relationship are wholly on the baby's part and that the parent is the sole provider. However, the mother has subtle emotional needs too, and the growing baby may or may not be able to fulfil these. The baby may reward the mother's care by, say, becoming quiet or content when fed; the older infant is able to reward behaviour it likes by smiles or vocalisations.

There is an *attachment* between mother and child, which may be secure or insecure. The secure infant will be able to make small explorations away from the mother. The insecure infant will cling and protest at any actual or threatened separation from mother. After necessary separations the secure infant will (after some protest) resume his secure behaviour while the insecure infant will continue to express its distress and anxiety that its mother will disappear again and may become very clingy or somewhat counter-intuitively avoidant of its mother. Ideally, securely attached children subsequently learn to use attachment figures as a secure base to explore from and return to. The child forms an internal working model of such relationships. Later in life when there are changing circumstances in the relationship (such as separation or loss) this internal working model (whether it is stable or unstable) may be evoked again.

The concept of attachment comes from the 20th-century work of John Bowlby, a child psychiatrist who had a psychoanalytic training.

If the overall personality could be considered like a planet, the *temperament* is the ancient and central molten core. The *personality* is built up in layers of sediment around this as a result of nurturing and life experiences and the outer mantle or coat is the *persona* – the planet's surface, which is what the individual features of the personality are that the individual chooses to present to the world, subject to conscious and unconscious influences. Persona is derived from the ancient use of masks in the theatre by classical actors.

JUNG

How outgoing people are and how easily they form relationships are reflected in Carl Jung's concepts of *extroversion* and *introversion*. Extroverts are people who socialise easily and enjoy company. They are the explorers of life, being outgoing and seeking new experiences and making their views about these known. Introverts prefer their own company or the company of a very restricted band of close friends. They tend to be loners, conservative in their tastes and often keeping their ideas to themselves. Whereas the extrovert seeks to invest in him- or herself in the outside world to get his or her rewards, often the rewards for an introvert are according to some internal system.

FREUD

Sigmund Freud's model of personality was that there were three distinct components: the id, the ego, and the superego. The id would be that portion which is driven by various forces such as hunger or sexual desire. Such biological imperatives create a tension which can only be discharged once the desired object is obtained. For instance, with regard to hunger this is the tension which can only be released when food is obtained. The ego is that rational part of the personality which can plan out how to achieve the id's object; for instance, in the case of hunger, planning how to get food. The superego is that part of the personality which judges the relative merits of the individual's behaviour in terms of conscience. The personality is therefore derived from an interaction between the id, ego and superego. It is thought that substance abusers are largely id driven; everything is directed towards satisfying an intense craving. Obsessional people, on the other hand, are directed by their superegos which demand a strict adherence to rules.

Sigmund Freud (1856–1939) and his daughter, Anna Freud (1895–1982) also described various psychological defence mechanisms used by the individual to minimise his or her own psychological discomfort or tension (*see* Table 12.1, p. 164). Everybody uses some of these defences to some extent at one time or another. However, when one or two defence mechanisms are used almost exclusively, the individual may run into problems. Substance abusers, for instance, often overuse the mechanisms of denial and projection. They deny to themselves the severity of their drug problem and often project the reasons for this behaviour onto others: 'I need this drink because my wife is so awful; it's her fault that I drink.' Repressed ideas or memories may sometimes be coded in dreams in a symbolic way. Sigmund Freud felt that the patient's dreams were a 'royal road' into their unconscious. Freud theorised that part of the mind and its thinking was conscious and part was unconscious. Various desires and memories could be held in the unconscious and repressed there. These ideas and desires may sometimes break out into the conscious mind through expression in dreams. Sigmund Freud often talked with his patients in psychoanalysis about their dreams to help them gain a better understanding of themselves and their inner fantasies and feelings. Psychoanalysis was very popular through the early part of the 20th century but has fallen into disregard, although some of its analytic concepts about transference and counter-transference in the doctor–patient relationship, the unconscious and dream therapy are sometimes found in updated therapies such as cognitive analytic therapy (CAT).

ADLER

Alfred Alder (1870–1937) said that there were four basic styles of coping with life's problems and that people tended to use one style in preference and this helped define their personality type. The four types he outlined were the dominant type; the getting type; the avoiding type and the socially useful type.

Table 12.1 Psychological defence mechanisms

- **Repression**: This is the person's own uncomfortable or unbearable ideas or feelings (such as intense aggression or sexual desires) being repressed from the conscious mind into the unconscious.

- **Denial**: In denial the individual often does not personally accept unpleasant thoughts, memories or emotions that he or she has. This is somewhat different to lying in a conscious manner; where the person is consciously aware of what the truth is but is intending to deceive someone else. In denial there is an internal deception of the conscious self in order to avoid psychological pain. For instance, a patient told of a terminal diagnosis may appear to fail to take in the information and act as if nothing has happened.

- **Projection**: In projection the person may project or attribute undesirable aspects of their own self onto other people. For instance, an alcoholic who might blame his habit on the actions of others or the thug who blames his own bad luck or incompetence on somebody from a persecuted minority.

- **Splitting**: In splitting there is a tendency to see others in either a very good or a very bad light; the possibility that another individual may have a mixture of traits is not considered. Other people are frequently idealised at first only to be cast down as fallen idols when they do not fit in with the person's needs or desires. Splitting is often seen in patients with borderline personality disorder.

- **Displacement**: In displacement feelings, usually of anger or fear, are displaced from one personal thing to another. So a man who feels anger towards his boss at work may 'take it out' on his wife when they meet for dinner, unaware of the fact that his anger is more about his boss than his wife, who may be blameless in any regard.

- **Rationalisation**: After the event reasoning may be used to justify actions and reduce hurt. For instance, a person who fails to attend a difficult appointment may justify his failure to himself on spurious grounds; for instance, 'I just missed the right bus'. The rationalisation may have an element of truth but can be confronted; for instance, it may be that the person who missed the bus did not want to get to the bus stop early enough to get to the appointment.

- **Reaction formation**: This occurs where people with various feelings develop opposite attitudes; for instance, people who feel chaotic and dirty may become obsessionally tidy and clean, or people who have a need to be cared for or a fear of decay and death become carers or healers.

- **Sublimation**: This is a sophisticated defence mechanism where a person may use the tension produced by an inner conflict to create art, for instance in writing or painting.

The dominant type rules without regard for others. The getting type gets other people to solve their problems for them. The avoiding type avoids difficulties and makes no attempt to face problems and the socially useful type cooperates with others and acts in accordance with their interests as well as their own.

Adler was also particularly interested in family structure and its effect on the development of personality. First-born, second-borns, youngest children, and only children all had certain characteristics depending upon their birth order as far as Adler was concerned. For instance, he viewed first-borns as having a problem, having received undivided parental attention until they are 'dethroned' by the arrival of the second-born. He felt that their life was dominated from then on by a battle to regain supremacy. Younger siblings have to develop language and motor skills quickly to compete with their elders. An only child generally does not learn to share and compete as well as a child with siblings.

BEHAVIOUR AND PERSONALITY

It is difficult to disentangle behaviour from personality. Learning theory suggests that some people behave in certain ways because they keep receiving rewards for that kind of behaviour. The rewards may be external and objective or they may be internal and difficult for doctors and therapists to perceive. For instance, people who find social situations very stressful may avoid them and stay on their own and this behaviour may be rewarded by an absence of anxiety which then reinforces their solitude. There is a continual feedback between the individual and the environment, much in the same way that in early life there was a continual feedback between the infant, his or her temperament, and the mother.

CATTELL AND TRAITS THEORY

Raymond Cattell, an English trait theorist born in 1905, looked at the traits that a personality might have. This trait approach contrasts with those of other theorists about personality who might classify personalities into different types, for instance Jung and his ideas about people being either extrovert or introvert types. Cattell believed that different people had various personality factors all acting to a certain degree and that the differences in personality could be accounted for by the various degrees that various personality factors manifest in different individuals. Over two decades he analysed various traits using statistical methods such as factor analysis. Cattell identified 16 or so *source* traits which form the core of the 16 personality factor (16PF) questionnaire. The traits are presented in Table 12.2.

MYERS-BRIGGS TYPE INDICATOR

Carl Jung, the Swiss psychiatrist, also investigated personality using novel approaches such as the word association test which he developed into the 1900s.

Disciples of his approach looking at personality types attempted to measure personality according to a type theory and looked at a more elaborate series of types which melded

Table 12.2 Cattell's 16 personality factors

Factor	A person with a low score on this factor is described as:	A person with a high score on this factor is described as:
A	Reserved	Outgoing
B	Less intelligent	More intelligent
C	Affected by feelings	Emotionally stable
E	Submissive	Dominant
F	Serious	Happy-go-lucky
G	Expedient	Conscientious
H	Timid	Venturesome
I	Tough minded	Sensitive
L	Trusting	Suspicious
M	Practical	Imaginative
N	Forthright	Shrewd
O	Self-assured	Apprehensive
Q1	Conservative	Experimenting
Q2	Group-dependent	Self-sufficient
Q3	Uncontrolled	Controlled
Q4	Relaxed	Tense

some of the ideas about traits into type theory as well. The Myers Briggs Type Indicator (MBTI) is a questionnaire which measures whether people are more introverted or extroverted; intuitive or sensing, thinking or feeling, or reliant on judgement or perception. Thus a personality can be assigned a four letter type and there are 16 types such as an INTJ or an ESTP. The approach is used quite successfully in career advice. An INTJ, for instance, may make an ideal designer consultant, physician or a psychiatrist, counsellor or lecturer. An ESTP may work well in human resources or as a marketing specialist or business analyst.

MINNESOTA MULTIPHASIC PERSONALITY INVENTORY

The MMPI was originally developed in the late 1930s and 1940s. The MMPI has over 550 items or questions; all are 'true or false' in format and the questionnaire may take about two hours to complete. The MMPI has been well researched in terms of reliability and validity. There are various scales embedded within the MMPI which may measure depression, anxiety, fears, negative emotionality, psychotocism, introversion and aggressiveness.

MASLOW

Abraham Maslow (1908–1970) described various needs that people have and put them into a hierarchy.

Maslow also reversed the kind of thinking that lay behind many descriptions of personality types and traits, and instead of looking for pathology, looks for ideals of personality that people could aspire to. He called the ideal a very rare personality type, a *self-actualising* personality. Self-actualisation was, according to Maslow, the realisation or fulfilment of all potentials and capabilities. He envisaged that such personalities were rare, being less than 1% of the population, and that they had

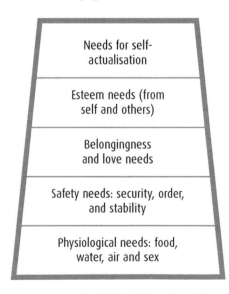

Figure 12.1 Maslow's hierarchy of needs

various characteristics such as an efficient person, a perception of reality, an acceptance of self others and nature, a spontaneous nature, a focus on external problems to the point of it being omission, a freshness of appreciation, a tendency to have mystic or peak experiences, profound interpersonal relationships, to be very creative and so on.

PERSONALITY DISORDERS

Personality disorders refer to extremes of personality and their expression. Some people dislike the term *personality disorder* because it can be used as an unpleasant label for people who are not superficially likeable and who are often denied help from professionals on this basis. The term *personality disorder* also implies that there are 'normal' personalities (you and me) and abnormal personalities (them). In fact, there is probably a spectrum of personalities and not just two categories of normal and abnormal. Although the term personality disorders is awkward there are sometimes rather extreme characters who do need some description and so the term continues to be used. Personality disordered people are therefore relatively extreme personalities who persistently behave in ways that are detrimental to themselves, to others, or to society as a whole. Nevertheless, before you could use the term about anybody you would need to be sure that their personality was fully developed as far as it could be (i.e. that they were not children or early adolescents), and that your assessment was thorough (including an informant history) and that the abnormal behaviours were not because of psychiatric or organic illness (e.g. hypomania or frontal lobe damage).

TYPES OF PERSONALITY DISORDER

The American Diagnostic and Statistical Manual (DSM) way of looking at personality disorders is grouped into three clusters. Cluster A includes odd or eccentric personality disorders such as paranoid, schizoid or schizotypal. These and personality disorders from the other clusters will be described in more detail later. Cluster B includes personality disorders which are seen as dramatic or erratic such as antisocial, borderline, histrionic and narcissistic. Cluster C includes personality disorders which characterise as anxious/fearful such as avoidant, dependent or obsessive-compulsive personality disorders.

Odd or eccentric personality disorders

A paranoid personality disorder is one where individuals are markedly distrusting and suspicious and interpret the motives of others negatively. It is important, obviously, to screen out paranoid psychoses and in terms of personality functioning we are looking for enduring problems.

Schizoid personality disorder is one where the individual is and always has been very aloof and separate from the rest of society. Others perceive schizoid personalities as being emotionally cold. They appear unable to express warm feelings and may not have friendships and may never have had sexual relationships. Often such people do not have even one close friend. They may be preoccupied with their own fantasies and ideas. There may be an overlap with Asperger's syndrome.

Schizotypal personality disorders are often seen as rather eccentric individuals who are uncomfortable in social situations and who may tend to think about the world in a 'magical' way, perhaps making associations between events which seem unusual to the people they describe them to.

Sometimes schizoid and schizotypal individuals are seen in other classification systems as being part of a schizophrenic spectrum.

Dramatic or erratic personality disorders

Antisocial personalities (or dissocial or sociopathic in some classifications) are personality disorders where there is a callous lack of concern for the feelings of others, a persistent and irresponsible disregard for social norms and rules (with them being broken by the individual), difficulty maintaining relationships (although they may find it easy to strike up an initial rapport) and an inability to learn from experience, particularly punishment. Sociopaths may therefore be persistent offenders who behave coldly and without regard to their victims' feelings. Dissocial personalities may have been noted to have a conduct disorder in childhood and adolescence.

Borderline personality disorders include people who have very unstable relationships, sometimes quite intense and explosive, often made more problematic by the borderline individual's extreme fear of being abandoned, which may paradoxically push the other individual in the relationship away. For instance, a borderline individual may find themselves so insecure in a relationship that they may take an overdose which partially expresses their desire to cling onto the other individual. The other individual, however, instead of responding with sympathy may be repelled by the act and the relationship may be broken down even quicker than either of the participants had wanted. Borderline individuals often have difficulty with their own identity and have rapidly fluctuating affect. They may be impulsive individuals and there is a pronounced propensity for self-harm. There is an overlap with affective disorder and the original concept indicated a borderline between neurotic and psychotic symptoms. Some people with borderline personalities may have brief episodes of psychosis.

Some people conceptualise antisocial and borderline personalities as being two sides of the same coin. Antisocial personalities tend to cluster in males and borderline personalities tend to cluster in females, leading to some concerns about gender stigmatisation of behaviour.

The narcissistic personality disorder has characteristics which include a lack of empathy, a tendency to be grandiose and a requirement for the admiration of others for achievements which are not seen as particularly remarkable by others.

Anxious/fearful personality disorders

Avoidant personality disorders are seen in individuals who feel somewhat inadequate, socially inhibited and are very sensitive to the negative evaluation of others.

Dependent personality disorders are seen as submissive individuals who often require other people to make decisions on their behalf and tend to comply with other people's wishes to an extreme degree, feeling helpless when they are left alone. A fear of abandonment allows these people to disregard their best interests and such dependent people may often seem to settle in relationships where their partner is excessively dominant or even cruel.

An obsessive-compulsive personality disorder (sometimes referred to as an anankastic personality) is one where there is excessive caution in a slavish attention to detail, order, timetables and rules. Colleagues of such people may be infuriated by their perfectionism and slowness. When urged to hurry or cut corners the anankastic individual can resort to stubbornness. There is an overlap with obsessive-compulsive disorder.

TREATMENT OF PERSONALITY DISORDERS

In terms of treatment, personality disorders are often lifelong in nature and relatively unresponsive to external alteration. A key requirement is that the individual themself wishes to change something about his or her behaviour or affect. Therapeutic communities can sometimes be useful in some cases of sociopathic or antisocial personality disorder.

Dialectical behaviour therapy (DBT) or cognitive behavioural therapy (CBT) can be useful in some cases of borderline personality disorder.

It is important to continually screen for other treatable psychiatric disorders which may be *comorbid* with the personality disorder. The coexistence of psychiatric disorder and personality disorder is quite high so that a third or so of personality disorder sufferers may have an affective disorder.

Personality disorder sufferers, being often prone to affective disorders, may also be particularly likely to take their own life.

Mood stabilisers such as lamotrigine may be useful in borderline personality disorder, particularly if there is an affective component. Borderline patients who have psychotic features may respond well to clozapine.

Apart from screening for suicide risk, it is important to screen for risk to third parties and dangerousness. One of the best predictors of future behaviour is past behaviour and a careful history of forensic difficulties should be taken during assessment, including all charges and past convictions. Some screening instruments, such as the HCR-20, are sometimes employed.

CASE HISTORY 1

Rachael had been seeing a psychiatrist since the age of 15. Her mother, unable to cope with her behaviours, threw her out when she was aged 18. At the age of 20 she was taken into the hospital with her seventh paracetamol overdose. The duty psychiatrist who saw her on a medical ward noticed that her forearms were so scarred from repeated cutting that there was more scar tissue than skin.

Rachael was unwilling to give a history to the doctor, but from her thick file of notes the psychiatrist noted several details about her past.

Rachael's father had left home when she was seven. After that age Rachael could only remember her parents' repeated rows and the fact that she lived in fear of her father beating her. Her mother married again when Rachael was 10. Rachael suffered sexual abuse at the hands of her stepfather. When her mother learnt about the abuse she accused Rachael of seducing her new husband, but she did insist on a divorce from him for which Rachael was grateful.

At the age of 13 Rachael had her first sexual intercourse with an 18-year-old fairground worker. She left home to stay with him in a caravan, but returned home three weeks later. She began drinking heavily at the age of 14 and started having a series of affairs with older men. Most of the affairs were short lived. The longest time that she saw anybody was two months. At the age of 15 she took an overdose of her mother's fluoxetine and saw her first psychiatrist.

What features about Rachael's history suggest an abnormal personality?

There is a long history of deliberate self-harm, impulsive behaviour – alcohol abuse, inappropriate sexual liaisons – and unstable relationships. The behaviours assume a repeating pattern. Presumably, at the start of each sexual relationship Rachael sees the other as desirable in some way but very soon they are rejected, possibly because they might be seen in a suddenly negative light. This might suggest the use of splitting as a defence mechanism. Overall there are features suggestive of a borderline personality disorder.

What Is there about Rachael's early life which may explain some of her personality and behaviour?

Nearly all her relationships are inconsistent ones, either because of others' actions or her own. Her parents' relationship was unstable and ended in failure at a critical point in her development. Children often blame themselves if their parents split up. More undeserved blame was laid at Rachael's door by her mother after her second marriage failed. In Rachael's position people often taken the blame on board and feel profoundly guilty even if they are not. They feel like a bad person. They see the people around them as either good or bad and view themselves in the same unforgiving way. Rachael may feel good about herself sometimes but this is always followed by feelings of guilt and badness. In helping such people it is difficult not to be sucked into being as inconsistent as previous figures in their life.

Consistency is something to be aimed for in terms of management. A long-term therapeutic relationship can help where sessions with the same person are given regularly but not necessarily over-frequently. Predictably, such therapy will revolve around issues of guilt, persecution and fear of rejection by the therapist.

CASE HISTORY 2

Ms Arbuthnot, 60, called her family doctor out to see her one weekend. She had never called a doctor out before. In fact she had not seen a doctor in 20 years. She was embarrassed at having to do so but had developed a chest infection and was feeling quite unwell.

Her family doctor was concerned that Ms Arbuthnot had pneumonia and had no one to care for her during her illness. She rejected his offer of a hospital admission because she could not face 'a ward full of strangers'. She would take anything he prescribed for her, but she would not leave her home nor allow any stranger in to give her help. For Ms Arbuthnot a stranger was just about anybody; even her closest relatives were strangers. She had only called the doctor because she felt desperate. It was clear that she resented his probing questions. It seemed that she had not one friend in the world. She occasionally went out to a local church and sat at the very back on her own. She fled if anybody asked her to stay for a coffee after the service. She shopped in the supermarket to avoid conversation. All her relatives had died, but it seemed that they were never a close family. She had worked briefly in insurance as a girl but found people to be 'busybodies'. She had never had a boyfriend, although somebody had asked her out once. Her hobbies included listening to the music of Liszt and Chopin and reading the works of Dostoyevsky.

She did not appear to be depressed, demented or psychotic and the doctor was unable to persuade her to go into hospital. Reluctantly, he gave her some antibiotics and said that he would return in a few days. She replied that he should not do this and that she would call if she needed to see him again. Having ushered the doctor out of her house she closed the front door and sighed with relief.

What features suggest an abnormal personality?

This lady has virtually no relationships at all beyond the superficial ones that are essential to daily transactions such as going to the supermarket. She avoids any deeper contact than this. There is no friendship or sexual relationship in her life. Such avoidant behaviour has characterised her behaviour all through her life. Even the superficial contact with the family doctor is resented. Her only interests are solitary ones. She could be described as a schizoid personality disorder. Helping her, as the family doctor tried to do, would be an uphill struggle unless she herself desired to change.

CASE HISTORY 3

Kyle, 22, was seen at a primary care clinic as a new patient. He had recently been in prison for a conviction of actual bodily harm and theft. It was his fifth conviction. Earlier convictions had included theft, assault and taking a car without permission. He had used cannabis and cocaine since the age of 13. He could not read or write. He was requesting methadone.

He disclosed a childhood where his alcoholic father beat him and he was frequently left alone in the house as a child without food. He had attended school infrequently. His mother had left the family home when he was small. He is himself angry with women in general and also described a quick temper. Kyle admitted he had wet the bed until the age of 15. He had once killed a neighbour's treasured pet with an airgun.

His most recent conviction had been for mugging a pensioner, which he had done many times to get money for drugs. When the practice nurse asked what had happened to the pensioner, Kyle shrugged and laughed. He said, 'They've got too much money these old people – they should all get euthanasia and pass it on to the next generation.' The nurse enquired whether he had thought at all about the feelings of the pensioner after the accident and said her own grandmother had once been mugged and had not been able to leave the house afterwards. Kyle looked at her and laughed and said, 'What do I have to do now? When can I get the prescription?' The nurse felt chilled by his attitude and also felt unsafe in the room with him.

What features suggest an abnormal personality?

Kyle has displayed antisocial behaviour since his early teens, possibly as a reaction to an emotionally deprived childhood where he suffered physical abuse. He shows little empathy with other people and a callous lack of concern or remorse for his behaviour.

What personality disorder would you consider in any differential diagnosis?

It would be inappropriate to label someone with a personality disorder diagnosis after only one consultation and without more evidence, but Kyle's presentation is redolent of an antisocial or dissocial personality disorder.

What features might predict dangerousness?

Dangerousness involves the propensity to cause harm to others, and the best predictor of dangerousness is past behaviour. Kyle's underlying antisocial attitudes, lack of empathy and remorse, history of experienced violence, coupled with immaturity, impulsivity, drug misuse and numerous acts of violence to animals and other human beings indicate that he is at high risk of further acts of violence to others.

LEARNING POINTS: PERSONALITY

➤ There are numerous theories of personality based on different types or different traits. Extroversion and introversion are two personality types often referred to and were first described by Dr Carl Jung.

➤ Dr Sigmund Freud described the personality as an interaction between id, ego and superego. He and his daughter defined various defence mechanisms such as denial, projection and sublimation. He also placed considerable emphasis on the concept of the unconscious mind.

➤ Dreams may sometimes highlight internal conflicts and repressed material in symbolic form.

➤ Personality disordered individuals have extreme personalities and may repeatedly behave in ways that are detrimental to themselves, the people around them and or society.

➤ Antisocial, dissocial and sociopathic personality disorders often show a callous lack of concern for others' feelings, difficulty in maintaining relationships in the medium or long term and are unable to learn from experience. This may lead to such individuals becoming persistent offenders. They may have a history of conduct disorder or cruelty to animals.

➤ Obsessional or anankastic personality disorders involve excessive caution, attention to detail, perfectionistic traits and slowness in completing tasks.

➤ Dependent personality disorders may get other people to make decisions on their behalf and comply with other people's wishes to the detriment of their own interests because of a fear of abandonment.

➤ Schizoid personality disorders are often emotionally cold and unable to express warm feelings. They lack close friendships and often have very limited psychosexual functioning.

➤ Paranoid personality disorders may be overly suspicious, bear grudges for a long time and will not forgive injuries or slights often when none was actually intended. Their focus on themselves is suggestive of a certain self-importance.

➤ Borderline personality disorders may have peaks of intense emotions like anger. They may act impulsively to harm themselves, sometimes in an attempt to forestall abandonment in a failing relationship. They have confusion about their own identity and may use defence mechanisms such as splitting or projection.

➤ Personality disorders benefit from treatment in the main, particularly if there is a coexisting physical or mental illness.

➤ Personality disorders have a risk of suicide and should always be screened sympathetically with regard to suicide risks, and risks to third parties.

SELF-ASSESSMENT
MCQs

1 Psychological defence mechanisms include:
   A denial
   B projection
   C displacement
   D materialism
   E mobilisation

2 Recognised personality traits include:
   A obsessionality
   B conscientiousness
   C suspiciousness
   D openness
   E submissiveness

3 The following individuals invented or pioneered these various concepts:
   A Freud and the id
   B Jung and attachment
   C Adler and sibling rivalry
   D Bowlby and introversion
   E Maslow and ego dystonia

SHORT ANSWER QUESTIONS

1 Describe the id, ego and superego. How do they work together to determine personality and behaviour?
2 What is the unconscious? How do we know whether there is an unconscious mind or not?
3 What is personality and how does it develop?
4 Describe how people with disordered personalities may present to medical care.
5 How can attachment affect a child's behaviour when admitted to hospital?

MCQ answers
1 A=T, B=T, C=T, D=F, E=F.
2 All true.
3 A=T, B=F, C=T, D=F, E=F.

EXPLORATIONS

Sources listed in the further reading and references section will help you with the following.

LINKS WITH PSYCHOLOGY

Find out more about the 16 personality factor questionnaire and the Myers-Briggs type indicator. Look at the personality types or factors that they use.

➤ Which category or categories do you think you might fit into best?
➤ What other personality tests are there?
➤ What research has been done to demonstrate their scientific validity?
➤ How reliable are they?
➤ What may they be used for in terms of society?
➤ What inappropriate uses may be found for such questionnaires?

Study the list of psychological defence mechanisms.
➤ Can you think of examples from your own experience that might illustrate each mechanism?
➤ Do you think that you have ever used any of these mechanisms?

LINKS WITH GENETICS

➤ What evidence is there to suggest that personality has an inherited basis rather than being a product of environment or upbringing?
➤ What studies have been done or could be done to establish a genetic contribution?

FURTHER READING AND REFERENCES

Abramson LY, Seligman MEP, Teasdale JD. Learned helplessness in humans: critique and reformulation. *Journal of Abnormal Psychology.* 1978; **87**: 32–48.

Ainsworth MDS, Blehar MC, Waters E, Wall S. *Patterns of Attachment: a psychological study of the strange situation.* Hillsdale, NJ: Erlbaum; 1978.

Bartholomew K. Avoidance of intimacy: an attachment perspective. *Journal of Social and Personal Relationships.* 1990; **7**: 147–78.

Beck AT, Rush AJ, Shaw BF, Emery G. *Cognitive Therapy of Depression.* New York: Guilford; 1979.

Bowlby J. *Attachment and Loss. Vol. 1: Attachment.* New York: Basic Books; 1969.

Bowlby J. *Attachment and Loss. Vol. 2: Separation, Anger and Anxiety.* London: Hogarth Press: 1973.

Eysenck HJ. Genetic and environmental contributions to individual differences: the three major dimensions of personality. *Journal of Personality.* 1990; **58**: 245–61.

Goldberg LR. The structure of phenotypic personality traits. *American Psychologist.* 1993; **48**: 26–34.

Grünbaum A. *The Foundations of Psychoanalysis: a philosophical critique.* Berkeley, CA: University of California Press; 1984.

Reiss D. Mechanisms linking genetic and social influences in adolescent development: beginning a collaborative search. *Current Directions in Psychological Science.* 1997; **6**: 100–5.

Soldz S, Vaillant GE. The Big Five personality traits and the life course: a 45-year longitudinal study. *Journal of Research in Personality.* 1999; **33**: 208–32.

Webster CD, Douglas KS, Eves SD, Hart SD. Assessing risk of violence to others. In: Webster CD, Jackson MA, editors. *Impulsivity Theory, Assessment and Treatment.* New York: Guilford; 1997. pp. 251–7.

Webster CD, Harris GT, Rice ME, Cormier C, Quinsey VL. *The Violence Prediction Scheme: assessing dangerousness in high risk men*. Toronto: University of Toronto: Centre of Criminology; 1994.

RESOURCES

http://en.wikipedia.org/wiki/Myers-Briggs_Type_Indicator

http://en.wikipedia.org/wiki/Big_Five_personality_traits

www.bbc.co.uk/science/humanbody/mind/surveys/personality/index.shtml

www.kirjasto.sci.fi/cjung.htm

www.freud.org.uk/

http://en.wikipedia.org/wiki/Alfred_Adler

www.pearsonassessments.com/tests/mmpi_2.htm

www.personalityresearch.org/

CHAPTER 13

Physical treatments

Physical treatments used in psychiatry today include antipsychotic and other drugs, electroconvulsive therapy, and psychosurgery.

CONTENTS

ADVANCES IN PHYSICAL TREATMENTS

It was the 1950s before *antipsychotic drugs* began to be introduced. Before that ECT, insulin coma and even psychosurgery were used for schizophrenia and severe depression. The new antipsychotics had fewer side-effects and unlike brain surgery – usually on the frontal lobes – antipsychotics were reversible.

Before the 20th century physical treatments were even more outlandish and basically ineffective. Patients could be condemned by mental illness to be psychotic for life. In the 18th and 19th centuries treatments included padded cells, straitjackets, cold wet blanket baths, spinning chairs, purges, emetics and magnetic fields. In the early 20th century deliberate infection with malaria, insulin-induced comas (developed by Dr Manfred Sakel in 1927) or intravenous metrazol-induced seizures (developed by Ladislas Meduna in the 1930s) and so on were used. No doubt some patients responded to these treatments either through a placebo effect or spontaneous recovery – just as with physical illnesses. These apparently good responses were probably used anecdotally to boost the claims of such odd treatments.

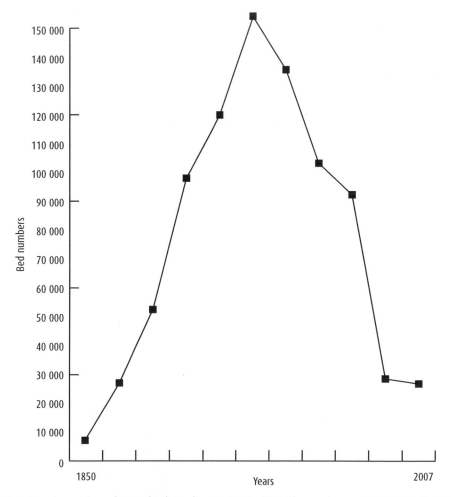

Figure 13.1 Numbers of psychiatric beds in the UK 1850–2007. The peak was 155 000 beds in 1955. At its inception in 1948 half of all NHS beds were in mental health. The introduction of the antipsychotics in the 1950s made a reduction in bed numbers possible.

The advent of the French drug chlorpromazine in 1950 showed that there could be a drug with a specific antipsychotic effect. Patients with schizophrenia who had been hospitalised in asylums for many years were sometimes transformed within weeks of the new treatment. Although chlorpromazine works on a variety of receptors in the brain including cholinergic and histaminergic receptors, it is felt to be its effects on dopamine receptors that are responsible for its antipsychotic effects. Chlorpromazine (a phenothiazine developed by Delay and Deniker) is seen as a *typical antipsychotic* or *first generation antipsychotic*. Other antipsychotics that emerged in the 1950s include haloperidol, a butyrophenone, which was developed in 1957.

Electroconvulsive therapy (ECT) was developed by the Italian Ugo Cerletti (1877–1963). Cerletti and Bini first used ECT in April 1938. At the time ECT transformed the treatment of depression. Before ECT old textbooks of psychiatry describe hospital inpatients with psychotic depression lasting for years.

Tricyclic antidepressants were introduced in the 1950s with the first example being imipramine (developed by Kuhn).

These new physical treatments enabled the decanting of thousands of patients from the old county asylums. Before these treatments existed, community care was impossible.

PSYCHOSURGERY

Psychosurgery is rarely used nowadays but was once very much in vogue following pioneering work on frontal lobe surgery by Egaz Moniz, who won the Nobel Prize in 1948 for the development of the concept. It became popular at a time when the antipsychotics were still years away. Psychosurgery was somewhat effective for aggressive patients with psychosis, but as it was irreversible any unwanted effects on mood or personality were unfortunately permanent.

Psychosurgery is still performed on a handful of patients each year whose illnesses are severe and unresponsive to drugs, for example in patients with persistent, severe, life dominating anxiety. Psychosurgery was certainly overused in the 1950s and acquired a frightening public image.

FUTURE DEVELOPMENTS

Research on the efficacy of physical treatments against placebos has enabled a process of continual refinement of drug molecules. Continuing research aims to replace established treatments with treatments that are safer, easier to comply with, more efficacious, non-addictive, more cost effective and quicker acting. For instance, new antidepressants were vigorously tested against the old 'gold standard' antidepressants amitriptyline and imipramine. Newer antidepressants such as fluoxetine are safer in overdose and offer a more acceptable treatment to the patient because of fewer side-effects.

In recent years an *atypical* or *second generation* antipsychotic, clozapine, has offered hope to patients with treatment resistant schizophrenia. About 20% of patients with schizophrenia do not respond to conventional antipsychotics, but a significant proportion of these do respond to clozapine. Based on this advance new safer, more effective antipsychotics are in development.

A safer, more acceptable alternative to ECT appeared to be *transcranial magnetic stimulation (TMS)*; however, efficacy studies have failed to prove any superiority of this treatment over ECT or other treatments such as antidepressants.

Further research into potential genetic causes of mental illness may yield radical new treatments in the future.

ANTIPSYCHOTIC DRUGS

Antipsychotic drugs are sometimes called neuroleptics or major tranquillisers. They are used in treating schizophrenia and in short-term control of disturbed psychotic states and abnormal behaviour. They are usually sedative.

MAIN PHARMACOLOGICAL ACTIONS

The main group of antipsychotic drugs exert their effect by blocking dopamine receptors (particularly D_2) in the brain. Blockade of dopamine receptors also leads to side-effects, and because cholinergic, histaminergic and noradrenergic receptors can also be affected, the side-effects can be varied.

ROUTE OF ADMINISTRATION

Antipsychotic drugs are usually given orally or intramuscularly (for emergency control of disturbed behaviour) and also by long-term depot injections (which allow the drug to leach into the bloodstream over a period of weeks, meaning that individuals can take their medication every few weeks or monthly). Antipsychotics are not usually given intravenously.

COMMON SIDE-EFFECTS

Side-effects often depend on the neurotransmitter system affected. Over-sedation may arise from activity at histaminergic receptors. Dry mouth, blurred vision, nasal stuffiness, constipation and tremor occur because of anti-cholinergic effects. Similarly, confusion can be a problem due to cholinergic effects, particularly in the elderly. Postural hypotension is particularly dangerous in the elderly and is due to peripheral and central alpha-adrenoceptor blockade. A reflex tachycardia and peripheral vasodilatation may lead to a concomitant hypothermia. Because of dopamine blockade in the hypothalamo-pituitary axis, prolactin levels may rise dramatically and lead to unwanted lactation in females.

Newer antipsychotics tend to have fewer of these problems, particularly in terms of *extra pyramidal side-effects* (EPSEs) and are by and large less sedative. Nevertheless they do have their own problems and newer 'atypical' antipsychotics like olanzapine are particularly associated with weight gain and there is debate over whether it may trigger early onset of diabetes mellitus.

OTHER SIDE-EFFECTS OF ANTIPSYCHOTICS

➤ Photosensitivity, e.g. with chlorpromazine.
➤ Movement disorders including acute dystonic reactions, restlessness (akathisia) tardive dyskinesia (repetitive, involuntary, purposeless movements such as grimacing, tongue protrusion, lip smacking, and movements of the arms, legs and trunk).
➤ Bone marrow suppression.
➤ Lowering of the epileptic threshold and stimulation of epileptic fits.
➤ Jaundice due to intrahepatic status.
➤ Pigmentary changes in the skin and eyes.

Acute Parkinsonian side-effects can be reversed by agents such as procyclidine (given 10 mg IV in acute dystonia, but otherwise given orally) or orphenadrine.

INTERACTIONS WITH OTHER DRUGS

These include interactions with:
➤ alcohol
➤ CNS depressants, e.g. benzodiazepines, barbiturates
➤ antihypertensives
➤ levodopa
➤ antiepileptics
➤ MAOI antidepressants.

CHLORPROMAZINE: THE FIRST ANTIPSYCHOTIC

Chlorpromazine was the first antipsychotic in widespread use. Its structure is that of a phenothiazine. Its main clinical effect arises from a blockade of dopamine (D_2) receptor sites. Chlorpromazine is sedative and particularly effective at controlling disturbed behaviour when given intramuscularly. Up to 80% of an oral dose of chlorpromazine is removed by the first pass hepatic metabolism, before it ever reaches the brain. There is no depot preparation. Intravenous administration may provoke a fatal arrhythmia. A typical dose regime for a young man with schizophrenia might be 150 mg of chlorpromazine four times a day. In an acute emergency where sedation is required a dose of 100–150 mg IM could be used. In older or smaller patients the dose must be altered.

OLDER TYPICAL ANTIPSYCHOTICS

Haloperidol (a butyrophenone) was another early antipsychotic. It is less sedating, more potent and more likely to induce extra-pyramidal side-effects (EPSEs) than chlorpromazine. There is a depot preparation. Other butyrophenones include benperidol, droperidol, and trifluperidol. Haloperidol is roughly 10 times more potent than chlorpromazine so that 10 mg of haloperidol produce the same effect as 100 mg of chlorpromazine.

Other phenothiazines include thioridazine and trifluoperazine. A phenothiazine which is sometimes used in psychiatric intensive care units (PICUs) is levomepromazine. This can be used orally or intramuscularly in 'rapid tranquilisation'.

Depot injections include flupenthixol and zuclopenthixol. Flupenthixol is a typical antipsychotic drug, a thioxanthene, and related to the phenothiazines. In depot form it is given as a decanoate ester, which lasts up to three weeks from a single injection. Risperidone is also available as a depot.

ATYPICAL OR NOVEL ANTIPSYCHOTICS

A second generation of antipsychotics was developed in the 1990s. This second generation includes olanzapine, risperidone, quetiapine, and paliperidone. Atypical antipsychotics cause fewer extra-pyramidal side-effects and tend not to increase prolactin levels. Atypical antipsychotics often have some dopaminergic effects but also work on serotonin receptors. Clozapine is the key example of an atypical antipsychotic but was actually developed in the 1950s. Clozapine has a tendency to produce white blood cell dyscrasias and bone marrow suppression. Its efficacy in treatment resistant schizophrenia seems unique, however, and despite its side-effects it was reintroduced into clinical practice. Clozapine is prescribed with caution with intensive monitoring of blood counts.

TREATMENT STRATEGY

In terms of a strategy for using antipsychotics the initial phase may, for example, begin with oral haloperidol or risperidone. Over the next few days or weeks the clinician will titrate the dose up or down to manage acute psychotic features such as hallucinations or delusions. Hallucinations typically become less frequent, less severe and less intrusive as treatment proceeds. Delusions recede to become overvalued ideas or unusual ideas that can be challenged and then eventually lapse. Maintenance of remission can be achieved using depot injections such as flupenthixol or risperidone depot. These depots are particularly important for patients who tend not to comply with long-term tablet regimes. Alterations to this strategy may occur when there are side-effects that require the use of anti-Parkinsonian drugs such as orphenadrine given concurrently or if there is treatment resistance (when ultimately clozapine might prove useful). Some units begin new patients on an initial short-acting course of oral medication and then move on to a longer depot injection of the same drug.

Table 13.1 Depot antipsychotics

Proper name	Dose	Frequency
Fluphenazine (Modecate)	up to 100 milligrams	every 1 to 6 weeks
Flupenthixol (Depixol)	up to 400 milligrams	every 1 to 6 weeks
Haloperidol (Haldol)	up to 300 milligrams	every 1 to 6 weeks
Pipothiazine (Piportil)	up to 200 milligrams	every 4 weeks
Zuclopenthixol (Clopixol)	up to 600 milligrams	every 4 weeks
Risperidone (Risperdal)	up to 50 milligrams	every 2 weeks

ANTIDEPRESSANT DRUGS
TRICYCLICS

Tricyclic antidepressants are so called because they all have a three ring structure. They can be expected to be successful in treating about 70% of depressive episodes compared with a 30–50% placebo response. Examples of tricyclics include amitriptyline (introduced 1961), imipramine and dosulepin. The tricyclic's main therapeutic effect is via inhibition of the reuptake of monoamines from the synaptic cleft by the presynaptic neuron. The monoamines involved include noradrenaline, serotonin and dopamine. The proven efficacy of tricyclics led to the monoamine theory of depression: that depression is secondary to a relative deficiency of monoamines in the synapse. Tricyclic antidepressants act by prolonging monoamine activity at the synapse.

Insomnia is resolved quickly (especially when a main dose of tricyclic is taken at bedtime) because of the tricyclic sedative properties (largely mediated by histaminergic side-effects). However, improvement in mood lags behind improvement in sleep by some weeks. Gradually raising the daily drug dose to a certain threshold also seems to be important before tricyclics work. Patients obviously require counselling as to the delay in effect and also the need for continued compliance.

Common reasons for the failure of tricyclic antidepressant therapy
➤ Inadequate dose.
➤ Not taken regularly by the patient.
➤ Wrong diagnosis.
➤ Wrong drug type.

Side-effects of tricyclics
Most side-effects are caused by indiscriminate actions on various neurotransmitter symptoms. These side-effects make tricyclics less acceptable to some patients, reduce patient compliance and increase dropout from therapy.

Anti-cholinergic side-effects
➤ Dry mouth.

➤ Blurred vision.
➤ Urinary retention.
➤ Constipation.
➤ Sweating.
➤ Confusion.

Adrenergic side-effects
➤ Postural hypotension.
➤ Tachycardia.
➤ Cardiac arrhythmias (may cause death in susceptible individuals and in overdose ECGs are required in older patients and in patients who might be suspected of having heart disease. Tricyclics used to cause 400 overdose deaths annually in the UK).

Antihistaminergic side-effects
Drowsiness and sedation (particularly important to those who operate dangerous machinery or who drive). Other side-effects include:
➤ Weight gain (by stimulating appetite).
➤ Hypomania.
➤ Restlessness.
➤ Rashes.
➤ Photosensitivity.
➤ Bone marrow suppression.
➤ Nausea.
➤ Impotence.

Contraindications to tricyclics
➤ Simultaneous prescription of irreversible monoamine oxidase inhibitors.
➤ Heart block and recent myocardial infarction.
➤ Prostatic hypertrophy (risk of precipitating acute urinary retention).
➤ Late pregnancy.
➤ Narrow angle glaucoma.

CASE HISTORY 1
A 48-year-old woman with a four week history of low mood and biological features of depression was prescribed dosulepin 75 mg nocte by her doctor. Her doctor noted that an improvement in the patient's sleep began immediately. Two weeks later the doctor

increased the dose of dosulepin to 100 mg nocte, and two weeks after this the patient's mood had lifted significantly. She was maintained on dosulepin for the next six months and then gradually the drug was withdrawn by reducing the dose by 25 mg at intervals in outpatients.

Research indicates that 70% of patients who stop their antidepressants within six months of starting them relapse. Current opinion suggests that antidepressant therapy should be maintained for up to a year after full recovery and only then gradually withdrawn (monitoring for signs of relapse).

CASE HISTORY 2

A 54-year-old man with a four week history of low mood, insomnia and weight loss attended the psychiatry outpatients clinic. Despite his GP's prescription of tricyclics two weeks previously the patient remained depressed. On mental state examination he revealed that he had been having suicidal ideas and was thinking of hanging himself. The ideas were suggested to him by derogatory second person auditory hallucinations. Organic causes of his depressed mood and hallucinations have been fully excluded by his general practitioner.

Why did the tricyclic antidepressants not work?

The tricyclics may not have worked because they have had only two weeks in which to improve matters. They were perhaps prescribed in too low a dose, and it may be that the patient is only taking them intermittently or not at all or because the patient is not responding to this particular drug.

What is the likely diagnosis now?

The patient is suffering from a severe depression with psychotic features. Given his suicidal ideation and the severity of his illness the doctor should consider whether it is in his best interests to continue on tricyclic antidepressants given their association with fatal overdoses.

What physical treatment might be more suitable now?

This gentleman may require inpatient admission. Consideration should be given to what level of home support he has. Home treatment teams, although popular with managers for economic reasons, may not be able to deliver the sustained level of monitoring that suicidal patients require. Treating a suicidal patient at home with professional staff being present for only part of the day is clearly illogical. An admission may allow more intensive analysis of his symptoms and his suicidal ideas. While he was in hospital his medication could be changed over to a less toxic antidepressant, and he could be considered for ECT, which has a swift mode of action. Patients with depression who exhibit psychotic features, particularly command hallucinations, are at high risk of suicide. They may require antipsychotic drugs in addition to an antidepressant regime.

Once this patient is euthymic, what physical treatment might be used to maintain his mental health?

In the long term he would need continued antidepressant medication and possibly treatment with mood stabilisers and antipsychotic drugs. He may benefit from cognitive behavioural therapy as an additional strategy to help avoid recurrence of his depressive illness.

MONOAMINE OXIDASE INHIBITORS

Monoamine oxidase inhibitors (MAOI) were introduced about the same time as tricyclic antidepressants. They are antidepressants themselves. In the past they were relegated to second line use after tricyclic antidepressants had failed, because they have interactions with other drugs and particularly with foods that contain high levels of tyramine. Because most of the monoamine oxidase inhibitors are irreversible a build up of tyramine can lead to hypertensive crises.

The advent of newer antidepressants such as the SSRIs relegated MAOIs into the hinterland of antidepressant therapy but they can still be useful sometimes in resistant cases. Some foods and drinks to avoid with irreversible MAOIs such as phenelzine and tranylcypromine include:

➤ mature cheese
➤ yeast extract
➤ textured vegetable protein
➤ dark beers
➤ Chianti wine
➤ game
➤ ripe avocado
➤ pickled herring.

In addition there are drugs to avoid while taking MAOIs, particularly drugs with sympathetic nervous system actions and pethidine.

Some drugs to avoid with irreversible MAOIs
➤ Tricyclic antidepressants.
➤ SSRIs.
➤ L-dopa.
➤ Amphetamines.
➤ Cough and cold remedies containing ephedrine and pseudoephedrine.
➤ Narcotic analgesics such as pethidine.
➤ Alcohol.

Moclobemide is a reversible inhibitor of monoamine oxidase A and doesn't have quite so many stringent safeguards with regards to its prescription.

SELECTIVE SEROTONIN REUPTAKE INHIBITORS (SSRIs)

In the late 1980s SSRIs such as fluvoxamine and fluoxetine were first introduced. Because they were relatively specific in reducing reuptake of serotonin and not affecting other neurotransmitter systems quite as much, SSRIs do not have many of the side-effects produced by tricyclic antidepressants. There are fewer anticholinergic and adrenergic side-effects and cardio toxicity is reduced so that SSRIs are much safer in overdose. Unwanted effects are largely due to serotonergic effects such as those of the gastrointestinal system (nausea, diarrhoea, appetite suppression). Critics of SSRIs point to an occasional tendency to increase anxiety and there is some controversy that they may increase suicidal ideation in the early days of prescription.

Examples of SSRIs in current use in the U.K. include fluoxetine, sertraline, citalopram, and paroxetine. SSRIs, particularly the shorter acting ones, are associated with a discontinuation syndrome which includes flu-like symptoms, dizziness, insomnia, nightmares, agitation and irritability. These symptoms may last several weeks after discontinuing the SSRI. They are more frequent with paroxetine and citalopram.

Discontinuation effects also occur with other antidepressants and it is a good general principle that all psychiatric drugs should be tailed off rather than stopped suddenly. A suggested withdrawal regime for paroxetine might be to reduce it by 10 mg every two weeks until the dose is 10 mg per day, and then to 5 mg per day for the last two weeks.

A suggested withdrawal schedule for sertraline might be to reduce it by 25 mg every two weeks until the dose is 25 mg a day and then a reduction of 12.5 mg every two weeks.

All SSRIs have differing clinical structures, unlike the tricyclics.

The dose titration seen with tricyclics is generally not needed for fluoxetine (20 mg daily) but other SSRIs such as sertraline and citalopram may require titration upwards. A starter dose for citalopram might be 10–20 mg daily raised according to response up to about 60 mg daily.

SSRIs usually begin to work within a month.

As with tricyclic antidepressants, patients may stop the treatment when they are feeling well again and need to be reminded that they must continue the course for six to 12 months after full improvement.

Caution is required where renal hepatic function is impaired. SSRIs may also reduce epileptic thresholds (as with other psychotropic drugs).

Fluoxetine may also be useful when treating bulimia nervosa.

MOOD STABILISERS: LITHIUM AND THE ANTIEPILEPTICS

Mood stabilising agents are often used in bipolar affective disorder and in recurrent depression.

Lithium carbonate has been used as a first line prophylactic agent in bipolar affective disorder for over 40 years.

It seems to be particularly useful where there is an excess of manic episodes in bipolar affective disorder. Other mood stabilisers appear to be more useful where there is an excess of depressive episodes in bipolar affective disorder or in recurrent depression. These other mood stabilisers appear to be mainly drawn from the antiepileptic class of drugs. They include sodium valproate, and lamotrigine. Carbamazepine used to be used as a mood stabiliser, but does seem to affect people's concentration, is a sedative, and often produces drug interactions by inducing hepatic enzymes.

LITHIUM

Lithium carbonate is used mainly in the treatment of bipolar affective disorder and is particularly useful where there are more manic symptoms. It is useful acutely in reducing hypomania and in maintaining remission.

Pharmacokinetics

The serum half-life of lithium carbonate is 18–20 hours in young adults and 36–42 hours in the elderly. It has a low therapeutic index which means that serum concentration must be regularly monitored to keep within a therapeutic range of, say, 0.6–0.8 mmol per litre. Above 1.2 mmol per litre toxic effects begin. Concentrations above 2 mmol per litre may be fatal. Twelve per cent of patients who overdose on lithium die.

The serum level of lithium is lineally related to the ingested dose.

Lithium in its ionic form is naturally hydrophilic and is distributed mainly in intra- and extracellular fluid (not body fat). It is excreted by the kidney and thus good renal function is essential to its prescription. If renal function is compromised then toxic levels of lithium can result.

Signs of lithium toxicity

These include:

➢ anorexia
➢ nausea and diarrhoea
➢ tinnitus
➢ ataxia
➢ dysarthria
➢ drowsiness
➢ convulsions
➢ coma
➢ death.

Management of high serum levels

The initial management of high serum levels may simply involve stopping lithium therapy for a few days and readjusting the doses but, with higher levels, osmotic or alkaline dieresis or peritoneal dialysis or haemodialysis may be necessary.

Baseline investigations

Before starting lithium therapy, various baseline investigations need to be done: full blood count, urea and electrolytes, serum creatinine (provides an indication of glomerular filtration rate), thyroid function tests, ECG.

Side-effects of lithium – early

These are:

➢ nausea
➢ diarrhoea
➢ thirst
➢ polyuria
➢ fine tremor
➢ metallic taste.

Side-effects of lithium – late

These are:

➢ weight gain

➤ leucocytosis
➤ renal damage
➤ ECG changes (T-wave inversion and QRS complex widening which may reverse once lithium is stopped)
➤ hypothyroidism – occurs in about 15% of women taking lithium. If hypothyroidism does occur it is sometimes better to add in thyroid hormone replacement rather than stop the lithium.

Lithium use in young women

Lithium may have teratogenic effects if administered during pregnancy, specifically Ebstein's anomaly (cardiac malformation) and neural tube malformations if given early during pregnancy. Nursing mothers on lithium secrete that lithium in breast milk. Patients at risk of becoming pregnant must be warned of these risks.

Interactions

Lithium interacts unfavourably with thiazide diuretics, other diuretics, aminoglycoside antibiotics and NSAIDs (because NSAIDs potentiate anti-diuretic hormone).

ANXIOLYTICS AND HYPNOTICS

Anxiolytics are those drugs such as benzodiazepines which are given to allay anxiety. Hypnotics are given to induce sleep and include such compounds as benzodiazepines, zopiclone, zolpidem and chloral hydrate. Chloral hydrate has been used since the 1890s but has fallen out of use in recent years. Barbiturates used to be used in the 1950s and 1960s but because of their addictiveness and toxicity they are rarely used nowadays.

Anxiolytics and hypnotics are less in vogue than they were in 1960s and 1970s. In 1981 it was estimated that 10% of men and 20% of women would use benzodiazepines at least once during the year. Problems with tolerance, dependence and withdrawal have led many doctors to reconsider their prescribing habits. Courses of these agents are usually short in nature now and often reviewed rather than being allowed to run off with repeat prescriptions. If the doctor suspects that there is an underlying depressive illness, insomnia may be better treated by antidepressants rather than hypnotics.

Other insomnias may respond to a 'sleep hygiene programme' which seeks to promote rest-inducing factors and reduce sleep-damaging factors.

Factors promoting sleep
➤ Exercise during the day.
➤ Warm bath at bedtime.
➤ Milky drinks.
➤ Bedtime snack.
➤ Soft music before bed.
➤ Relaxation tapes / exercises.

Factors adversely affecting sleep
➤ Caffeine in tea, coffee and soft drinks.
➤ Alcohol (although it may induce sleep, alcohol withdrawal later in the night promotes wakening).
➤ Street drugs, e.g. amphetamines.
➤ Heavy meals.
➤ Withdrawal from short-acting benzodiazepines.

BENZODIAZEPINES

Benzodiazepines act by making nerve cells more receptive to gamma-amino-butyric acid (GABA). GABA is an inhibitory neurotransmitter. Benzodiazepines therefore damp down neural activity and reduce cerebral excitation. They are useful in pre-anaesthetic sedation and in aborting epileptic fits.

Benzodiazepines are well absorbed when given orally, rectally or intravenously. Virtually all of them are metabolised by the liver by oxidation conjugation. Benzodiazepine metabolites are often pharmacologically active too and indeed may have longer half-lives.

Diazepam has a half-life of 20–30 hours but its active metabolite desmethyl diazepam has a half-life of 30–200 hours.

Benzodiazepines produce tolerance and dependence. The shorter the half-life of the benzodiazepine, the more addictive it is. Once courses of benzodiazepines are stopped there is often a rebound anxiety and rebound insomnia (as the brain tries to adjust to the sudden absence of a cerebral depressant). Withdrawal effects also include epileptic fits. Benzodiazepines suppress rapid eye movement sleep (REM sleep) and patients in withdrawal may complain of very vivid dreams as a rebound REM phenomenon. Other withdrawal symptoms include depersonalisation, perceptual distortions, panic attacks, craving, headache, muscle stiffness, formication, hypersensitivity, ataxia, muscle twitches, dysphagia, diarrhoea, nausea, vomiting, palpitations, hyperventilation, flushing, sweating, skin rash and itching and influenza-like symptoms among others. In order to reduce these effects, patients are often weaned off short-acting benzodiazepines onto longer acting ones which are gradually tailed down to zero.

Discounting the many negative attributes of benzodiazepines and the many negative attitudes of doctors and patients towards them, they are potent anxiolytics and no compound or psychological therapy comes close in rapid alleviation of anxiety. They are rarely fatal in overdose.

ELECTROCONVULSIVE THERAPY (ECT)

Doctor-induced seizures have been used to treat depression since the early years of the 20th century. Fits induced by smelling camphor or through injections of metrazol had been noted to abort depressive episodes. Such methods, though, were not without risk and it was not until Cerletti and Bini introduced ECT in Rome in 1938 that the way opened for a safer method of inducing fits. ECT is used to induce modified fits (modified in that muscle relaxants and short-acting anaesthetics are also used). To induce the fit, electrodes are placed on the surface of the scalp, either bilaterally or just on one hemisphere. A small pulsed current is passed through the skull and brain. A modified generalised fit follows.

Without 'modification' simultaneously contracting opposing muscle groups can cause fractures of long bones and crush fractures of vertebrae during the tonic phase of the fit. Modification involves the use of muscle relaxants to stop such fractures and short-acting anaesthetics are used to induce unconsciousness to make the procedure more tolerable.

ECT is rapidly effective in severe depression, and is often the treatment of choice for a depression with psychotic features. For such cases it is superior to antidepressants. The rapidity of its therapeutic onset is valuable since acutely depressed individuals may stop eating and drinking (secondary to nihilistic delusions, for example) and their lives may consequently be at risk. ECT also rapidly reduces very real suffering. ECT treatment may be given in a course of two sessions a week for six to eight weeks. Resolution of depression is rapid, but further improvement often continues through the course. The induced fit is crucial to the therapeutic properties of ECT. Drugs which increase fit threshold, such as diazepam, impair its efficacy. Modified fits should be bilateral, monitored by EEG, and it is generally held that they should last for about 30 seconds. EEG monitoring is important to ensure that continued (otherwise unnoticed) partial fit activity does not occur in the brain. Prolonged fit activity in the brain post ECT may need to be dampened down by intravenous benzodiazepines.

In terms of efficacy ECT has been shown to resolve depressive illnesses more quickly than conventional antidepressants. It is, however, associated with a relapse rate which is quite marked after therapy has ended. This problem of relapse can be averted by concomitant prescription of antidepressants in the long term. There is also some anecdotal evidence to suggest that maintenance ECT with one or two sessions a month may also be an effective strategy of keeping depression at bay. Given that there is a high mortality in untreated severe depression, ECT can be considered a life-saving treatment in some cases.

ECT may also be safer in the elderly than tricyclic antidepressants because it lacks cardio-toxicity. It is not without risk, though, and there is a mortality rate but this is primarily due to the anaesthetic component of the treatment.

Cerebral systolic blood pressure rises up to about 200 mmHg during the fit and so recent cerebrovascular accidents and myocardial infarctions are contraindications. Raised intracranial pressure is an absolute contraindication.

ECT has effects on memory formation, causing a retrograde amnesia and a confused phase following the convulsion with a period of anterograde amnesia. Conventional wisdom suggests that these effects are minor and reversible, but some patients complain of losing larger portions of memory.

Large scale research comparing the effects of depression on memory and ECT on memory and comparing the two are not available, however. On balance, considering the potentially devastating effects of major depression, ECT seems a more than worthy treatment.

SELF-ASSESSMENT
MCQs
1 Lithium carbonate:
    A is mainly metabolised by the liver
    B interacts with non-steroidal anti-inflammatory drugs (NSAIDs)
    C is lipophilic
    D is most therapeutic when serum levels are greater than 3 mmol per litre
    E sometimes causes hypothyroidism

2 The following drugs are tricyclic antidepressants:
    A phenelzine
    B dosulepin
    C tranylcypromine
    D sertraline
    E olanzapine

3 Chlorpromazine:
    A affects anticholinergic receptors
    B causes photosensitivity
    C is a butyrophenone
    D is a second generation antipsychotic

E is regularly given intravenously

MCQ answers
1 A=F, B=T, C=F, D=F, E=T.
2 A=F, B=T, C=F, D=F, E=F.
3 A=T, B=T, C=F, D=F, E=F.

SHORT ANSWER QUESTIONS
1 What are the side-effects of amitriptyline?
2 How does the pharmacology of lithium carbonate differ from the pharmacology of a serotonin reuptake inhibitor?
3 Which foods and drugs must a patient taking phenelzine avoid?
4 What investigations need to be performed on a patient before and during lithium therapy?

FURTHER READING AND REFERENCES
Anderson IM. Lessons to be learnt from meta-analyses of newer versus older antidepressants. In: Lee A, editor. *Recent Topics from Advances in Psychiatric Treatment*. London: Gaskell Press; 1999. pp. 45–51.

Anderson IM. Drug treatment of depression: reflections on the evidence. *Advances in Psychiatric Treatment*. 2003; **9**: 11–20.

Fink M. *Electroshock: healing mental illness*. Oxford: Oxford University Press; 2002.

Green B. *Focus on Antipsychotics*. Newbury: Petroc Press; 2003.

Haddad P, Dursan S, Deakin JFW. *Adverse Syndromes and Psychiatric Drugs: a clinical guide*. Oxford: Oxford University Press; 2004.

Healy D. *Psychiatric Drugs Explained*. Edinburgh: Churchill Livingstone; 2004.

Meyer J, Quenzer L. *Psychopharmacology: drugs, the brain and behavior*. Sunderland, MA: Sinauer Associates; 2004.

Taylor D, Paton C, Kerwin D. *The Maudsley Prescribing Guidelines*. 9th ed. London: Informa Healthcare; 2007.

UK ECT Review Group. Efficacy and safety of electroconvulsive therapy in depressive disorders: a systematic review and meta-analysis. *Lancet*. 2003; **361**: 799–808.

RESOURCES
Cochrane Reviews
www.cochrane.org/reviews/

Dr Ivan Goldberg's Depression Central
www.psycom.net/depression.central.html

Electronic Medicines Compendium
http://emc.medicines.org.uk/

National Institute for Clinical Excellence
See pages on 'Mental health and behavioural
conditions':
www.nice.org.uk/

Pharmacy On-Line
www.priory.com/pharmol.htm

CHAPTER 14
Psychotherapy

Psychotherapy and counselling are 'talking cures' where mental disorders can be treated over time and in which the relationship with the therapist is often of vital importance. Although psychotherapy is often a viable alternative to physical treatment, physical and psychological treatments can also be combined. In depression, patients may have a better prognosis if both kinds of treatment are used.

CONTENTS

PSYCHOLOGICAL TREATMENTS

Psychotherapies include:

- Behavioural therapy
- Cognitive therapy
- Cognitive behavioural therapy (CBT)
- Cognitive analytic therapy (CAT)
- Dialectical behaviour therapy (DBT)
- Group therapy
- Family therapy
- Interpersonal psychotherapy
- Psychoanalysis
- Counselling
- many others.

There are so many different types of psychotherapy and counselling that it is impossible to describe them all.

The differences in style, content and duration of therapies means it is very difficult to research the effectiveness of different therapies for specific conditions. This also makes it difficult to generalise from published research on any particular form of therapy. In prescribing psychotherapies doctors must be careful to find a therapy that matches the illness and refer to a therapist who has the necessary experience and qualifications.

Cognitive behavioural therapy (CBT) has become very popular in recent years and is recommended by the government agency NICE (National Institute for Health and Clinical Excellence) for mild to moderate depression and PTSD as a first line treatment. Nevertheless the popularity of CBT and long waiting lists on the NHS have led to a mushrooming of the number of independent CBT therapists. Some of these therapists have as little training as a few days and others have higher degrees in therapy, nursing and psychology with extensive clinical backgrounds. In most cases it is appropriate to refer patients to a person who has some years of experience in a professional background such as nursing, social work or psychology, plus a higher degree plus the necessary qualifications and years of experience in therapy.

Talking cures have been used for centuries, which is a testament to their popularity. Soranus of Ephesus, a physician working in the 1st century AD, talked to his patients and challenged the false ideas of people with depression. Nowadays in cognitive therapy therapists look for erroneous ways of thinking in depressed people and teach them to challenge these themselves. Holy men in all kinds of cultures have listened to the troubles of people who came to consult them and these people often derived comfort and reassurance from pouring out their heart.

At the end of the 19th and the beginning of the 20th centuries there was considerable interest in and popularity of the ideas of Sigmund Freud. He believed that many mental disorders, particularly neuroses, arose from the unconscious where they were attached to ideas, memories or desires that couldn't be accepted by the conscious mind and were therefore repressed into the unconscious. In psychoanalysis, the therapy invented by Freud, patients used to lie on his couch in Vienna for an hour a day, five days a week for many years and recount whatever came into their minds (the method of so called *free association*). Free association often led the patient to talking about traumas in their childhood that accounted, in part, for their current distress. Since the unconscious was thought to work on a symbolic level Freud also explored this by means of dream analysis. Patients would recount their dreams in detail and together the patient and Freud would explore the symbolic meaning of the dreams' content often by asking the patient what ideas they associated with elements of the dream. Sigmund Freud regarded dreams as the 'Royal Road to the Unconscious'.

CASE HISTORY 1

In her third session of therapy Ann brought up a dream that she had had in the previous week. She had dreamt of entering a big house with a large hall and a wide staircase. Room by room Ann began exploring the place with the help of a guide. The ground floor and the first floor boasted quite comfortable rooms with dark wood panelling and deep red curtains. The rooms were nonetheless cheery and bright and the sun streamed in through the windows. However, in some dark corridors sections of flooring were sagging and her guide referred to rot in the fabric of the floor. On the first floor landing the guide pointed out the top floor which he couldn't take her to. She tried to see up some stairs and saw a brighter place where some golden girl was singing. Next the guide showed her some steps that led into the basement. A man and a woman lived there in the gloom. Ann felt that she did not want to go downstairs 'because of the things that happened there'.

What do you think the therapist might make of this dream? Is it an optimistic dream or a pessimistic one? What could parts of the dream symbolise?

It is difficult to interpret dreams without knowing the patient and the context of the dream. Dreams sometimes merely seem to repeat the previous day's events. In this case Ann could have been looking around an old house with an estate agent the day before and that might help explain elements of her dream. However, in this case the therapist discussed the dream's contents with Ann and together they decided that the dream was on the whole an optimistic one that was about Ann and her therapy. In her dream the house represented Ann's life, with the ground and first floor as her current life which is largely a happy one although occasionally spoilt by periods of low mood (symbolised by the rot in dark corridors). The basement was her past shrouded in darkness and unclear in detail. The top floor seemed to be a possible future. The language describing the top floor is optimistic: 'golden' and 'singing'. The guide in the dream house was probably a representation of the therapist. If the therapist was to ask for more details about the guide this might give

a chance to find out what Ann felt about him. In psychotherapy much attention is focused on these feelings which are often held to be the patient's *transference*. Transference involves the patient bringing their past experiences and emotions into therapy and transferring the qualities of significant past relationships onto the therapist. When these are recognised correctly and interpreted properly it can help the patient gain control over feelings and ways of relating to other people that may always have seemed overwhelming and mysterious before. Alexander and French (1946) called this 're-experiencing the old, unsettled conflict, but with a new ending' – a corrective emotional experience.

CASE HISTORY 2

Mrs Davenport had been referred by her doctor to a psychologist. Mrs Davenport complained that she felt she was a worthless person and that she felt guilty and that she could not be a better mother. The psychologist asked exactly why Mrs Davenport felt she was worthless. She replied, 'I was putting the washing out to dry this morning when the clothes line broke and all the washing fell onto the ground. It's the kind of thing that happens to me.' When asked why she needed to be a 'better mother' Mrs Davenport said, 'My 20-year-old son got his girlfriend pregnant but he's not sorry about it. I should have taught him some old fashioned values.'

How are events that Mrs Davenport described linked to the way she feels?

It's difficult to see exactly how. Some events happen (the washing falls down, her son gets his girlfriend pregnant) and Mrs Davenport thinks about these, draws some very large conclusions ('I am worthless' and 'I should be a better mother') and feels low because of these ideas (or cognitions). Cognitive behavioural therapy seeks to work on this link between cognitions and emotions. The work of the

American psychiatrist Aaron T Beck and colleagues focused on people with anxiety and depression. They concluded that in these disorders people have various negative automatic thoughts based on various cognitive errors. For instance, Mrs Davenport makes a giant leap of thought from her washing getting dirty to her being 'worthless'. This way of thinking may have routes in the past but it can be challenged in the present and hopefully leave Mrs Davenport to draw different conclusions about herself in the future. CBT would help her become skilled at finding alternatives to negative automatic thoughts. For example, in the case of the washing line Mrs Davenport might think, 'The wind was strong and the washing line was old, which was why it broke. I can buy a new washing line and I can wash the clothes again. I can cope with the unexpected.' A therapist might ask her to keep a diary of her thoughts and feelings and ask her to record what alternatives thoughts she found to her original negative ones. The diary could be reviewed during therapy sessions.

THE STRUCTURE OF INDIVIDUAL THERAPY

Psychotherapists generally give a structure to the therapy by ensuring that sessions are all of a similar length (usually about 50 minutes), are given regularly (say once a week), and conducted in the same room at the same time of day by the same therapist. This agreement to form a structure for a course of therapy is known as the *therapy contract*. Contact between the therapist and client between sessions or after therapy has ended is generally discouraged in most models, although in some it is encouraged (DBT). A course of psychotherapy may be brief, e.g. eight weeks or so (in the case of CBT) or long term, e.g. three years (in the case of psychoanalysis).

The structure of therapy sets in place some *boundaries*. Boundary setting is an important aspect of therapy. Sometimes the relationship between therapists and patients can become intense. The boundaries can contain anxiety

and give a sense of momentum, purpose and security.

Generally, people regard psychotherapy as being without side-effects and thus compare it with physical treatments in a favourable light. Unfortunately, psychotherapy does have side-effects and these can include dependence on the therapist and upon therapy and in certain cases a fallout of an abusive relationship.

It is difficult to estimate the amount of abuse that goes on, but in therapy where boundaries are not respected abuse is more likely. Some estimates are that sexual abuse occurs in up to 12% of psychotherapy in the United States. In such cases psychotherapy can be seen as having much more severe and long-lasting side-effects that may be much more dangerous than routine side-effects of physical treatments such as drugs.

CASE HISTORY 3

Ms Trentham is a 45-year-old woman who works as a postwoman. She walks many miles a day and was concerned when she developed some panic attacks doing her post round some three years ago. She recalled the first one where she was breathless, her heart beat fast and irregularly and she felt very hot and flushed. Her doctor thought she was very anxious and trembly when he saw her and referred her to the psychiatric nurse. The psychiatric nurse saw her on behalf of the psychiatric team and thought Ms Trentham was anxious as a result of the breakdown of her relationship with her civil partner, Jenny. Ms Trentham was keen not to have any 'tablets' and readily agreed to be referred to the psychotherapy service. After waiting a year for therapy she was seen there every week for two years by a consultant psychologist for 'interpersonal therapy'. The symptoms of anxiety never settled down, though, and her panic attacks became more frequent. This was interpreted by the psychologist as an 'unconscious resistance to therapy'. Her weight loss was interpreted as 'borderline anorexia nervosa'.

A new GP saw her for a cervical smear and was alarmed to see her marked tremor and on examination found a tachycardia. He noted some characteristic eye signs.

What is the likely diagnosis?

The case has key features of hyperthyroidism – tachycardia, anxiety, weight loss, tremor, irregular pulse and some eyes signs, which could be lid retraction, exophthalmos and lid lag. A full physical examination might find others such as brisk reflexes and a goitre. The failure to diagnose hyperthyroidism at an earlier stage in the illness' presentation is inexcusable and the patient could well sue for clinical negligence and blame could be placed at the door of primary and secondary care services.

Although the multidisciplinary team can offer patients some benefits it may also be the case that the patient is not seen by the most relevant or appropriately trained individuals – which may increasingly be the case where managers cynically seek to save costs by using less expensive staff on the frontline of 'specialist' services. Unfortunately, this is a problem not only in psychiatry.

Nevertheless it is only fair to point out that highly trained staff may also miss some diagnoses, although it is difficult to see how less trained staff (and staff not trained in diagnosis) can be expected to make correct diagnoses more often.

This cautionary tale could also be said to illustrate another adverse effect of psychotherapy – wrong diagnosis. Some conclusions of therapists may be incorrect – here for instance that weight loss is anorexia nervosa, or that a failure to respond to therapy is somehow the 'fault' of the patient. Similar problems may occur when patients are seen for 'hysteria' and their physical symptoms are seen as the result of unconscious conflict, when in fact there may be an obscure underlying physical illness.

BEHAVIOUR THERAPY

Behaviour therapy is usually employed when specific goals can be established, e.g. in a phobia of flying where the patient really wants to fly on holiday but cannot face the journey. In such phobias therapists often use *systematic desensitisation* using a *hierarchy* of stimuli. For instance, a person with a phobia of spiders may be presented with a dead spider in a jar at the end of the room (an aversive stimulus). At this stage the person is taught how to relax in the presence of the spider. Having achieved this, the next most severe aversive stimulus in the hierarchy of presented, e.g. a live spider in a jar at the end of the room. Relaxation is repeated at each step and so on until the final step in the hierarchy is presented, for instance handling a spider or – in the case of the flying phobia – taking a plane journey.

More complicated behaviour therapy programmes can be used to reward certain desired behaviours, e.g. hygiene or self-presentation skills in patients with negative symptoms in chronic schizophrenia; or appropriate seeking of help in deliberate self-harm patients and deliberately not rewarding undesirable behaviours, e.g. violence or self-harm.

In obsessive-compulsive disorder systematic desensitisation may be used. For instance, in compulsive hand washing the patient may be encouraged to handle increasingly dirty things and to postpone washing by attempting to relax. The prevention of compulsions is often called *response prevention*. Clinical psychologists are often expert in the construction of behavioural therapy programmes.

COGNITIVE BEHAVIOURAL THERAPY (CBT)

CBT originated (in its 20th-century incarnation) with the work of American psychiatrist Aaron Beck. It is useful for depressive disorders, panic disorder, agoraphobia, generalised anxiety disorder, post-traumatic stress disorder, bulimia, and chronic fatigue. Treatment usually takes between eight and 20 sessions.

The therapist helps the patient break each

problem down into separate parts, often through asking the patient to keep a diary to identify patterns of thoughts, emotions, bodily feelings and actions.

Table 14.1 Examples of cognitive errors

1	Filtering – focusing on the negative aspects of a situation, while filtering out any positive aspects (sometimes called 'selective abstraction').
2	Polarised thinking – thinking of things as very good or very bad with no middle ground (sometimes called 'dichotomous reasoning').
3	Overgeneralisation – making sweeping judgements on the basis of single instances: a single mistake becomes extrapolated to 'I do everything wrong'.
4	Arbitrary inference – jumping to conclusions based on inadequate evidence.
5	Mind reading – feeling you know what people are feeling or thinking about you without objective evidence.
6	Catastrophising – expecting absolute disaster from minimal situations or news.
7	Personalisation – thinking that everything people do or say is some kind of reaction to you.
8	Shoulds – having unchanging rules about how you and other people 'should' act.

The therapy often seeks to correct various cognitive errors that are postulated to lead to depressive states. Automatic negative thoughts are challenged and alternatives encouraged – see below.

The patient is then set 'homework' to practise new tasks and ways of thinking.

CBT is popular and public systems cannot meet the demand with long waiting lists that make the therapy impractical for acute psychiatric conditions where it could be most useful. However, CBT can be delivered by computer. For example 'Beating the Blues'

Table 14.2 Example of a CBT diary entry

Situation:	I was having a bad day at work, felt bullied by my boss, so at lunchtime I went out shopping – retail therapy. As I walked down the street, an old school friend walked by and, just ignored me.	
	Automatic	**Possible helpful alternatives**
Thoughts:	She ignored me – she doesn't like me	She looks a bit preoccupied – maybe she was worried about something herself?
Emotional feelings:	Even more rejected	Worried about my old friend
Physical:	Started to get a headache	No physical discomfort
Action:	Go home, sulk, and make sure I avoid that friend in future	Phone the friend up and check if she's OK

is a programme for people with mild and moderate depression and 'FearFighter' is a programme for people with phobias.

COGNITIVE ANALYTIC THERAPY (CAT)

CAT is a 1:1 psychotherapy originally devised by Anthony Ryle. It was developed nearly 30 years ago from Ryle's work with Student Health patients. It merges analytic theory about transference and relationships with cognitive models.

CAT is most often offered in an outpatient package of 16 sessions and is deemed to be relatively cost effective.

The therapist and client work together to examine the clients' life and problems using questionnaires and diagrams of parental figures, feelings and how they affect feelings and behaviours and 'reformulate' the client's life experiences in a written and diagrammatic form. The reformulation re-tells the patient's history and describes currently damaging procedures within it. Because the reformulation is worked on side by side with the therapist this can be quite a powerful element of the therapy and more likely to be 'owned' by the patient.

This reformulation is then used throughout remaining therapy sessions to develop patient homework about transference-countertransference interactions. The reformulation helps the patient recognise, challenge and revise old patterns that do not work well

The fact that therapy is clearly time-limited means that patients are naturally working towards a conclusion and at the end of therapy both the therapist and client write 'goodbye' letters, reviewing what has been achieved. This is quite a powerful and emotional technique.

DIALECTICAL BEHAVIOUR THERAPY (DBT)

DBT was developed by the psychologist Marsha Linehan (b. 1943) as a psychotherapeutic technique to help people with borderline personality disorder and who deliberately self-harm. It blends cognitive techniques with some Zen philosophy. Linehan starts with the assumption that people with borderline personalities have a defective emotion regulation system. Linehan postulates that such people have deficits in skills needed to regulate emotions and that they can be taught to develop sufficient interpersonal skills, develop emotional and self-regulation capacities and start to tolerate distress better. In individual and group session DBT focuses on 'mindfulness' – developed from Zen tradition, interpersonal effectiveness, distress tolerances and emotional regulation. The process may take some 12 months or so.

FAMILY THERAPY

This may be conducted by a family therapist who may work with the family together in a room separated from one another by a one-way screen. Behind the screen a colleague or supervisor can watch the family and its members' interactions with each other and the interactions with the therapist and feedback to the therapist in the next room via a telephone or an earpiece.

Although psychiatric illness mainly affects an individual within a family, the family is usually affected by the consequences of the illness or may affect the prognosis of the illness by their actions. Hostile, over-involved and critical families may adversely affect the relapse rate of patients with schizophrenia (so-called *high expressed emotion* families). Bulimia nervosa has been associated with families where there is excessive conflict and anorexia nervosa has been linked to rather repressed, controlled families, sometimes with distant or uninvolved fathers. Various mental disorders have also been linked to abusive relationships within families, although evidence for this is often contested.

Family therapy seeks to establish and reflect back the family structure and style of interacting and to change this style if it appears to be a problem. As the family is a system of individuals rather than a single individual with a disorder, it has proved difficult to assess the effectiveness of family therapy but it has been considered successful in a variety of mental disorders.

GROUP THERAPY

In group therapy a group of about six to eight people meet regularly with one or two therapists. Group therapy may involve a variety of therapeutic styles. Some groups may be supportive or educational; others may be interpretive and analytical. Groups may be formed of people with differing disorders, e.g. a day hospital group, or of people with similar problems, e.g. an eating disorder. Patients in such groups often derive a feeling of mutual support and hope. New coping styles may be learnt. From their own self-knowledge patients are particularly able to challenge other group members' defences. For instance, if a member of an alcohol abuse group projects all the blame for his heavy drinking onto his absent wife, a group peer may be more able than a therapist to confront him with the fact that it is he who is drinking too much, not his wife.

LEARNING POINTS: PSYCHOTHERAPY

➢ Defence mechanisms are psychological devices used to prevent or reduce psychological discomfort. They include denial, projection, displacement and repression.

➢ Transference is a mechanism whereby people transfer emotions from one past setting or relationship to another. For instance, we may feel comfortable with a stranger because he or she reminds us of someone we previously knew and liked who was very similar in appearance.

➢ Dreams can be useful tools in psychotherapy. They contain messages from the unconscious mind often in symbolic form. They need to be interpreted with care, though, according to the context and experience of the patient.

➢ Cognitive behavioural therapy focuses on the thoughts associated with various emotions – for instance, depression may be associated with various negative automatic thoughts such as 'I can't cope' or 'I'm useless'. Cognitive therapy seeks to challenge such thoughts and restructure them.

➢ Family therapy is used in a variety of mental disorders and focuses on the impact that they have on the family and the way that families can affect the illness. Family therapy seeks to identify dysfunctional interactions between family members and suggests alternative ways of behaving that may be tried within therapy sessions.

➢ Group therapy occurs in a group of about eight patients together with one or two therapists. Members of the group support, encourage and challenge each other while the experienced therapist shapes the group's progress. Group therapy is useful in restructuring personal relationship behaviours and attitudes and can be used in a variety of disorders such as alcoholism or eating disorders.

SELF-ASSESSMENT
MCQs

1 Appropriate psychotherapies for people with learning disability include:
   A group therapy
   B family therapy
   C psychoanalysis
   D behaviour therapy
   E cognitive therapy

2 Classical ingredients of cognitive therapy include:
   A focusing on the transference
   B dream analysis
   C exposing psychological defence mechanisms
   D challenging erroneous ways of thinking
   E use of a diary

3 Behaviour therapy
   A is not of use in obsessive-compulsive disorder
   B is used almost exclusively by approved social workers
   C may involve systematic desensitisation
   D may involve relaxation training
   E focuses on thoughts

SHORT ANSWER QUESTIONS

For the following vignettes think what you would say next to the patients during a long interview.

1 (A 47-year-old man with alcohol dependency) 'I went on a binge last weekend. I couldn't stop myself. I went in to celebrate a win on the horses and I just had one after the other and before I knew it I was down again. Thinking about what I was going to do in the future. Thinking about how it's all my wife's fault. If she hadn't insisted that we move here I wouldn't have started work at Taylors and I wouldn't have been made redundant. And then I wouldn't have an alcohol problem . . .'

2 (A 20-year-old woman who presents with anxiety attacks) 'I never told anybody this

[pause] . . . I am so ashamed about it . . . I . . . promise me that you'll never tell anybody . . . Please?'

3 (A 40-year-old woman recalling her father who died during her childhood) 'So I never really knew him when I grew up . . . he was just this smiling face when I was little . . . ice creams and trips out. I remember him rowing me down the river on a boat . . . [tears begin to form in her eyes] . . . and . . . [she pauses and cannot continue speaking].'

MCQ answers
1 A=T, B=T, C=F, D=T, E=T.
2 A=F, B=F, C=F, D=T, E=T.
3 A=F, B=F, C=T, D=T, E=F.

EXPLORATIONS

Sources listed in the resources and further reading sections will help you with the following.

LINKS WITH PUBLIC HEALTH

Local health purchasers are keen to set up a variety of therapies for primary care including a psychotherapy and counselling service. They have only a limited budget for mental health. Investing in psychotherapy and counselling would mean that some resources will have to be diverted from elsewhere. Imagine you are an adviser to the purchasers.

➤ What evidence is there that psychotherapy is an effective treatment for a mental disorder like depression?

➤ Is any therapy particularly useful?

➤ Which therapy style might be the most cost effective?

➤ How might this therapy be implemented in the local community so that as many people as possible can benefit from the investment of the purchasers?

LINKS WITH MEDICINE

➤ How many cases referred to general medical clinics have a strong psychological component?

➤ What is somatisation?

➤ How can psychotherapy or counselling

skills help doctors manage these patients sympathetically and effectively?

➤ What percentage of people on general medical wards have depressive symptoms?

➤ How might these symptoms be detected and treated?

➤ What contribution to recovery might psychotherapy or counselling make?

FURTHER READING AND REFERENCES
TEXTS

Alexander F, French T. *Psychoanalytic Therapy: principles and applications.* New York: Ronald Press; 1946.

Balint M. *The Doctor, His Patient and the Illness.* 2nd ed. Edinburgh: Churchill Livingstone; 2000.

Beck AT. *Cognitive Therapy of Depression.* New York: Guilford; 1979.

Bennet E, Storr A. *What Jung Really Said.* London: Abacus; 2000.

Bergin AE, Garfield SL. *Handbook of Psychotherapy and Behaviour Change.* 4th ed. London: Wiley; 2003.

Bowlby J. *Attachment and Loss: Vol. 1 Attachment.* London: Pimlico; 1997.

Bowlby J. *Attachment and Loss: Vol. 2 Separation – Anxiety and Anger.* London: Pimlico; 1998.

Dallos R, Draper R. *An Introduction to Family Therapy: systemic theory and practice.* Maidenhead: Open University Press; 2005.

Green BH. Creating rapport. In: Green BH, editor. *Psychiatry in General Practice.* London: Kluwer Academic Publishers; 1995.

Haley J. *Uncommon Therapy.* New York: WW Norton; 1993.

Hawthorne K, Salkovskis P, Kirk J, Clark DM. *Cognitive Behavioural Therapy for Psychiatric Problems: a practical guide.* Oxford: Oxford Medical Publications; 1989.

Hobson RF. *Forms of Feeling: the heart of psychotherapy.* London: Tavistock; 1985.

Peck MS. *The Road Less Travelled.* New York: Simon and Schuster; 1990.

Ryle A, Kerr I. *Introducing Cognitive Analytic Therapy: principles and practice.* Chichester: Wiley; 2002.

Stafford-Clark D. *What Freud Really Said.* Harmondsworth: Penguin Books; 1967.

Storr A. *Art of Psychotherapy.* London: Routledge; 1999.

Yalom I, Lezszcz M. *Theory and Practice of Group Psychotherapy*. 5th ed. New York: Basic Books; 2005.

PAPERS

Green B. Pain and Somatisation. A Lecture given at the Royal College of Physicians, 1 February 2007. www.priory.com/psych/pain.htm

Sarkar SP. Boundary violation and sexual exploitation in psychiatry and psychotherapy: a review. *Advances in Psychiatric Treatment*. 2004; **10**: 312–20.

Slater E. Diagnosis of hysteria. *BMJ*. 1963; **1**: 1395–9.

Slater E, Glithero E. Follow up of patients diagnosed as suffering from 'hysteria'. *J Psychosom Res*. 1965; **9**: 9–13.

RESOURCES

Association for Cognitive Analytic Therapy
PO Box 6793, Dorchester DT1 9DL
www.acat.me.uk/

Beating the Blues
www.ultrasis.com/products/product.jsp?product_id=1

British Association for Behavioural and Cognitive Psychotherapies (BABCP)
Victoria Buildings, 9–13 Silver Street,
Bury BL9 0EU
www.babcp.com/

British Psychological Society
www.bps.org.uk/

Computerised CBT
www.nice.org.uk/TA97

Dialectical Behaviour Therapy (DBT) for Borderline Personality Disorder by Marsha Linehan
www.portlanddbt.com/pages/linehan.html

Institute of Psychoanalysis
www.psychoanalysis.org.uk/

Overview of Dialectical Behaviour Therapy in the Treatment of Borderline Personality Disorder by Barry Kiehn and Michaela Swales
www.priory.com/dbt.htm

Society of Analytical Psychology
http://jungian-analysis.org/

CHAPTER 15

Mental retardation

Mental retardation involves an impairment of intellect and learning ability of congenital origin. Causes may be genetic or environmental and have major implications for preventive medical practice and the ethical behaviour of health professionals. The relevance to psychiatry is the demonstration of how brain function can be affected by various congenital factors, how these may make psychiatric illness more likely, e.g. through epilepsy, and the impact on family function.

The term 'learning disability' is sometimes substituted for mental retardation, but the ICD-10 and DSM-IV classification systems use the term 'mental retardation'. Patients with learning disability have historically been described using various terms over the years, such as idiot or imbecile, many of which have fallen into general misuse and understandably have been discarded.

CONTENTS

EPIDEMIOLOGY

About 2% of the UK population have a learning disability. Sixty per cent of people with a learning disability live at home. They have higher rates of physical and mental illness and particularly have higher rates of epilepsy. Most adults with learning disability are not known to learning disability services. Of those known to learning disability services only a third live in special accommodation. Seventeen per cent have paid work.

Table 15.1 Epidemiology of mental retardation

Condition	Incidence
Foetal alcohol syndrome	1–7/1000 live births
Down's syndrome	1/1000 live births in mothers <20
	1/30 live births in mothers >45
Fragile-X syndrome	1/1000 men
Klinefelter's syndrome	1/1400 live births
XXX syndrome	1/1600 live births
Turner's syndrome	1/3300 live births
Edward's syndrome	1/3500 live births
Patau's syndrome	1/7600 live births
Phenylketonuria	1/14 000 live births
Tuberose sclerosis	1/20 000 live births

CAUSES

General intelligence, as measured by such things as IQ tests, is normally distributed in the population, and as a continuum may be assumed to have a polygenic inheritance. However, environmental and genetic factors may act to reduce intelligence to abnormally low levels. Other factors may impair specific skills like reading or language development.

GENETIC CAUSES

The classical chromosomal cause of mental retardation is Down's syndrome, first described by Dr Langdon Down's in 1866. The syndrome is usually caused by trisomy 21, but rarely may be due to a translocation (parts of damaged chromosomes are rejoined in an abnormal way). Table 15.2 shows the clinical features of Down's syndrome. Other autosomal causes include trisomy 13 (Patau's syndrome), trisomy 18 (Edward's syndrome), and deletion of part of chromosome 5 as in the cri-du-chat syndrome. Sex chromosome abnormalities are also associated with retardation. Fragile-X syndrome, Klinefelter's (XXY), Turner's (XO), the XYY and the XXX syndrome are examples. Fragile-X syndrome is the second commonest known cause of mental retardation in males (1/4000). Table 15.3 shows the clinical features of Fragile-X. Fragile-X carrying women may have some symptoms – reduced intellectual ability, poor muscle tone, prominent ears and long faces. Single genes are causes of such conditions as tuberose sclerosis (autosomal dominant inheritance). In tuberose sclerosis tumours in the brain may cause epilepsy and

Table 15.2 Clinical features of Down's syndrome

Oblique eye folds
Small, flattened skull
Large tongue
Broad hands with stumpy fingers
Single transverse palm crease
High cheek bones
Small height
Squint
Brushfield's spots on the iris
Abnormal finger prints
Crypto-orchidism
Straight pubic hair
Congenital cardiac defects
Early dementia
Hypothyroidism

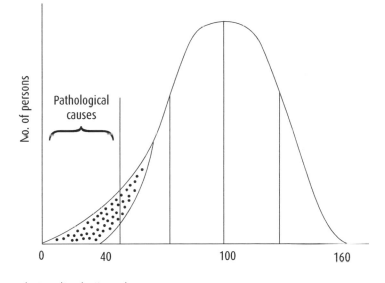

Figure 15.1 Population distribution of IQ

cognitive impairment. Other autosomal dominant causes include Sturge-Weber syndrome (angiomatous malformation within the skull) and neurofibromatosis where intracranial neuromas may occur. There are numerous autosomal recessive conditions such as phenylketonuria, galactosaemia, Hurler's disease and Niemann-Pick disease.

OTHER CAUSES

The causes of some conditions are as yet unknown. Intrauterine infection with syphilis, rubella, toxoplasmosis, influenza and cytomegalovirus can cause retardation. HIV infection acquired perinatally may present with a dementing-like illness in the early years of life. In this the fruits of early developmental milestones may be lost, or never gained at all. Other causes include kernicterus, obstetric instrumental brain damage, perinatal hypoxia, and hydrocephalus.

The specific causes of retardation are numerous and well studied. Nevertheless, the majority of people with retardation cannot be given a specific cause for their condition. Why do you think this is?

Table 15.1 shows some how common various causes of retardation are in the population.

Table 15.3 Clinical features of fragile-X syndrome

Large, floppy ears
Protruding jaw
Macro-orchidism
Elongated face
Hypotonia
Autism
Gynaecomastia
High-arched palate
(Female carriers may have variable mild presentations of the syndrome)

Among patients with IQs less than 50 about a third have Down's syndrome. About 10–20% of retarded males have fragile-X syndrome.

FOETAL ALCOHOL SYNDROME (FAS)

Foetal alcohol syndrome probably affects some 7/1000 live births. This is comparable to rates of Down's syndrome and spina bifida. About 60 per cent of women drink alcohol during pregnancy. As alcohol consumption per capita rises then inevitably there will be a growing number of babies born with FAS. The classic presentation in childhood involves altered facial characteristics, but not all children with FAS have these, and other behavioural changes can be more subtle. Many cases are missed. The more subtle presentations can be a foetal alcohol spectrum disorder (FASD).

BOX 15.1 CLINICAL FEATURES OF FAS

> Small birth weight
> Reduced head circumference
> Small eye openings
> Smooth, wide philtrum
> Thin upper lip
> Delayed milestones
> Heart defects
> Irritability
> Muscle tone abnormalities
> Anomalies of ears, eyes, liver, or joints

The relationship between late presentation of FASD through behavioural problems and maternal alcohol consumption may never be appreciated or only be appreciated much later on and probably only as a result of careful history taking and clinical suspicion.

FAS is associated with microcephaly and structural abnormalities on brain imaging including increased grey matter density, frontal lobe and basal ganglia problems, displacements in the corpus callosum and abnormalities in the hippocampus.

Most children with FASD have an IQ in the normal or above normal range – only 15% have an IQ less than 70.

Neurobehavioural problems associated with FASD include:
> attention deficits
> memory deficits
> hyperactivity
> difficulty with abstract concepts
> inability to manage money
> poor problem solving skills
> difficulty learning from consequences
> immature social behaviour
> inappropriate friendliness to strangers
> lack of control over emotions
> poor impulse control
> poor judgement.

AUTISM

Autism has been linked to fragile-X syndrome, but this can account for only a small percentage of boys with the condition. Early childhood autism is characterised by autistic aloneness, failure to make relationships, difficulties perceiving certain sounds and images, overactivity or hyperkinesis in childhood and hypoactivity in adolescence, an 'obsessive desire for the maintenance of sameness', ritualistic behaviour, echolalia, pronoun reversal (e.g. using 'you' in sentences instead of using 'I').

An autistic spectrum disorder is a complex lifelong developmental disability that affects the way a person communicates and relates to people around him or her. The autistic triad combines impairment of social interaction, impairment of social communication and impairment of social imagination.

Impaired imagination may lead to concentration of repeated stereotyped activities such as watching things that spin, or feeling special textures, or rocking, or flicking the fingers. More complex activities may involve intense preoccupation with objects or rituals, or fascination with obscure topics.

The autistic spectrum includes the syndromes described by Leo Kanner (1943) and by Asperger (1944).

Eighty per cent of individuals with autism have a significant intellectual disability and also autistic 'traits' are very common among people with intellectual disability.

An autistic spectrum disorder is a lifelong disability and children with the disorder grow up into adults with the disorder. Appropriate interventions early in life and specialised education and support can help a child optimise his or her skills and achieve higher potential as an adult.

Table 15.4 Levels of mental retardation and IQ

Level of mental retardation	IQ	Percentage of learning disabled population
Mild	50–70	80%
Moderate	35–49	12%
Severe	20–34	7%
Profound	Below 20	1%

PSYCHIATRY AND MENTAL RETARDATION

The organic brain abnormalities that underlie mental retardation also predispose to epilepsy and to psychiatric illness. Whereas epilepsy only affects less than 1% of all children, children with IQs of less than 50 are 40 times as likely to suffer from fits. About 10% of

mentally retarded adults have had a fit in the previous year. Rates of psychiatric illness are also higher in the retarded compared with the general population. Maybe as many as 30% of mentally retarded adults have a mental disorder. Alcoholism and drug abuse are very rare.

Failing to make the correct diagnosis of a mental illness and attributing abnormal speech and behaviour to the mental retardation itself may lead to a person not receiving the necessary and correct treatment for his or her illness. Drug treatment in this population is just as useful as in any other. The presentation of the illness may be modified by the degree of mental impairment, however. Affective disorders may present in terms of increased or reduced motor activity, rather than specific complaints of sadness or elation. Altered eating and sleeping patterns, sexual indiscretions, mood lability, self-harm and attacks on others may all be signs. Schizophrenia may present with bizarre behaviour, poverty of thought, thought blocking, mannerisms and preoccupation with internal fantasy (although care is needed to distinguish this from normal fantasy). Various organic processes can overlie the original mental retardation. Cognitive decline in a Down's person must raise the suspicion of a superimposed dementia. Epilepsy (or antiepileptics!) may cause confusional states. Self-harm may be a manifestation of out-of-control phenylketonuria.

TREATMENT OPTIONS

Most people with mental retardation live at home. The family is their main support. Community resources, including highly trained teachers in regular schools, special schools, community adult training day centres, community nurses, specialist social workers and occupational therapists, may help support the family in their caring task. Because retarded people are significantly more vulnerable to psychiatric disorder than non-retarded people, access to psychiatric treatment is of a high importance. Family doctors have a key role in coordinating medical care for this group of people. Conventional antidepressants and antipsychotics may lead to significant improvement in mood and behaviour in psychiatrically ill retarded people. Relatively selective serotonergic antidepressants (such as fluoxetine and clomipramine) have proved particularly useful in the treatment of compulsive and stereotyped behaviour in autistic patients. Difficult behaviours, such as aggression, may respond to psychological interventions designed to find out triggers for such behaviour. Drug treatments with antipsychotics, antidepressants, and mood stabilisers such as sodium valproate and lithium may be useful if coexisting psychiatric disorder is present. Aggression, particularly episodic aggression, may be a feature of epileptic activity and may require antiepileptic medication. Paradoxically, hyperactivity disorders in retarded children may respond to stimulants such as methylphenidate.

CASE HISTORY 1

John was taken to his family doctor by his mother when he was aged 19. His mother had become concerned about him because for the past two months he had refused to leave the house and had started hoarding old newspapers and magazines. He kept these in strict date sequence on top of and behind cupboards, radiators and wardrobes. He had also taken to giggling inappropriately and making faces at thin air. He had attended a comprehensive school and been in a class of 35. He left school at the age of six but he had never learned to read or write properly and he could only do simple mental arithmetic. He enjoyed watching cartoons or motoring programmes on television. He had an amazing ability to recall details of vehicles and enjoyed talking about them at length, although other people found his conversation repetitive and dull. He had no friends and only a few acquaintances. He had never been able to find a job, although he dreamt of being a racing driver.

In what way is John different from most people?

John differs in two ways: he has a persistently low level of intelligence and recently has developed signs of mental illness. The details of his case are incomplete, but they do point towards various difficulties: coping with schoolwork, socialising with peers and restricted areas of interest. These would be consistent with mild mental retardation, although the history above gives no hint as to the aetiology of this. (It is possible for mildly retarded people to make their way through regular school, although they perhaps do not progress to such levels as their peers and may find difficulties in gaining employment in a very competitive and technologically orientated job market. In school it is important to recognise learning difficulties so that teaching strategies can be adjusted to maximise the individual's potential. It is important to distinguish between specific learning difficulties, e.g. numerical skills, and more global cognitive disabilities.) Against this background of mild mental retardation, John is exhibiting some signs of mental disorder such as social withdrawal, compulsive hoarding and possible hallucinations which might make a doctor consider whether John was developing schizophrenia or had an affective disorder. Certainly a referral would be appropriate to either an adult psychiatrist or a psychiatrist specialising in learning disability.

CASE HISTORY 2

Anne was brought to her family doctor by her foster mother and her social worker who had been increasingly concerned about her for some weeks. Anne was now aged four. She had begun to walk and talk at the appropriate ages. Six months ago she had even begun to read simple texts. Now, however, she had stopped speaking in sentences and seemed to have difficulty comprehending speech. Her foster mother found it increasingly difficult to get Anne to concentrate on anything for more than a few minutes, whereas previously her concentration had been very good. The doctor watched Anne playing with the toys in her surgery and noticed that Anne was really quite clumsy. This too was something new.

What is the main problem described here?

Anne is a four-year-old girl who was making good progress developmentally. In recent months this progress has not only been halted but has actually reversed.

How does this differ from conventional mental retardation?

Conventionally, in mental retardation certain skills and abilities are either never acquired or acquired with great difficulty. Anne's problem almost reverses this situation. Here skills once acquired are being lost, as in a dementia.

What could be causing Anne's cognitive decline?

Normal development sometimes ebbs and flows. There may be a plateau in the development of new skills or the child may even revert or regress to more childish ways when stressed or physically unwell. In Anne's case, though, the reversal is alarming. Good receptive and expressive language skills seem to have disappeared, and the conjunction with motor signs such as clumsiness suggests a process affecting the CNS in some way.

The doctor enquired about Anne's family history from the social worker and learnt that Anne's father was unknown. Her mother, though, was known to social services as an intravenous drug addict who had shared needles with others. On the basis of this information the doctor formed a hypothesis as to what was wrong with Anne. What hypothesis do you think this was and how would you investigate this hypothesis?

CASE HISTORY 3

A 16-year-old girl was referred to a psychiatrist after her parents became concerned at her repeated attempts to meet much older men off the Internet. Her parents confiscated her mobile phone and were horrified to learn she had run up a bill of hundreds of pounds. After she had been counselled once as to the extreme danger of the practice, she did not appear to learn from her mistake and kept giving out the home phone number to men she met online and arranging meetings. At first the interviewing psychiatrist could find no psychiatric cause to this behaviour, which initially looked like inappropriate risk taking in a naive adolescent. However, a detailed history included a family history of maternal early death at the age of 36 through alcoholic liver disease and catastrophic haemorrhaging. Corroborative history obtained from her father confirmed that his ex-wife had drunk very heavily through pregnancy. He also revealed that his daughter had limited language skills and although she could read short segments of text, she could not read a book or follow the plot of a film. Mental State Examination demonstrated she had difficulty explaining simple proverbs.

What features of FASD are present in the assessment?

At first glance the initial referral letter regarding risky behaviour did not immediately suggest any mental disorder, but in context the inappropriate relationship seeking could be construed as being inappropriately friendly with strangers and the failure to curtail such behaviour after counselling could be seen as difficulty learning from consequences associated with poor judgement. The history of maternal alcohol abuse is marked and there are also hints of difficulty in processing abstract concepts, e.g. in interpreting proverbs and following the plot of a film or book.

Table 15.5 Causes of dementia in childhood

HIV encephalopathy (commonest worldwide cause of childhood dementia)
Wilson's disease (autosomal recessive inheritance, associated with abnormal movements, potentially reversible)
Huntington's chorea (autosomal dominant inheritance, abnormalities of chromosome 4, predictive testing available)
Leucodystrophies
Subacute sclerosing panencephalitis (late complication of measles, more common in boys, typical EEG changes)
Rett's syndrome
Pervasive developmental disorders

LEARNING POINTS: MENTAL RETARDATION

➤ General intelligence, as measured by IQ tests, is roughly normally distributed in the population.

➤ One of the most common identified causes of retardation is Down's syndrome – about a third of moderately retarded people have it.

➤ About 10–20% of retarded males have fragile-X syndrome.

➤ About 30% of mentally retarded adults have a mental disorder.

➤ About 30% of mentally retarded adults have epilepsy.

SELF-ASSESSMENT
MCQs
1 Causes of mental retardation that affect more than 1/10 000 live male births include:
   A Down's syndrome
   B Huntington's chorea
   C fragile-X syndrome
   D enteroviruses
   E Wilson's disease

2 Compared with people with an IQ of 100 or more, people with learning disability:
   A have an equal chance of developing mental illness
   B are several times more likely to have epilepsy
   C when mentally ill require smaller doses of psychotropic medication
   D are more likely to be infertile
   E are significantly more likely to be violent

3 Active prevention of mental retardation in first pregnancies is currently possible for:
   A phenylketonuria
   B cytomegalovirus
   C toxoplasmosis
   D Hurler's syndrome
   E trisomy 18

4 In Down's syndrome:
   A the 'severity' of facial stigmata predicts poor intelligence and reduced self-sufficiency later in life
   B epileptic phenomena are exceedingly rare
   C the majority of births occur in mothers aged 30–39
   D receptive language ability declines with age

5 Learning disability:
   A is present in about 3% of the population
   B caused by trisomy 18 is known as 'cri-du-chat'
   C due to phenylketonuria is caused by a deficiency of phenylalanine
   D is associated with an increased tendency to epileptic fits
   E in a person means that psychotherapy cannot be offered as a treatment option

SHORT ANSWER QUESTIONS
1 List *five* causes of foetal malformations (other than alcohol or prescribed drugs).
2 List clinical features of foetal alcohol syndrome.

3 List *three* different mechanisms by which genetic abnormalities are transmitted and types of mental retardation associated with these.

MCQ answers

1 A=T, B=F, C=T, D=F, E=F.
2 A=F, B=T, C=F, D=T, E=F.
3 A=T, B=F, C=T, D=F, E=F
4 A=F, B=F, C=F, D=T.
5 A=T, B=F, C=F, D=T, E=F.

Short answer questions answers

1 Ionising radiation; maternal disease, e.g. diabetes mellitus; maternal infection e.g. rubella; pollution e.g. dioxins; genetic, and dietary deficiencies or excesses, among some others.

2 Intrauterine growth retardation, failure to thrive, short stature, mild to moderate mental retardation, microcephaly, thin upper lip, small eyes, maxillary hypoplasia, hyperactivity and some others.

3 Dominant gene, e.g. tuberose sclerosis. Deleted autosome, e.g. 'cri-du-chat'. Trisomy, e.g. Edward's syndrome. Others include: recessive gene, extra autosome, extra sex chromosome, deleted sex chromosome and sex linked recessive gene.

EXPLORATIONS

Sources listed in the further reading and references section will help you with the following.

LINKS WITH OBSTETRICS

➤ What routine aspects of antenatal care are designed to prevent mental retardation?
➤ What aspects of perinatal and post-natal care are designed to prevent mental retardation?

LINKS WITH PAEDIATRICS/MEDICINE

➤ Besides the CNS, what other organ systems can be affected in Down's syndrome?
➤ How can this be treated?
➤ What are the main causes of mortality in Down's syndrome?

LINKS WITH RESEARCH

➤ What other conditions in psychiatry might feasibly be related to parental alcohol abuse or substance abuse?
➤ How could research be designed to reliably investigate any hypothesis you generate?

MEDICO-LEGAL LINKS

➤ What is 'mental capacity'?
➤ How does the Mental Capacity Act (2005) affect people with learning disability?
➤ How can mental capacity be assessed?
➤ What is the purpose of the associated Code of Practice?

LINK WITH PSYCHOLOGY/SOCIOLOGY

➤ How do parents react to their own mentally retarded offspring, (a) before, (b) just after, and (c) years after the diagnosis is confirmed?
➤ How does the arrival of a mentally retarded child affect its siblings?

FURTHER READING AND REFERENCES

Asperger H. Autistic pyschopathy in childhood. Reprinted in Frith U. *Autism and Asperger Syndrome.* Cambridge: Cambridge University Press; 1991. pp. 37–92.

Berney TP. Autism – an evolving concept. *British Journal of Psychiatry.* 2000; **176**: 20–6.

Collacott RA, Cooper SA, McGrother C. Differential rates of psychiatric disorders in adults with Down's syndrome compared with other mentally handicapped adults. *Br J Psychology.* 1992; **161**: 671–4.

Dupont A, Voeth M, Videbech P. Mortality and life expectancy of Down's syndrome in Denmark. *Journal of Mental Deficiency Research.* 1968; **30**: 111–20.

Gath A. The school-age siblings of Mongol children. *British Journal of Psychiatry.* 1973; **123**: 161–7.

Gath A. The impact of an abnormal child upon the parents. *British Journal of Psychiatry.* 1977; **130**: 405–10.

Hall SM. Congenital toxoplasmosis. *BMJ.* 1992; **305**: 291–7.

Huang T, Watt HC, Wald NJ, *et al.* Birth prevalence of Down's's syndrome in England and Wales

1990 to 1997. *Journal of Medical Screening.* 1998; **5**: 213–14.

Kanner L. Autistic disturbances of affective contact. *Nervous Child.* 1943; **2**: 217–50

Kanner L, Eisenberg L. Notes on the follow-up studies of autistic children. In: Koch PH, Zubin J, editors. *Psychopathology of Childhood.* New York: Grune & Stratton; 1955.

Langdon Down J. Observations on an ethnic classification of idiots. *Clinical lectures and reports of the London Hospital.* 1866; **3**: 259–62.

Multidisciplinary Working Group. *Pre-natal Screening for Toxoplasmosis in the UK.* London: Royal College of Obstetricians and Gynaecologists; 1992.

Murdoch JC. Congenital heart disease as a significant factor in the morbidity of children with Down's syndrome. *Journal of Mental Deficiency Research.* 1985; **29**: 147–51.

Niccols A. Fetal alcohol syndrome and the developing socio-emotional brain. *Brain and Cognition.* 2007; **65**(1): 13–42.

Patau K, *et al.* Multiple congenital anomaly caused by an extra autosome. *Lancet.* 1960; **1**: 790–3.

Reid AS. *The Psychiatry of Mental Handicap.* London: Blackwell Scientific Publications; 1982.

Thompson C, Westwell P, Viney D. Psychiatric aspects of human immunodeficiency virus in childhood and adolescence. In: Rutter ML, Taylor E, Hersov L, editors. *Child and Adolescent Psychiatry.* Oxford: Blackwell Scientific Publications; 1994. 711–19.

Turk J. The fragile-X syndrome: on the way to a behavioural phenotype. *British Journal of Psychiatry.* 1992; **160**: 24–35.

Vernon PE. *Intelligence and Attainment Tests.* London: University of London Press; 1960.

Wing JK. *Early Childhood Autism.* London: Pergamon Press; 1966.

Wing L. Classification and diagnosis – looking at the complexities involved. *Communication.* 1998; **Winter**: 15–18.

WEB SOURCES

Epilepsy in Learning Disability: www.epilepsy.org.uk/info/learning.html

Symptoms of Foetal Alcohol Spectrum Disorders: www.come-over.to/FAS/faschar.htm

FASAware UK: www.fasaware.co.uk/

Statistics on Learning Disability: www.learningdisabilities.org.uk/information/learning-disabilities-statistics/

Learning about Intellectual Disabilities and Health: www.intellectualdisability.info/home.htm

Mental Capacity Act: www.publicguardian.gov.uk/mca/mca.htm

Fragile-X Research Organisation: www.fraxa.org

RESOURCES

British Epilepsy Association
New Anstey House, Gate Way Drive, Yeadon
Leeds LS19 7XY
Tel: 0808 800 5050
Email: helpline@epilepsy.org.uk
www.epilepsy.org.uk/

Down's Syndrome Association
Langdon Down's Centre, 2a Langdon Park,
Teddington TW11 9PS
Tel: 0845 230 0372
Email: info@Down'ss-syndrome.org.uk
www.Down'ss-syndrome.org.uk/

National Autistic Society
393 City Road, London, EC1V 1NG
Tel: 020 7833 2299
Email: nas@nas.org.uk
www.nas.org.uk/

Foundation for People with Learning Disabilities
9th Floor, Sea Containers House, 20 Upper Ground, London SE1 9QB
Tel: 020 7803 1100
www.learningdisabilities.org.uk/welcome

CHAPTER 16

The history of psychiatry

The history of psychiatry is surprisingly lengthy and this reflects the long time that humankind has suffered with symptoms of mental illness.

CONTENTS

INTRODUCTION

The position of psychiatry as a medical discipline has been largely affected by tensions between various beliefs about mental illness held by the prevailing culture.

1 Madness could be perceived as an internal bodily illness or it could be projected externally on supernatural causes. In the past people with mental illness have been seen as prophets, shamans, to suffer from a 'sacred disease' or to be witches. The attribution of mental illness to a medical model has been relatively recent and could be seen by some to be jeopardised by the introduction of community mental health teams rather than hospital-based care.

2 A second tension is the contribution of personality to the illness. At one extreme of the spectrum the personality could be seen as affected by illness, at the other end of the spectrum the illness itself can be seen as a manifestation of personal sin or even a degenerative family process.

3 A third tension is the culture and whether it thinks scientifically, i.e. whether society as a whole regards things in a rational light and takes a logical view of cause and effect. The views of people of learning in the Enlightenment, for instance, could be contrasted with the lack of logical thinking by people in the Dark Ages with their emphasis on magical constructs.

4 The final tension on the position of psychiatry in society is a conflict between a community model of looking at mental health and an idea of containment. Should patients be special people with special staff treating them in a special place outside society? In this model doctors and nurses dealing with the mentally ill are very much 'alienists' possibly seen as protecting society. The alternative could be a community model where people with psychological problems are seen as members of a community and that all members of society have an active input into their welfare and well-being.

The current model could be expressed as seeing insanity as an illness rather than resulting from a supernatural cause; that personality factors have a place in the form of mental illness and how patients can be engaged in therapy but that they are not personally totally responsible for their illness. Society adopts a logical approach to mental illness rather than approaching it from the point of view of magical thinking. At present our society has moved away from a hospital model towards a community care model and there is a demedicalisation of mental illness. Whether this matters will be considered further in this chapter by referring to historical eras where madness was not seen as a medical entity.

MENTAL ILLNESS IN ANCIENT TIMES

The early great cultures of Egypt and Mesopotamia viewed mental illness very differently from how we view it today, often ascribing a supernatural rather than a natural aetiology. The patients with mental illness were then sometimes seen as oracles or as divine conduits from the gods, rather similar to the position of a shaman in North American Indian tribes.

The views of Greek physicians progressed beyond external projection. Hippocrates himself certainly recognised the simple phobia as an example of mental illness and had experience in treating depression. With regard to epilepsy, Hippocrates (460–377 BC) wrote, 'The position regarding the so-called sacred disease is as follows: It seems to be no more divine and no more sacred than other diseases, but like other affections it springs from natural causes . . . those who first connected this illness with demons and described it as sacred seem to be no more different from the conjurers, purificators, mountebanks and charlatans of our day, who pretend to great piety and superior knowledge. But such person are merely concealing . . . their perplexity and inability to afford any assistance.'

Galen (AD 129–216), a Greek physician who treated five Roman Emperors, wrote about melancholia, which he said was due to a localisation of vapours or humours in the brain, blood or gut.

Soranus of Ephesus (AD 100) described a condition called 'phrenitis' in which thinking was predominantly affected. He distinguished it from mania and melancholia. Other features of phrenitis that he described, beyond affected thinking, were acute fever, foolish gesticulations and a small, full pulse. It may be that he was perhaps describing an acute confusional state or condition similar to lethal catatonia. Soranus was also interesting in terms of his philosophy in that he thought that the process of thinking was localised to the head where others favoured the heart. He also described delusions in mania, that people saw themselves as perhaps sparrows, cockerels, gods, orators, actors or the centre of the universe. He also wrote about a form of cognitive therapy and with manic patients he would adopt a 'serious demeanour' and with depressives he would adopt a 'cheerful demeanour' to try to alter their mood. He would also try to 'strengthen their reasoning powers by asking them questions or getting them to read and criticise text which contained false statements'.

The concept of hysteria was recognised by the Greek physician Aretaeus of Cappadocia, who ascribed hysteria to a wandering uterus but recognised that the same clinical picture could occur in men, which perhaps defies logical thinking. As regards his philosophy of mental illness, Aretaeus stressed the frequency of relapses that he saw in cases of mental illness, the incurability of mental illness and also asserted the right of the physician not to treat incurables.

Some Roman archives suggest that the mentally ill were essentially warehoused in prisons but that they were able to receive medical care. The use of chains is documented in Roman literature. A pious Roman lady, Fabiola, went so far as to found a dedicated institution for the care of the mentally ill in the 4th century AD. The Emperor Constantine, a Christian, started many hospitals but no specific mental asylums.

The 4th century also saw the first record of a specific house for lunatics in Byzantium and another in Jerusalem in AD 491.

AD 560 TO THE MIDDLE AGES

Some monasteries specialised in the care of the mentally ill, e.g. in Cologne in AD 560. There are records of Islamic asylums from the 7th century, for instance at Fez, and an early Caliph founded an asylum in Cairo where the inmates were daily entertained by music. There are some records of private charitable asylums in England in AD 700 but by and large care of the mentally ill and their cure was ignored and relegated to a supernatural realm.

There are progressively more records of establishments as time goes on and one notable one is of an asylum in Baghdad called the House of Grace in 1173 where the insane were brought from all over Persia to receive medical care. Patients were essentially detained until they were well but it is of note that every month the asylum was visited by a magistrate who examined the patients and discharged those who had recovered. There was also a community care system in that patients who had returned home received medical attention for a few months in order to prevent relapse. There is also a reference to music and storytelling as therapies.

In England in 1369 a hospital was founded by Robert Denton, Chaplain, for poor patients and other men and women that were 'sick of the phrenzie to remain there until whole or restored to good memorie'.

In 1377 the Bethlem Hospital (Bedlam) started to receive lunatics – it had been founded earlier in 1247, but had a general medical remit. The therapeutic armamentarium of the Bethlem Hospital at that stage included the manacles, stocks and padded rooms.

A Royal Commission looked into the running of the hospital in 1403 and criticised the Janitor, Peter Tavener, for purloining the patients' goods and for running a bawdy house at the gate of the hospital where his wife sold beer. The Commission further commented that the nuns who ran the hospital were 'looking through the windows a little too earnestly at the world' and that the prioress was commanded to 'sleep in her own bedroom'.

Elsewhere in Europe there were other asylums such as one in Spain in 1409 which was established 'because the maniacs were hooted by the crowds and otherwise persecuted by the people'. At Granada in the 15th century the Hospital De Los Locos was completed under the command of Charles VI. This specifically admitted the insane, but specifically excluded cases of senile dementia.

MIDDLE AGES AND THE RENAISSANCE

Medieval medicine saw a fragmentation into various specialities. Barber surgeons and their assistants looked after surgical cases, childbirth was looked after by midwives and the mentally ill were looked after by exorcising priests, the church and, most unfortunately, witch finders. The Middle Ages period was also infamous for the resurgence of the idea that mentally ill were possessed; that their hallucinations were apparitions and the work of the devils. There are numerous accounts of patients who were hallucinating being put to death as they were consorting with the devil. In 1486 a handbook for witch hunters called the *Malleus Maleficarum* was put together by the Dominicans Kraemer and Sprenger, who were also Inquisitors. This book includes quite clear descriptions of psychopathology which were misconstrued by society and used as a basis for executions and the stake in a period running from the 15th to 17th centuries. In one paragraph the monks Kraemer and Sprenger brush aside the whole mass of such psychiatric knowledge as had been collected and preserved over the previous thousand years or so by medical investigation and say, 'The devil has extraordinary powers over the minds of those who have given themselves up to him so what they do in imagination is they believe they have actually and really done it in the body.' Even illusions acknowledged as such do not excuse

a woman from the crime of being a witch. Kraemer and Sprenger believed that the soul afflicted by mental illness in terms of hallucinations and illusions could be set free again if the body was destroyed, and to the men of those days the destruction of the witch was therefore an act of mercy salvaging a soul from corruption. The possessed were collected together and condemned in groups of 10, 15, or even as large as 150. Examples of those destroyed by fire included a 60-year-old priest who for 30 years had heard the voice of a woman lusting for him and acting as a succubus to him. This sounds very much like a possible combination of auditory and somatic hallucinations. Another example was an old woman 'of such ugliness and deformity as must be a witch'. A further example is an old priest who in great sadness admitted that he had sucked the blood of many babies. This sounds very much like a delusion of guilt and a depressive psychosis. A further example is a young girl who while playing at her father's tomb saw a 'black man' who admitted that he was Satan and wanted to violate her. He suggested to her that she scream or jump into a well or strangle herself. This sounds like an unfortunate case of second person auditory hallucinations and a visual hallucination possibly in somebody with a depressive psychosis.

In the reign of Francis I it is possible that 100 000 people lost their lives through such inquisitions and misconceived beliefs about mental illness. The culture was such that in medieval times physicians had to be particularly careful what they termed or treated as a disease. It could be a distinctly political exercise. In considering the aetiology of syphilis a physician called Von Mellerstadt in 1496 had to be very careful in his phrasing with regard to balancing his view that syphilis was a disease and the church's view that it was the manifestation of sin. Despite this the hold of the Church on the mentally ill was slipping. Psychiatric wings were developed in most of the general hospitals in Europe including Paris, Lyon, London, Zurich and Basle.

Sin and mental illness became equated in men's minds. Inspired by Kraemer and Sprenger's *Malleus Maleficarum* and the *Codex Theodisianus*, witch hunts began after a Papal Bull was issued in 1484: 'in some parts of Northern Germany and other dioceses . . . many people have abandoned themselves to devils, incubi and succubae . . . have slain infants yet in the mother's womb . . . have blasted their harvest . . . hinder women from conceiving . . . committing and perpetrating the foulest abominations and filthiest excesses to the deadly peril of their own souls'.

The Pope appointed Inquisitors to purge the land, punishing as they thought fit. The *Malleus Maleficarum* began to be applied throughout Europe with great zeal. In the first part of the *Malleus Maleficarum* the authors prove the existence of witches and in the second part they give clinical reports on how to identify a witch. In the third part they describe how to examine and then sentence a witch. The punishment was usually death. Doctors who spoke out against the *Malleus Maleficarum* were labelled as heretics and received due punishment. At the beginning of the Renaissance increasing numbers began to speak out, for instance see Reginald Scott's book *The Discoverie of Witchcraft* dated 1584. Paracelsus in 1567 was writing of 'diseases which lead to a loss of reason' and stated quite clearly that mental illnesses were not caused by spirits but by natural causes. He was able to differentiate cases of epilepsy, mania, 'true insanity' and melancholia. He thought epilepsy rose from either the brain, heart, liver or intestines or limbs and that it began very early in life, possibly from intrauterine causes. He also thought epilepsy was a phenomenon in animals and also plants! In terms of treating mental illness he asked apothecaries to make up specific prescriptions incorporating camphor, skull shavings, unicorn and herbs.

In 1624 Robert Burton wrote the *Anatomy of Melancholy* which considers the nature of depression. Felix Plater (1536–1614) was a Swiss physician who produced a classification of psychiatric diseases, distinguishing mental impairment from mental illness and was also the first to describe an intracranial tumour (a meningioma). He also described alcoholism (the distilling process itself was invented in the Middle Ages).

In France in the mid-17th century society's answer was to incarcerate all mentally ill in special insane wings where they were chained. In Britain there was a developing system of 'houses of correction' and early workhouses.

Thomas Sydenham, born in 1624, was a Puritan and a sometime officer in Cromwell's army. He qualified as a physician aged 39 in 1663, escaped the plague in 1665 and died in 1689. He recognised the condition of hysteria which he thought was primarily a female disease and he also thought that men who tended to lead a sedentary life could also succumb to it. He did mention problems with the condition and was also aware of the difficulties that could be caused by diagnostic errors. He said that people with neurotic illnesses such as hysteria often held their reason but were often depressed as well. In terms of treatment he recorded using phlebotomy, iron preparations, milk diets and horse riding.

Thomas Willis (1621–75) (of Circle of Willis fame and co-founder of the Royal Society) saw the brain, not the womb, as the site of hysteria. He advocated strenuous treatment for chronic mania, and changes including changes of scene and work on the land. He also made observations of cases of mental deficiency, epilepsy and a schizophrenia-like illness. He also described patients with clear manic-depressive mood swings. Besides describing the arterial supply of the brain he also described cranial nerves, the autonomic nervous system and originated the concept of the reflex. He was also aware of cerebral localisation as a phenomenon and was responsible for the description of the condition myasthenia gravis.

Napier, the English physician, working around 1660, thought that purges were extremely useful for the mentally ill and advocated laxatives and emetics. He had a thriving private practice nevertheless.

In 1761 Morgagini distinguished himself by particularly looking at the pathology of the brains of deceased mentally ill patients. Nevertheless treatments were often of a rather desperate quality predicated by the apparent incurability of mental illness despite therapeutic endeavour. Examples include the grandfather of Charles Darwin (Erasmus Darwin) and his infamous spinning chair in which the insane were rotated until blood oozed from their mouths, ears and noses. It had, apparently, anecdotal success. Other dramatic interventions included castration, starvation, and the use of camphor to induce fits.

A series of textbooks began to be published at the end of the 18th century, for instance William Battie's *Treatise on Madness*, dated 1758; Benjamin Rush produced the first American book on mental illness, but also invented the restraining chair of great fame.

The conditions that the mentally ill were warehoused in continued to be of concern to a certain number of individuals. Haslam, the apothecary to Bedlam until 1861, was dismissed because of appalling conditions that prevailed there. Philip Pinel struggled with the tension in the system which threatened to see the mentally ill as people who should merely be locked up. He published the *Philosophy of Medicine for Mental Alienation*. This noted physician, born in 1745 in the south of France, developed an interest in psychiatry only when he was aged 40. Pinel tried to bring order into the chaos of the plethora of unpleasant and often ineffective treatments. In terms of his observations on the causation of mental illness he thought heredity was the primary cause but that secondly harmful social factors, for instance poor education, were of distinct importance. His other important causative areas were thirdly an irregular way of life, fourthly spasmodic passions (for instance rage and fright), fifthly inactivity and, sixthly, a melancholic constitution. Pinel taught eminent psychiatrists

including Esquirol, who later went on to develop a system of classification.

There were advances made towards the end of the 18th century particularly in terms of an approach towards the mentally ill. Key players included aforementioned Philip Pinel of Paris, William Tuke the Quaker of York and Langerman in Bayreuth. Their philosophy of mental illness was that it was precisely that, an illness, and that it should not be treated in workhouses or prisons and that the use of chains was unethical. They worked to produce a system of care, which did not rely on physical restraint but created humane asylums. Pinel saw the hospital itself as the main therapeutic tool and was very keen on the organisation of mental hospitals, which he thought should apply a vigorous, hopeful and liberal attitude to the treatment of mental illness.

Before the modern 'medical model' of mental illness, the place of the lunatic was dire indeed. Esquirol wrote to the Minister in Paris describing their plight in 1818: 'I saw patients naked, with rags or nothing more than straw to protect them against the cold, damp weather. I saw how in their wretched state they were deprived of fresh air to breathe, of water to quench their thirst, and of the basic necessities of life. I saw them turned over for safekeeping to brutal jailers. I saw them chained in damp, cramped holes without light or air; people would be ashamed to keep in such places the wild animals which are cared for at great expense in our large cities. That is what I observed almost everywhere in France, and that is how the mentally ill are treated almost everywhere in Europe.'

Pinel thought that the institution should be large enough so that different types of patient could be segregated from one another. For instance, Salpêtrière hospital had separate departments for idiots and thieves, dements, senile dements, incurable agitation and curable agitation. He rejected using chains in treatment but did advocate the use of straitjackets for short periods. He also advocated the use of cold baths but straitjackets and cold baths were only to be used on the orders of the doctor (to prevent abuse). He recommended a constant routine in the asylum and that this should fit the patient's personality. He thought that there should be a physical exercise and mechanical work programme and he advocated a separation of patients from their families since the family (a) could not look after the patient properly and (b) was often a source of unnecessary strain. Therefore he advocated reduced contact with the outside world as a 'therapeutic measure', thinking that too early a resumption of contact might lead to a dangerous relapse. In cases of food refusal, Pinel introduced tube feeding.

He warned against suicide as an ever present danger both for staff and for patients. He also began to record the results of statistical investigations into various conditions and observed that mania tended to occur predominantly between puberty and 45, that melancholia began between the ages of 20 and 40 often after setbacks in love or property and that it was often linked to amenorrhagia and to puerperium in females. He said that he had a 'cure rate' of 51% for mania, 62% for melancholia, 19% in dementia and 0% in idiocy.

It is important to note that in his early dementia category he would also have been coping with undifferentiated alcoholic dementia, thyroid disease, and other currently reversible causes of dementia.

The average length of treatment he required for melancholia was six and a half months and for mania five and a half months.

Esquirol was Pinel's pupil. He was the son of a doctor and in 1811 joined the staff of the Salpêtrière. His basic attitudes were very similar to his mentor Pinel's but he was a great gifted teacher and responsible for the then pre-eminence of the French school of psychiatry in the first half of the 19th century. He was a better statistician than his mentor and he gave clearer descriptions of progressive paresis and epilepsy. He threw away Pinel's idea that mania was sited in the abdomen and adopted Gall's theory of cerebral localisation.

He differentiated between hallucinations and illusions in psychopathology and helped design the French legal code of 1838 to administer the mentally ill. This was used subsequently as the model for legislation in Switzerland, England (1842) and Norway. He designed various asylums in France.

Not all of the reform of the treatment of mental illness was by doctors. The layman Quaker William Tuke and subsequent generations of his family were angered by conditions in which the English mentally ill lived and died, and spent their lives reforming their care. Tuke founded the York Retreat, which was then used as a model for several American hospitals. He inspired his family for generations to come with the same aim of helping the mentally ill. His son, Henry, and his grandson, Samuel, and finally his great-grandson, Daniel Hack Tuke (psychiatrist) were all involved in the treatment of the mentally ill. Daniel Hack Tuke developed a new classificatory system based upon the idea of the presenting complaint. He worked as a medical student at Barts and the Royal College of Surgeons, received a doctorate from Heidelberg and visited institutions in France, Germany and Holland to pick up their best practices. He went on to edit the *Journal of Mental Science*. He was interested, for a while, in Braidism. James Braid was a Manchester doctor who was interested in hypnotism and operated on patients under its influence. Eventually, Daniel Hack Tuke became the Professor of Psychiatry at Charing Cross.

Unhappily coinciding with Darwinian Theory was the Degeneration Theory in the 19th century. This emphasised the family history of mental illness and proposed that certain families became progressively more degenerate as the years went on; for instance, there might be a neurotic grandfather, producing a depressed mother who might then produce insane offspring; i.e. the theory was that the mental illness became more severe with each successive generation. A main proponent of this theory was Benedict Morel

(1809–73), who wrote the treatise 'Traité des dégénérescences physiques, intellectuelles et morales de l'espèce humaine et des causes qui produisent ces variétés maladives'. He said that 'degenerations are deviations from the normal human type which are transmissible by heredity and which deteriorate progressively towards extinction'. The causes of this degeneration could be very much the 'sins of the fathers' in terms of intoxication, the social milieu, moral sickness within the family, inborn or acquired damage or heredity. He found numerous followers in Germany, for instance Baron Richard von Krafft-Ebing, a psychiatrist who went on to describe various sexual perversions (in the book *Psychopathia Sexualis*). He thought homosexuality and criminality were caused by degeneration. Cesare Lomborso (1836–1909) saw criminals as an evolutionary leftover of a primitive race. Some psychiatrists, including Kraepelin, expressed reservations about the degeneration theory but the idea caught on and became popular. The seed would grow into the Nazi mental health policy in the 1930s that would see a similar number of mentally ill (100 000) killed to that killed by the medieval inquisitions.

In the second half of the 19th century German psychiatry very much took the lead academically. Psychiatrists like Emil Kraepelin published textbooks and assiduously audited their care of patients, but despite their clinical research some doctors persisted in believing that illness was secondary to sin and a disease of the soul or inherited as some kind of genetic leftover of a primitive race. Nevertheless there was some good research by physicians such as Meynert (Professor of Brain Psychiatry at Vienna) who believed that external stimuli set up cerebral cortical excitation at specific points. He thought that various psychological states had anatomical correlates within the brain. Professor Wernicke was famous for his studies on aphasia and also described Wernicke's psychosis. In 1857 the physicians Esmarch and Jessen in Germany proposed a link between general paresis of the insane (GPI) and syphilis. This view was not generally accepted.

Alzheimer found that 30% of the mental hospital population had a demonstrable disease of the brain on post mortem, emphasising the medical aspect of mental illness.

Eugene Bleuler (1857–1939) demonstrated that dementia praecox did not always end in a dementing state and preferred the term schizophrenia.

The undifferentiated nature of some of the psychosis proved problematic but people were beginning to get a handle on the organic causes. Conditions such as general paresis of the insane (GPI) and *tabes dorsalis* still were not recognised as being caused by a single microorganism. A heated debate went back and forth. Pinel in 1858 had talked of an illness with tremor of the tongue, difficulty in articulating speech and abnormal gait with poor balance, which he differentiated out from the morass of other mental illness. Neuropathologists noted a 'softening of the brain' associated with GPI but postulated that this was due to 'cerebral congestion causing inadequate nutrition to the brain'; i.e. they had a circulatory hypothesis for GPI rather than an infective one.

In vain doctors were looking for a cause. Bayle thought that GPI and *tabes dorsalis* had a multi-factorial model with moral and physical causes. He thought that the association of the condition with the male sex was 'easily explained because males were more subjected to mental shocks, excessive drinking, suppression of the haemorrhoidal flow and injuries to the head'. He also noted that the condition was most common between the ages of 30 and 60 but thought that personality might be important and that those who suffered were previously of a sanguine temperament or choleric and passionate. He noted that 50% of cases had a family history and that in terms of an occupational association, soldiers were often seen because of 'privation and excessive drinking associated with Napoleonic wars'. He thought that a half of the cases followed disappointment, violent love, profound jealousy, or excessive intellectual endeavour. He did note that a fifth of the patients had had venereal excesses but these excesses are 'common anyway' and so he thought there was no role in the aetiology.

Lumbar puncture had been developed in 1890 by Quirke and in studies Babcock showed (in 1896) that there was an increased protein level in the cerebral spinal fluid of patients with GPI. In 1906 the German, August von Wasserman, developed a test for blood serum and CSF which was proved to be 90% positive in people with GPI. In 1912 Lange found that the abnormal protein in the CSF precipitated the colloidal gold from a solution and this represented a further test for GPI.

Although people now began to see that there might be an infective cause of general paresis and *tabes dorsalis*, i.e. syphilis, caused by *Spirochaetes*, there was no specific treatment. Mercury and potassium iodide were used. In 1910 Paul Ehrlich advised the use of salvarsan (arsphenamine) given intravenously; it was an organic arsenical compound. Later on the drug was given into the subdural space via trephine and subsequently even into the lateral ventricles themselves. None of these desperate measures worked particularly well. Some people advocated malarial therapy. Only later during the 20th century did proper antibiotic treatment produce dramatic effects.

20TH CENTURY

The final recognition that syphilis was caused by a specific micro-organism and that there was a specific treatment allowed the decanting of almost 10–20% of patients from asylums.

Around the same time there was increased interest in neurotic illness and adherents of psychoanalytic theory, led by Sigmund Freud (Austrian physician, 1856–1939), were spreading their theories around the Western world. Sigmund Freud had started as a neurologist (he made observations about the potential use of cocaine as a topical anaesthetic). Freud then went to Paris and saw Charcot (the noted

French physician–Charcot's joint and Charcot's triad) demonstrating patients with hysteria.

Freud became interested in this illness and moved away from neurology into the field of psychiatry and built up a private practice of patients with hysteria. Initially he used hypnosis to treat them but found the sometimes alarming effects (positive transference in patients) unsettling and resorted to using pure talking treatments (psychoanalysis). In psychoanalysis patients were allowed to talk at length for a considerable time until their 'resistance' was broken. He used dream therapy and regarded dreams as the 'royal road to the unconscious'. Freud's contributions to psychological theory include the id, the ego and the superego and the ideas regarding the unconscious. His daughter Anna developed various concepts including psychological defence mechanisms. His many followers, including Jung, took his ideas further. Jung contributed concepts such as word association, extroversion and introversion, and rebelled against Freud's theories that the primary drives of human beings included *eros* and *thanatos*. Freud often employed a notion of spirituality in his therapy and regarded one of the life aims of people as being to 'individuate' and develop spiritually in life. Jung was also responsible for the ideas of archetypes and symbol and worked very much in terms of symbols in dreams.

Germans made such a contribution to psychiatry in the late 19th and early 20th centuries, but the advent of the Nazis launched a tidal wave of destruction as far as German psychiatrists and German psychiatric patients were concerned.

The National Socialist Party in 1933 passed the Law of 'Erb-Gesundheitsgesetz' to 'protect the race' by introducing the forced sterilisation of the incurably mentally ill and handicapped. Psychiatric doctors and institutions were required to make card registers of all psychiatric patients. Dissenting doctors (e.g. 61 psychiatry professors), were removed from office and from then on only 'reliable members' of the Nazi Party were allowed to be appointed. The editorships of medical journals and the presidencies of medical associations were manipulated by the Nazi Government. Between 1936 and 1939 psychiatrists who were employed were involved in administrating 'Racial Hygiene Policies' rather than necessarily treating illness. The youngest reported victim of psychiatric sterilisation was a two-year-old girl. In 1939 there was a change in policy, but not for the better; from then on only 'life worthy of life' was allowed to continue and 'life unworthy of life' ('Lebensunwertes Leben') was eliminated. Both fiction and non-fiction cinema were used to put over the doctrine of euthanasia for the mentally ill as a 'kindness'.

There are echoes here again of the 'kindness' meted out to the socially inadequate and ill in the Middle Ages by putting witches to death and thereby saving their souls.

A board of psychiatrists and pharmacologists was put together in Nazi Germany and consulted on the most 'humane' way of killing the mentally ill and carbon monoxide was decided upon as the killing agent of choice, but to their questionable credit doctors refused to have anything further to do with the policy.

In November 1939 the heads of all the German asylums were required to notify which patients were curable and which patients were incurably ill. 'Special treatment centres' were set up and incurable patients were sent there. The majority of psychiatrists unfortunately did nothing to stop this process. Some did, but they were arrested, interrogated and executed by guillotine. Other psychiatrists protested to the Church which denounced the murders in turn. Nevertheless the policy continued in secret. In 1941 some medical students from the University of Munich and a philosophy professor formed an opposition group called 'The White Rose'. They wrote pamphlets denouncing Hitler's regime and his policy of exterminating the vulnerable. As a result of this resistance campaign, the core students and their professor were beheaded in 1943. Some 100 000 mentally ill or disabled patients were murdered and only a fifth of all psychiatric inpatients survived the Nazi regime.

ENGLISH PSYCHIATRY IN THE 20TH CENTURY

A 20th-century English psychiatrist, Dr William Sargent, was a pioneering doctor with a belief that physical treatments would relieve much of the suffering of mental illness:

In the early 1930s, when I took up this speciality, the usual medical approach to the treatment of the mentally ill was almost a wholly negative one. In Great Britain most patients were obliged to enter a 'lunatic asylum' as they were still often called, the majority of them were compulsorily certified as insane and many of them were detained for very long periods under the old Poor Law and Lunacy Acts. Discharges were much rarer than today. At the famed Maudsley Hospital, even where all entries were voluntary, and the best available treatments were tried out on cases specially chosen for having a good prognosis, only a third, for instance, of our patients suffering from schizophrenia were back home and reasonably well three years after admission. Roughly two-thirds of all the other half-million schizophrenics were either kept locked up in mental hospitals, or stayed at home more or less incapacitated from work. The suffering involved was fearful. Few patients, however, died of this mental disease; most of them lingered on, imprisoned with their often agonizing delusions and hallucinations under jail-like conditions for as long as forty years or more.

Sufferers from anxiety states and depression fared little better; the more depressed patients often died earlier than schizophrenics because of their continued distress of mind, extreme agitation, loss of weight and final refusal to eat. Tens of thousands of such patients tried to commit suicide, thousands succeeded before they could be brought to hospital. Even today, depression accounts for nearly one-third of all patients with psychological illnesses who apply for treatment from their general practitioners. Depression accounts for nearly a quarter of all those who go to general hospitals for medical investigation and physical check-ups (and who are too often informed after medical examinations that 'nothing wrong is found').

At one British mental hospital before World War II, the average duration of a severely depressed patient's stay – unless he quickly died of agitation or managed somehow to kill himself – was 381 days, in addition to all the time off work before going into hospital and after being discharged. A severe attack of depression or anxiety – to which some hundreds of thousands in Britain are still liable today – could last anything from two to twenty years. Minor depressions and anxiety states, though almost too numerous to assess, can involve weeks or months of incapacity and suffering. After World War II, Paul Wood suggested that of those patients who had 'anxious hearts' or suffered from a purely functional heart disorder named 'effort syndrome', no more than one-third ever really recovered; the rest were either liable to frequent attacks or remained permanently ill. 'Creaking doors hang long': a relative of my own, though otherwise well and married to a professor interested in psychology, confirmed Paul Wood's findings. She was incapacitated by a functional heart disorder from going out by herself from the age of twenty-five right up to her death at ninety-three. The incidence of mental illness, mental defect, psychopathic personality, and of all minor and major neuroses, is as cruel now as it ever was, but treatments are at last being discovered that relieve, even if they do not always cure, some of these many varied disorders.

Freudian techniques of psychotherapy and its derivatives were tried out in World War I and came into increasing use in the 20s. These techniques with those of Adler and Jung were the sole special forms of psychotherapeutic treatment then available to British psychiatrists. If they had proved efficacious at a time when they constituted a practical monopoly of the specialized treatment of mental ills, everybody would very soon have recognized it.

The Unquiet Mind, William Sargent, 1967

LEARNING POINTS: HISTORY OF PSYCHIATRY

➤ Madness has existed since ancient times.
➤ The view that madness was mental illness delivered the mentally ill from the hands of the witchfinders, the superstitious and those who would imprison them in prisons.
➤ The asylums were intended as a therapeutic environment.
➤ Scientific data collection and classification of mental illness allowed doctors to separate out causes of mental illness, e.g. neurosyphilis.
➤ Political systems have used mental health legislation to distort the public perception of and treatment of the mentally ill and have led to abuses in various countries including Germany, America and the USSR.
➤ In the 20th century more specific and more effective treatments began to be developed.
➤ Specific treatments enabled the decanting of thousands of mentally ill from the asylums and prepared the ground for community treatment.
➤ There are cycles in the history of psychiatry that tend to repeat.
➤ Cheap and inadequate community care and the demedicalisation of mental illness contain intrinsic threats for the mentally ill, allowing them to perhaps be portrayed in the future as other than 'ill' – maybe as dangerous, or responsible for all their actions, or even as immoral.

Table 16.1 NHS admissions for schizophrenia – all ICD-10 types

Admissions	Years			
	2002–03	2003–04	2004–05	2005–06
Male total	14 391	13 968	14 677	13 558
Female total	7262	7169	7434	6776

Source: HESONLINE Statistics.

EXPLORATIONS

Use the resources and further reading suggestions for help with the following.

The government invested hundreds of millions of pounds in creating teams for treating severe mental illness in the community in the early years of this millennium. One of the promises made for such teams was that they would prevent hospital admissions. Using the figures in Table 16.1 of the admissions for schizophrenia, describe any trend you observe. Next use search engines to find up to date admission statistics and continue the table for 2006–07, etc. What trend do you find?

Find out the figures for total NHS mental illness beds for the years above. Express the admission figures in terms of percentages of the total NHS mental illness beds available. What trend do you find?

FURTHER READING AND REFERENCES

Craddock N, Antebi D, Attenburrow MJ, Bailey A, Carson A, Cowen P. Wake-up call for British psychiatry. *Br J Psych*. 2008; **193**: 6–9.

Fish F. The diagnosis of acute schizophrenia: instructions on the use of the acute schizophrenia diagnostic checklist (ASDC). *Psychiatric Quarterly*. 1969; **43**(1): 35–45.

Graeber MB, Kosel S, Egensperger R, *et al.* Rediscovery of the case described by Alois Alzheimer in 1911: historical, histological and molecular genetic analysis. *Neurogenetics*. 1997; **1**: 73–80.

Kraepelin E. *One Hundred years of Psychiatry*. New York: Philosophical Books; 1962.

Meyer-Lindenberg J. The Holocaust and German psychiatry. *Br J Psych*. 1991; **159**: 7–12.

Sargent W. *The Unquiet Mind: the autobiography of a physician in psychological medicine*. London: Heinemann; 1967.

Shorter E. *A History of Psychiatry: from the era of the asylum to the age of Prozac*. New York: John Wiley & Sons; 1997.

Zilboorg G, with Henry GW. *A History of Medical Psychology*. New York: Norton; 1941.

RESOURCES

Case histories from psychiatry
http://bms.brown.edu/HistoryofPsychiatry/hop.html

Hospital Episode Statistics (NHS) – HES Online
www.hesonline.nhs.uk/

'Life Unworthy of Life' and other Medical Killing Programmes – Dr Stuart D. Stein
www.ess.uwe.ac.uk/genocide/mord.htm

CHAPTER 17

Sexual aspects of psychiatry

Human sexuality is a vital and integral part of behaviour and personality. Sexual dysfunction is a source of great distress to individuals and couples. Sexual dysfunction may lead to a failure to form relationships or the break-up of existing relationships and families.

CONTENTS

MALE SEXUAL PROBLEMS
PROBLEMS OF DESIRE

The sexual drive or libido is inherent in all human beings. Most often a male's sexual drive is directed towards appropriately aged heterosexual partners, but sometimes there can be problems with the drive in terms of its amount or direction. Loss of libido implies a diminution in the sexual drive and can be caused by psychological disorders such as depression and anorexia nervosa, and physical illnesses such as carcinomatosis or heart failure. Excess libido can be associated with psychological disorders such as hypomania or frontal lobe syndrome or, rarely, physical illnesses such as tuberculosis.

Less often the libido may be directed towards the same gender, as in homosexuality. Homosexuality was once, but is no longer, classed as a psychiatric disorder. Less socially acceptable objects of desire include children (*paedophilia*) and animals (*bestiality*). Arousal may also be associated with objects (*fetishism*), such as high-heeled shoes and leather, or be associated with inflicting pain (*sadism*) or having pain inflicted upon one (*masochism*). *Transvestism* is a behaviour where arousal is produced by dressing in clothes appropriate to the opposite sex (*cross-dressing*). Transvestites may be heterosexually or homosexually oriented.

PROBLEMS OF GENDER

Apart from biological intersex conditions, gender is generally appropriately assigned by society according to the normal male's genitalia. The social gender given to the newborn male is usually followed by a core male gender. In other words the male looks *and* feels that he is a male. In *male transsexuals*, although male genitalia are fully developed, the core gender is female. Although phenotypically male, the male transsexual feels that he is female and should have female genitalia. There is a fundamental difference with male homosexuals who both look male and feel that they are males. Male transsexuals may cross-dress and seek hormonal and surgical means of adopting feminine attributes.

PROBLEMS OF PERFORMANCE

Because of social taboos, the sexual act is shrouded in a certain aura of mystery. The sexually naive individual or couple may lack the necessary knowledge and skills to perform sex. Doctors sometimes do not help this process, because they often overestimate their patient's knowledge of sexual anatomy and function, and often fail to explain sexual matters clearly.

Lacking the confidence that experience can bring, the younger male may suffer with *premature ejaculation*, where semen is ejaculated before penetration, or before sex has properly got under way. The problem may lead to an avoidance of the sexual act (a bit like the avoidance associated with a phobia) and thus to problems in relationships.

CASE HISTORY 1

Simon came to his family doctor twice before he said what he wanted to say. The first time he spoke to the female partner in the general practice and came away red-faced, clutching a prescription for a sore throat. The second time Simon attended he saw a young male doctor who spent some time trying to understand Simon's anxiety. Simon told him that he was having problems with his girlfriend and that she had told him to 'get it sorted out, because there must be something wrong with you'. Amid some embarrassment the teenager told the doctor that when he tried to have sex with his girlfriend 'it didn't last very long'. On careful questioning about what Simon meant it transpired that Simon always ejaculated during foreplay. He had never managed to penetrate his partner. The closest that they had both got to intercourse was when he managed to put a condom on. Unfortunately, he ejaculated immediately afterwards.

What can the doctor do to help?

Talking about the problem in a straightforward way will help defuse some of the anxiety that Simon feels. People are often greatly troubled by sexual problems, but wonder whether their doctor can help, or will even be prepared to listen. In this case the doctor is careful to find out exactly what Simon means when he says 'it didn't last very long' doctors are used to taking long histories about pains and other presenting complaints, but are all too often prepared to take statements about sexual problems at face value.

Feeding back what the doctor understands the problem to be (i.e. premature ejaculation) will enable Simon to correct any misapprehensions on the doctor's part and will begin to help explain matters. Education about sex using explanations, diagrams, videos or books may help as may further practice. Engaging both partners in helping each other with the problem often reduces anxiety, improves the relationship, and allows other issues to be discussed between the couple. Giving permission for the couple to experiment may defuse tension. The female partner may be asked to help the male ejaculate outside the vagina, and they may work together in prolonging the sexual encounter by stimulating so far then stopping before male orgasm ('stop-start technique'). Once control is established in this way, then the couple might progress on to vaginal penetration. Such simple psychological management is often all that is required, but the doctor needs to follow the case up. Individuals may go away from the doctor and the doctor may wrongly assume that the problem is solved when they do not return. People may be too embarrassed to return, so the doctor needs to make things easier for them to do so, by making a further appointment.

What if the problem doesn't get better?

Some simple physical techniques can be used by the couple, such as the 'squeeze technique' in addition to the 'stop-start' technique. A behavioural programme which relies on 'sensate focus' could be used, as set out in Table 17.1. In the sensate focus technique the doctor prescribes a total cessation of attempts at sexual intercourse and instead introduces a series of graded tasks. These graded tasks slowly lead from simple caressing to full penetration. The effect of initially prohibiting intercourse enhances this as a goal, but also reduces anxiety associated with the performance. Couples can focus on simple ways of giving each other pleasure that do not rest upon penetration.

Table 17.1 An example of a sensate focus programme

- Therapist asks couple to take it in turns to touch each other's body, when in private, comfortable and unclothed. Therapist forbids couple to have sexual intercourse or touch each other's genitals.

- Partners tell each other only if some touching is unpleasant. The touching is then changed.

- In the next stage the couple is asked to touch each other and say what they like as well as what they find uncomfortable.

- Problems with 'assignment' are discussed.

- Genital touching is allowed and stages 2 and 3 are repeated. The 'stop-start' technique is incorporated. Orgasm is allowed, but is not the prime aim of touching. Communication is stressed.

- Subsequent stages involve brief vaginal entry, or different positions, leading to sexual intercourse.

There may be underlying problems in the relationship that need to be resolved and relationship counselling as provided by organisations such as RELATE may be helpful.

Pharmacological means of retarding ejaculation can be tried. A side-effect of fluoxetine can be to delay ejaculation, and a short course of the drug may be sufficient to restore confidence. Other SSRI antidepressants may also have this effect (and sexual side-effects will need to be discussed when prescribing these drugs for depression).

Male *impotence* is either a complete failure to attain an erection, or an inability to maintain an erection. Classically, the problem is seen in older men, but it can affect all ages. When the erection commonly occurring on waking is also absent, thought must be given to an underlying organic cause (such as diabetes mellitus or alcoholism). Anxiety is a common psychological cause of impotence. Often a mixture of physical and psychological factors may interact to produce impotence.

Table 17.2 Physical causes of male impotence

Illness and disease

- Alcoholism (neuropathy)
- Diabetes mellitus
- Arterial disease, e.g. Leriche's syndrome
- Renal failure
- Carcinomatosis
- Neurosyphilis
- Hypothalamo-pituitary dysfunction
- Liver failure
- Multiple sclerosis, and many others

Drugs

- Beta-blockers
- Thiazide diuretics
- Tricyclic antidepressants
- Phenothiazines
- Spironolactone
- Cimetidine
- Cannabis
- Antiepileptics

CASE HISTORY 2

Graham, 34, attended his family doctor after his wife left him. He had been married for only two months. His initial complaint was that he was not sleeping. He asked for some sleeping tablets. His doctor, who did not know about the separation, asked him about his wife, because she knew that he had only just got married. Graham became tearful and said that he had been responsible for his wife's leaving. He was reluctant to say why, but eventually admitted that they had been unable to consummate the marriage. Despite his wanting to have sex and his enjoyment of foreplay to a limited extent, he felt somehow threatened by the idea of entering his wife. He was, he said, frightened of what would happen. His wife had been understanding at first, but had grown angry with him. Now he was even more afraid. With tactful questioning the doctor elicited some important facts from his psychosexual history. Graham had never had a girlfriend before his wife and they had never attempted sex before marriage. Graham also disclosed (for the first time in his life to anyone) that he had been sexually abused by an uncle when he was 10. He had deep feelings of regret about this and the whole area of sexual behaviour was clouded by the feeling that it was dirty and forbidden.

What can the doctor do to investigate a diagnosis?

There are strong pointers to a psychological cause for Graham's impotence – his avoidance of sex in the past, his fear of penetrating his wife, and continuing feelings about childhood sexual abuse (which he has been unable to disclose to his wife). The doctor needs to ask more questions about Graham's normal sexual functioning – is he able to get an erection in other circumstances? Can he masturbate to orgasm? These questions are not intended to pry, but to establish whether Graham has the ability to function physiologically (*see* Table 17.2 for organic causes of erectile dysfunction). The hypothesis would then be that psychological factors are inhibiting normal physiological functioning.

If the doctor suspects that organic factors may be playing a part in the impotence (although there are no particular features in the case above) a variety of investigations is open to her. Most cases of impotence have physical causes, and a physical examination followed by simple screening blood tests may alert the family doctor to problems. Suitable first-line investigations may be a full blood count, serum urea and electrolytes, thyroid function tests (if indicated), and serum testosterone.

Graham has found it possible to confide in his family doctor, and the relationship is probably therefore an important one to him. If the family doctor can manage the case herself, then this might be useful – the management would consist of excluding organic causes and counselling Graham about sexual function and exploring his feelings about the past abuse. The family doctor may not wish to undertake this counselling or therapy herself, but refer Graham on to a psychiatrist who specialises in psychosexual medicine, or an experienced counsellor.

Physical treatments are available which can promote erections. Once the erection is attained, sexual intercourse can occur. Successful intercourse hopefully leads to increased confidence and a short course of such treatments can break the cycle of low self-esteem and performance anxiety.

Physical treatments can include phosphodiesterase type 5 inhibitor drugs such as sildenafil (Viagra), tadalafil or vardenafil. The doctor needs to exclude cardiovascular disease prior to prescription. Other treatments involve intrapenile injections of prostaglandin E_1 or papaverine given into the corpora cavernosum. Cases of neurogenic impotence and psychogenic impotence respond with erection, but where arterial insufficiency is a problem erection may be impossible even with intracavernosal injections. External vacuum devices can help produce erections and are sometimes seen as more acceptable than self-administered injections.

LEARNING POINTS: MALE SEXUAL PROBLEMS

➢ The most common male sexual problems that present to specialist clinics are impotence (or erectile failure) and premature ejaculation.

➢ Psychogenic impotence is a diagnosis of exclusion. Physical causes account for the majority of cases, underlining the importance of medical training and diagnostic skills.

➢ Where organic causes of sexual dysfunction have been excluded, management consists of improving the individual's and couple's knowledge about sex, enhancing their communication skills and teaching simple behavioural techniques to use during sex.

➢ Intensive psychotherapy is reserved for patients in whom internal conflicts about gender identity can be identified, or in whose lives there are repeating patterns of relationship behaviours that can be changed.

➢ Erections can be produced by oral preparations such as sildenafil, or intracavernosal injections of prostaglandin E_1, papaverine or the use of external vacuum devices.

FEMALE SEXUAL PROBLEMS
PROBLEMS OF DESIRE

The most common female sexual problem presenting to specialist clinics is one of low sexual interest sometimes associated with impaired arousal (female sexual arousal disorder – FSAD). This problem is relatively difficult to treat, because it may require psychotherapy looking at reasons for ambivalence about sexual behaviour, caused by, say, childhood sexual abuse. There is limited evidence that drugs such as sildenafil (Viagra) or topical prostaglandins may assist with local arousal problems, e.g. lubrication or engorgement. Organic causes such as endocrine disturbance (hypothyroidism, hyperthyroidism, Cushing's disease, pituitary adenomas and others) need to be excluded as do psychiatric disorders like depression. Hysterectomy and mastectomy seriously affect self-image and appropriate counselling may help patients overcome difficulties in resuming sexual behaviour after such operations. Hysterectomy and mastectomy patients often need to mourn the loss of their uterus or breast. Their partners often need to be involved, although they commonly resist inclusion and 'deny' problems. Fear of recurrent disease does not help matters. Appropriate exploration of fears and reasonable reassurance may help, but a depressive reaction and treatment for this must be considered.

PROBLEMS OF GENDER

Transsexualism occurs in women, but is probably about three times less common than in men. Transsexual behaviour can manifest as early as middle childhood. There is no good current evidence of a genetic mechanism, but some studies suggest that some female-to-male transsexuals may have raised testosterone levels and a higher incidence of polycystic ovarian disease. Even so, environmental and cultural factors are thought to be more important than biological factors.

PROBLEMS OF PERFORMANCE

Dyspareunia is pain felt during sexual intercourse. Although dyspareunia can occur in men it is 10 times more common in women. Organic causes such as vaginal infection or irritation and post-menopausal dryness and atrophic vaginitis are common and must be either treated or excluded before too much reliance is placed on a purely psychological hypothesis. Table 17.3 shows some causes of dyspareunia. Despite this it must be recognised that even where there are organic causes of dyspareunia, psychological factors may have a part to play; for instance, difficulties in the relationship may lead to inadequate foreplay,

resulting in inadequate vaginal lubrication before penetration, leading to discomfort during and after intercourse and a resulting cycle of anger and disharmony in the couple. Alternatively the memory of past sexual trauma or damage done during childbirth may account for a change in the perception of the experience.

Similar ambivalent feelings about sex in general or the partner in particular may lead to *vaginismus*, an inability to allow penetration of the vagina associated with spasm of the perineal muscles, *sexual aversion, lack of enjoyment, and anorgasmia* (the lack of orgasm).

CASE HISTORY 3

A teenager called Clare was referred to a female gynaecologist because she had pain when her boyfriend tried to make love to her. She had refused to let her male family doctor examine her then, just as she had refused to allow him to examine her when she had requested the contraceptive pill a few months before. The family doctor had felt unable to issue a prescription for the pill and the relationship between him and Clare was strained.

The gynaecologist took a careful and sensitive history from Clare. It transpired that she had never been able to allow any of her boyfriends to enter or even touch her vagina. She was sure that her vagina was too small, and would burst if she allowed anything inside it. When her boyfriend put on a condom and tried to enter her she 'froze rigid', and all her muscles went tense.

What can the gynaecologist do?

She can assess what knowledge Clare has about female anatomy and what her sex education was like. What beliefs or fears does she have about the size of her vagina? What are Clare's feelings about sex? Is she very worried about becoming pregnant without the contraceptive pill? Her anxieties are probably contributing to an increased pelvic muscle tone which would

Table 17.3 Causes of dyspareunia

Female

- Failure of vaginal lubrication
- Failure of vasocongestion
- Failure of uterine elevation and vaginal ballooning during arousal
- Oestrogen deficiency leading to atrophic vaginitis
- Radiotherapy for malignancy
- Vaginal infection, e.g. *Trichomonas vaginalis*, or herpes
- Vaginal irritation, e.g. sensitivity to creams or deodorants
- Abnormal tone of pelvic floor muscles
- Scarring after episiotomy or surgery
- Bartholin's gland cysts/abscess
- Rigid hymen, small introitus

Male

- Painful retraction of the foreskin
- Herpetic and other infections
- Asymmetrical erection due to fibrosis or Peyronie's disease
- Hypersensitivity of the glans penis

make entry painful or impossible (vaginismus), therefore reinforcing the idea that she cannot accommodate an erect penis. Simple education and a gradual and gentle vaginal examination by the gynaecologist (perhaps using Clare's own fingers first) may change some of Clare's ideas about her own body and be all that is required. Sometimes the use of graded dilators by the patient and then her partner may help.

LEARNING POINTS: FEMALE SEXUAL PROBLEMS

➢ The most common female sexual problem seen in specialist clinics is one of low sexual interest/arousal (female sexual arousal disorder – FSAD), which may have physical and psychological causes.

➢ Most non-organic problems can be relieved by open discussion, education and involvement of the partner.

➢ Doctors should also seek to improve communication between the partners so that each partner's desires and needs begin to be clearly expressed and listened to.

➢ Underlying psychiatric disorders, such as depression, require treatment.

SELF-ASSESSMENT
MCQs

1 Common sexual problems include:
  A transsexualism
  B erectile dysfunction
  C male dyspareunia
  D premature ejaculation
  E vaginismus

2 Causes of a reduction in libido or erectile dysfunction include:
  A antihypertensive drugs
  B haemochromatosis
  C diabetes mellitus
  D hypothyroidism
  E hyperthyroidism

3 Useful treatments for:
  A erectile dysfunction include intrapenile injections of paroxetine
  B premature ejaculation include the squeeze technique
  C homosexuality include aversion therapy
  D vaginismus include the 'stop-start' technique
  E premature ejaculation include fluoxetine

MCQ answers
1 A=F, B=T, C=F, D=T, E=F.
2 All true.
3 A=F, B=T, C=F, D=F, E=T.

EXPLORATIONS
LINKS WITH GENETICS, EMBRYOLOGY AND ANATOMY

➤ How do problems with male and female genotypes express themselves phenotypically?

➤ What causes do you know for intersex states?

➤ What psychological reactions might occur in children with anatomically abnormal sexual organs?

LINKS WITH PHYSIOLOGY

➤ How is sexual function linked in to the female reproductive cycle?

➤ How is the reproductive cycle controlled?

➤ How might psychological stress interfere with gonadotrophin production?

➤ What sensory inputs lead to male arousal?

➤ How can cortical activity modulate arousal?

➤ What changes in penile blood flow lead to erection?

➤ How can damage to pelvic nerves affect this process?

LINKS WITH COMMUNICATION SKILLS

➤ How might patients with sexual problems present to their family doctor?

➤ What communication skills of the doctor will enable him or her to pick up these problems?

➤ What kind of language should be used in exploring sexual problems and explaining proposed management of these problems?

LINKS WITH GYNAECOLOGY

➤ How common is dyspareunia?

➤ What is the age distribution of women presenting with the problem?

➤ What effect does age have on sexual function?

FURTHER READING AND REFERENCES

Bancroft J. *Human Sexuality and its Problems.* 2nd ed. Edinburgh: Churchill Livingstone; 1989.

Claret L, Cox EH, McFadyen L, Pidgen A, Johnson PJ, Haughie S, Boolell M, Bruno R. Modeling and simulation of sexual activity: daily diary data of patients with female sexual arousal disorder treated with sildenafil citrate (Viagra). *Pharmaceutical Research.* 2006; **23**(8): 1756–64.

Cranston-Cuebas MA, Barlow DH. Cognitive and affective contributions to sexual functioning. *Annual Review of Sex Research.* 1990; **1**: 119–62.

Green R. Gender identity in childhood and later sexual orientation: follow-up of 78 males. *American Journal of Psychiatry.* 1985; **142**: 339–41.

Hatzimouratidis K. Sildenafil in the treatment of erectile dysfunction: an overview of the clinical evidence. *Clinical Interventions in Aging.* 2006; **1**(4): 403–14.

Kinsey AC, Pomeroy WB, Martin CE. *Sexual Behaviour in the Human Male.* Philadelphia: Saunders; 1948.

Kinsey AC, Pomeroy WB, Martin CE, Gebhard PH. *Sexual Behaviour in the Human Female.* Philadelphia: Saunders; 1953.

Lipsius SH. Prescribing sensate focus without proscribing intercourse. *J Sex Marital Ther.* 1987; **13**(2): 106–16.

Makhlouf A, Kparker A, Niederberger CS. Depression and erectile dysfunction. *Urologic Clinics of North America.* 2007; **34**(4): 565–74.

Masters WH, Johnson VE. *Human Sexual Inadequacy.* London: Churchill; 1970.

Mathers N, Bramley M, Draper K, Snead S, Tobert A. Assessment of training in psychosexual medicine. *BMJ.* 1994; **308**: 969–72.

Pollack MH, Reiter S, Hammerness P. Genitourinary and sexual adverse effects of psychotropic medication. *Int J Psychiatry Med.* 1992; **22**(4): 305–27.

Walbroehl GS. Sexuality in the handicapped. *Am Fam Physician.* 1987; **36**(1): 129–33.

Wyatt GE, Peters SD, Guthrie D. Kinsey revisited, Part I: comparisons of the sexual socialization and sexual behavior of white women over 33 years. *Arch Sex Behav.* 1988; **17**(3): 201–39.

SEXUAL PROBLEMS IN LITERATURE

Earthly Powers (1980) by Anthony Burgess.
Lolita (1955) by Vladimir Nabokov.
The Old Devils (1986) by Kingsley Amis.
The Rebel Angels (1981) by Robertson Davies.
Portnoy's Complaint (1969) by Philip Roth.

RESOURCES

Institute of Psychosexual Medicine
12 Chandos Street, Cavendish Square, London
W1M 9DR
Tel: 020 7580 0631
Email: admin@ipm.org.uk

Relate
Premier House, Carolina Court, Lakeside,
Doncaster DN4 5RA
www.relate.org.uk (Look on webpage for local
addresses and telephone numbers or phone 300
100 1234.)

Association of Psychosexual Nursing
www.wanstead.park.btinternet.co.uk

The Balint Society
www.balint.co.uk

**British Association of Sexual and
Relationship Therapy**
www.basrt.org.uk

**British Society of Psychosomatic Obstetrics,
Gynaecology and Andrology**
www.bspoga.org

**Faculty of Family Planning and Reproductive
Healthcare**
www.ffprhc.org.uk

Family Planning Association
www.fpa.org.uk

Lovelifematters
www.lovelifematters.co.uk/

Royal College of General Practitioners
www.rcgp.org.uk

Royal College of Obstetrics and Gynaecology
www.rcog.org.uk

Sexual Dysfunction Association
www.sda.uk.net/

CHAPTER 18

Psychiatry: ethics and the law

Most countries have mental health legislation to enable the state to provide care and treatment to severely mentally disordered individuals who for one reason or another refuse treatment. Such treatment is arranged for these individuals in the interests of their own health and the well-being of society as a whole. However, such legislation attracts controversy because it interferes with the autonomy of an individual. When is this kind of intervention justified? Is what is legal always ethical?

CONTENTS

THE NEED FOR MENTAL HEALTH LEGISLATION

There are perhaps six key points that we can learn from the history of psychiatry:

➤ Mental illness has occurred throughout history and we can predict from this that it will occur in the future of humankind as well and that there needs to be some provision to treat and prevent as much suffering as possible.

➤ Without treatment mental illness can persist for many months or even years, thereby blighting the life of the individual, his or her family and society.

➤ Some mental disorders rob their sufferers of insight and consequently they may fail to take treatment or care for themselves and rarely they may present a danger to others.

➤ There needs to be some means of giving adequate and justified treatment to patients who need it but are unable to make a clear judgement about their own mental state and health needs.

➤ In some countries in the past mental health legislation has sometimes robbed individuals of their ability to reproduce and even cost them their lives. Legislation should be as reasonable, humane and open to scrutiny as possible.

➤ There needs to be a carefully monitored means of providing care under such legislation, i.e. there have to be adequate treatments together with trained people and regularly inspected places to administer that treatment properly.

DANGEROUSNESS

Apart from potential self-harm through self-neglect or suicide, a particular concern of the media in society is the potential for dangerousness or harm to third parties. Such harm is rare, but may occur in a variety of mental disorders. Severely depressed people may see no future for themselves and others. Depressed mothers and fathers may kill themselves and their children in such circumstances. People with schizophrenia in response to hallucinatory voices and suffering from persecutory delusions may act on their psychotic symptoms to kill those they see as the root of their problems. Other individuals with personality disorders may actually enjoy harming other people or setting fires, which may kill many people. One of the objectives of a mental state examination is therefore to assess a risk of harm to third parties.

MENTAL HEALTH LEGISLATION

The Mental Health Act (2007) amended the previous Mental Health Act (1983).

The phrasing of such acts is the key to their success or failure. The 2007 Act concerns the assessment and 'appropriate' treatment of people with *mental disorder,* (defined as 'any disorder or disability of the mind'). Mental health laws in England and Wales in past centuries have referred to mental illness in terms such as lunacy, psychopathic disorder, and so on. The 2007 term *mental disorder* brings these terms together. The 2007 phrase *'learning disability'* replaced the 1983 phrase 'mental impairment'.

The 2007 Act excludes some conditions from being considered a mental disorder. The 1983 Act excluded alcoholism, drug dependence and immoral conduct, sexual deviancy or promiscuity. The 2007 Act merely excludes dependence on alcohol or drugs which *'is not considered to be a disorder or disability of the mind'.*

People with mental disorder of a nature or degree to warrant it can be detained for appropriate treatment and this would include *'medical treatment the purpose of which is to alleviate, or prevent a worsening of, the disorder or one or more of its symptoms or manifestations'* and *'psychological intervention and specialist mental health habilitation, rehabilitation and care'.* The detention would have to be *'necessary for the health or safety of the patient or for the protection of other persons that he should receive such treatment and it cannot be provided unless he is detained under this section'.*

Detention for treatment of patients who have learning disability alone requires that there is also 'abnormally aggressive or seriously irresponsible conduct'. It is possible, though, for people with learning disability to have mental illness and to fulfil the criteria for detention under that umbrella.

Recommendations that persons are detained under Section 2 or 3 of the Act for assessment or treatment can be made by *registered medical practitioners* and the application is made by an *approved mental health professional*. The *approved mental health professional* may be someone like a specially trained social worker, occupational therapist or psychologist.

Some patients with mainly psychological problems such as personality disorder are intended to be admitted under a *'responsible clinician'*, who may or may not be medically qualified – these specially trained individuals could include psychologists, nurses, social workers or occupational therapists. They would have the 'overall responsibility for the patient's case' and should have the 'most appropriate expertise to meet the patient's main treatment needs'.

RELEVANT SECTIONS OF THE MENTAL HEALTH ACTS (1983 AND 2007)
Sections 135 and 136

This is an emergency section under which a police constable can remove a mentally disordered person from a public place to a place of safety, for a maximum period of 72 hours. Section 135 covers the removal of patients from their home or other private premises. Section 135 requires a warrant from a justice of the peace.

Section 4

This is an emergency section designed to detain individuals not yet admitted to hospital for a maximum period of 72 hours, until they can be more formally assessed for detention under Section 2 or Section 3, or discharged. Detention under Section 4 is based on a recommendation by a *registered medical practitioner* and applied for by an *approved mental health professional*.

Section 5.2

This is an emergency section designed to hold previously informal hospital inpatients for a maximum period of 72 hours, until they can be more formally assessed for detention under Section 2 or Section 3, or discharged. It might be used for, say, a suicidal patient who wished to take their own discharge. It is applied by a *registered medical practitioner* or 'approved clinician' or his or her nominee.

Section 5.4

This is an emergency section designed to grant registered mental nurses the power to hold a previously admitted patient for up to six hours until a doctor or approved clinician can be found to assess the patient for possible further detention.

Section 2

This is a section allowing for detention of a patient for 28 days, primarily for assessment where there are grounds to suspect a mental disorder of a sufficient nature or degree. Treatment can be given under this section, though. The detention must be in the interest of the patient's own health or safety or with a view to the protection of others. The recommendations must come from two registered medical practitioners and the application is usually made by the *approved mental health professional*. Therefore an assessment by three professionals is required. Patients may appeal to the Mental Health Review Tribunal and/or the hospital managers to be discharged. The patient can be discharged before the 28-day period has elapsed if the clinician in charge of the case rescinds the section.

Section 3

This is a section allowing for detention of a patient for six months, primarily for treatment of a mental disorder which has been assessed and diagnosed. The recommendations must come from two registered medical practitioners and the application is usually made by the *approved mental health professional.* Therefore an assessment by three professionals is required. Patients may appeal to the Mental Health Review Tribunal and/or the hospital managers to be discharged. The patient can be discharged before the period of six months has elapsed, if the clinician in charge of the case rescinds the application for detention under the section.

Sections applying to patients involved in criminal proceedings or in prison

Section 35 allows for the court to remand accused persons to hospital for a psychiatric report. This does not give the authority to treat without consent.

Section 36 allows for the court to remand accused persons to hospital for psychiatric treatment.

Sections 37 and 38 allow convicted prisoners to be detained in hospital for appropriate medical treatment.

Occasionally the court may impose a further *restriction order* on these forensic patients for public safety reasons – the order controls the movement of the patient and regulates any leave and similar conditions.

COMMUNITY TREATMENT ORDERS

These exist to allow monitoring of patients in the community and for recall to hospital if their illness deteriorates or they fail to take medication or comply with other treatment packages. Treatment can then be enforced on recall. Forced treatment in the community is not possible. Patients can appeal against such orders.

DISCHARGE BY NEAREST RELATIVE

Unless Home Office/Court restrictions apply, the patient's nearest relative can discharge a patient from hospital by giving 72 hours' notice to the managers of the hospital. This discharge can be barred by the responsible clinician if the patient is considered liable to act in a manner dangerous to other persons or to him- or herself.

MENTAL HEALTH REVIEW TRIBUNAL (MHRT)

The MHRT is an independent tribunal that is set up specifically to assess a patient's appeal against detention under a section of the Act. The tribunal consists of a medical member, a legal member and a lay member. They can consider the case by interviewing the patient, and through seeking reports from clinicians and by questioning them during the tribunal. They can discharge the patient from hospital if they are not satisfied the criteria for detention are still fulfilled.

COMMON LAW

The Mental Health Act covers specifically psychiatric or psychological treatments for mental disorders. It does not necessarily govern physical treatments for physical illnesses suffered by mentally disordered patients. Treatments outside the Mental Health Act are governed by the body of common law, the Mental Capacity Act (2005) and other relevant legislation.

ETHICS AND PSYCHIATRY

There are four main ethical principles underpinning good medical care:
- autonomy
- beneficence
- non-maleficence
- justice.

Autonomy literally means self-rule and would involve the patients' right to be informed about their health and to be able to use that information to make their own decisions about whether or not to accept any particular treatment.

Beneficence is a principle which hopefully lies behind the doctors' motives for helping the individual, i.e. a desire to do the best they can to help the patient. Behind it lies the idea that one ought to prevent or remove harm or evil and do or promote good.

Non-maleficence would be a principle guiding the health professional to do no harm by his or her actions, i.e. not to cause damage to the patient by intervening or by failing to intervene.

Justice involves a sense of fair play regarding, say, the appropriate and fair distribution of resources or ensuring that third parties come to no harm.

Health professionals use these principles to weigh up their actions or proposed actions to determine whether these are ethical or not. The ethical standards of a group, society or country are known as its *ethos*. Clearly, the ethos of any particular group changes with the individuals in that group, the prevailing social beliefs and many other factors – including the passage of time.

HIPPOCRATIC OATH
HIPPOCRATES 460–370 BC

The Hippocratic Oath was an oath supposedly originating with the ancient physician Hippocrates who founded a school of medicine in Kos. The oath was taken on graduation from medical school. The oath prescribed certain behaviours to protect the professional and his or her patients. Medical graduates no longer automatically swear the oath. Reference to modern ethical behaviours against the standards of this past code of conduct can be made, but only if the reference is clearly placed in a historical setting or as part of descriptive ethics (where the ethos of past civilisations or the ethics pertaining to another country are considered).

The original version is:

I SWEAR by Apollo the physician and Aesculapius, and Health, and All-heal, and all the gods and goddesses, that, according to my ability and judgement, I will keep this Oath and this stipulation – to reckon him who taught me this Art equally dear to me as my parents, to share my substance with him, and relieve his necessities if required; to look upon his offspring in the same footing as my own brothers, and to teach them this art, if they shall wish to learn it, without fee or stipulation; and that by precept, lecture, and every other mode of instruction, I will impart a knowledge of the Art

to my own sons, and those of my teachers, and to disciples bound by a stipulation and oath according to the law of medicine, but to none others. I will follow that system of regimen which, according to my ability and judgement, I consider for the benefit of my patients, and abstain from whatever is deleterious and mischievous. I will give no deadly medicine to any one if asked, nor suggest any such counsel; and in like manner I will not give to a woman a pessary to produce abortion. With purity and with holiness I will pass my life and practise my Art. I will not cut persons labouring under the stone, but will leave this to be done by men who are practitioners of this work. Into whatever houses I enter, I will go into them for the benefit of the sick, and will abstain from every voluntary act of mischief and corruption; and, further, from the seduction of females or males, of freemen and slaves. Whatever, in connection with my professional service, or not in connection with it, I see or hear, in the life of men, which ought not to be spoken of abroad, I will not divulge, as reckoning that all such should be kept secret. While I continue to keep this Oath unviolated, may it be granted to me to enjoy life and the practice of the art, respected by all men, in all times. But should I trespass and violate this Oath, may the reverse be my lot.

Some contemporary medical schools impose a revised version of the oath as an admonition and an affirmation to which their graduating classes assent. One version, approved by the American Medical Association, is as follows:

You do solemnly swear, each by whatever he or she holds most sacred:

That you will be loyal to the Profession of Medicine and just and generous to its members

That you will lead your lives and practice your art in uprightness and honor

That into whatsoever house you shall

enter, it shall be for the good of the sick to the utmost of your power, your holding yourselves far aloof from wrong, from corruption, from the tempting of others to vice

That you will exercise your art solely for the cure of your patients, and will give no drug, perform no operation, for a criminal purpose, even if solicited, far less suggest it

That whatsoever you shall see or hear of the lives of men or women which is not fitting to be spoken, you will keep inviolably secret

These things do you swear. Let each bow the head in sign of acquiescence

And now, if you will be true to this, your oath, may prosperity and good repute be ever yours; the opposite, if you shall prove yourselves forsworn.

The British Medical Association updated the oath and produced this version in 1997:

The practice of medicine is a privilege which carries important responsibilities. All doctors should observe the core values of the profession which centre on the duty to help sick people and to avoid harm. I promise that my medical knowledge will be used to benefit people's health. They are my first concern. I will listen to them and provide the best care I can. I will be honest, respectful and compassionate towards patients. In emergencies, I will do my best to help anyone in medical need.

I will make every effort to ensure that the rights of all patients are respected, including vulnerable groups who lack means of making their needs known, be it through immaturity, mental incapacity, imprisonment or detention or other circumstance.

My professional judgement will be exercised as independently as possible and not be influenced by political pressures nor by factors such as the social standing of the patient. I will not put personal profit or advancement above my duty to patients.

I recognise the special value of human life but I also know that the prolongation of human life is not the only aim of healthcare. Where abortion is permitted, I agree that it should take place only within an ethical and legal framework. I will not provide treatments which are pointless or harmful or which an informed and competent patient refuses.

I will ensure patients receive the information and support they want to make decisions about disease prevention and improvement of their health. I will answer as truthfully as I can and respect patients' decisions unless that puts others at risk of harm. If I cannot agree with their requests, I will explain why.

If my patients have limited mental awareness, I will still encourage them to participate in decisions as much as they feel able and willing to do so.

I will do my best to maintain confidentiality about all patients. If there are overriding reasons which prevent my keeping a patient's confidentiality I will explain them.

I will recognise the limits of my knowledge and seek advice from colleagues when necessary. I will acknowledge my mistakes. I will do my best to keep myself and colleagues informed of new developments and ensure that poor standards or bad practices are exposed to those who can improve them.

I will show respect for all those with whom I work and be ready to share my knowledge by teaching others what I know.

I will use my training and professional standing to improve the community in which I work. I will treat patients equitably and support a fair and humane distribution of health resources. I will try to influence positively authorities whose policies harm public health. I will oppose policies which breach internationally accepted standards of human rights. I will strive to change laws, which are contrary to patients' interests or to my professional ethics.

BOUNDARY VIOLATIONS

The original Hippocratic Oath is perhaps the most explicit of the three oaths in terms of forbidding inappropriate sexual relations. Boundary violations concern danger to the security of the relationship between patient and health professional. The boundaries are held to keep both the professional and the patient safe. The prevalence of the problem is surprisingly high with some estimates that up to 10% of psychotherapists and psychologists indulge in sexual involvement with patients. The problem is predominantly between male therapists and female patients, but up to 4% of female therapists may also be at fault. The ethical stance of psychiatric professional bodies is that sexual activity with a patient is absolutely unacceptable. The American Psychiatric Association stated in 2001: 'Sexual activity with a current or former patient is unethical.' Note that former patients are also included.

The path towards such a serious boundary violation is held to be a 'slippery slope' with small infringements leading to more severe ones.

BOX 18.1 THE 'SLIPPERY SLOPE' (BASED ON THE WORK BY SIMON 1995)

➤ Erosion of therapist's neutrality in little ways.
➤ Therapist and patient use first names.
➤ Therapy sessions become more social and less clinical.
➤ Patient is treated as 'special' or a confidant.
➤ Therapist self-disclosures occur, e.g. about personal problems or fantasies about the patient.
➤ Therapist touches patient or uses hugs or embraces.
➤ Patient transference is manipulated.
➤ Contacts outside therapy occur.
➤ Therapy sessions are scheduled near the end of the day.
➤ Sessions become extended in time.
➤ Therapists have drinks/dinner; dating begins.
➤ Therapist/patient sex begins.

GROUP WORK ON ETHICS: WHAT WOULD YOU DO?

Form a group of colleagues. Ask them to read and then discuss the brief psychiatric case histories that follow. Ask them to decide precisely what they would do and then ask them to justify their actions using the four ethical principles listed on page 234. Try not to influence their discussion or their decisions but record their deliberations. This experiment should give you an idea of that group's ethos. Repeat the experiment using a different group of people and record their deliberations. What do you think accounts for the differences in the ethos of these different groups?

CASE HISTORY 1

You are a junior doctor in general medicine. Your consultant is consistently late for ward rounds. In the mornings he has a marked tremor and his breath continually smells of alcohol. He appears to be getting forgetful and is always mixing up his patients and their illnesses. Other more senior doctors on your team desperately try to cover for him.

What do you do?

CASE HISTORY 2

You are a consultant psychiatrist. There is a change of government. The incoming government favours the policy of eugenics. Using the latest discoveries in science (that major psychoses have a high genetic component) as justification it passes a law to the effect that proven sufferers of psychotic illness and their first degree relatives must submit to sterilisation. You are asked to provide the Home Office with a list of your patients.

What do you do?

CASE HISTORY 3

You are an Accident and Emergency Doctor. A 24-year-old man is brought in by his brother. Earlier that evening he had tried to hang himself after his marriage broke down. His brother cut him down and talked him round; however, the patient had a change of heart immediately afterwards and took 24 tricyclic antidepressant tablets and 50 paracetamol tablets to kill himself. His brother found out an hour later just by chance. You see the patient but before you can physically do anything the patient refuses to cooperate. You try to persuade him but he says he is a law student and any treatment by you without his consent is an assault. Unfortunately, he lapses into unconsciousness as you argue your case.

What do you do?

CASE HISTORY 4

You are a consultant psychiatrist. An outpatient's family doctor asks you to visit her. She is aged 40. She is not eating and has not drunk anything since the day before. She says that there is nothing inside her and that she has no future. She wants to die and is lying immobile in a darkened room, 'waiting for death'. You assess her and think that she has features of severe depression and ask her whether she will come into hospital for treatment. She refuses your offer.

What should you do? Is this in the patient's best interests?

CASE HISTORY 5

An 80-year-old lady is refusing to see her family doctor for routine screening which he is paid to do. He presses the point since his contract stipulates he should screen all elderly patients. She reluctantly agrees and in the course of a physical examination he discovers that she has a carcinoma of the vulva. He arranges an appointment with a gynaecologist with a view to surgical treatment. She refuses to comply.

What can or should the family doctor do?

CASE HISTORY 6

You are a general practitioner. A 24-year-old man has been coming to see you 'in confidence' for puzzling trivial minor complaints. Now he tells you that he has been unsure of whether to tell you something he has been ashamed of all his life. Can you promise that you will treat it in absolute confidence? You reassure him that you will treat his remarks confidentially. He tells you that he was sexually abused by his father until the age of 17. As a consequence he is now worried about his own sexuality. However, while he is talking to you, you realise with some discomfort that his 13-year-old brother is now being abused by his father.

What do you do? Do you respect the confidentiality of the discussion or do you do something else?

CASE HISTORY 7

You are a general practitioner. A 21-year-old woman comes to see you about starting a family. Her husband is worried and has not accompanied her. His father died in his thirties of a movement disorder characterised by unintentional choreiform movements. His grandfather died in his fifties of a dementing illness and similar odd movements. Her husband is aged 23 and is asymptomatic.

What would your advice be?

CASE HISTORY 8

You are a trainee cognitive behavioural therapist. A patient is halfway through their therapy with you. You find that the patient is very attractive and the patient spends a large portion of the session flirting with you, which you enjoy. Near the end of the fifth session the patient goes so far as to ask you out on a date. You are tempted to agree.

What do you do? What is the ethical justification for your actions?

CASE HISTORY 9

You are a professor of psychiatry. Your department is under pressure to publish as much research as possible. A senior trainee brings you a review paper that she has spent much time writing. You can see some elementary but small errors which need correcting and are tempted to ask for your name to go on the paper so the department (and you) can gain extra credit when the paper is published.

What do you do? Should ethical problems in medical publishing (e.g. plagiarism) be considered part of professional life that should be regulated by professional bodies such as the General Medical Council?

CASE HISTORY 10

You are a locum doctor working in a country where the law regarding sexual behaviour is very strict. Homosexuality is illegal and homosexuals are generally held to be mentally ill and often given 'therapy' including behavioural conditioning in hospitals under compulsion. Doctors who do not comply with the laws regarding treatment for known 'cases' face short-term prison sentences of a few weeks. A mother brings her 16-year-old son to you for 'treatment'.

What do you do? Is something which is legal always ethical? Is ethical behaviour always legally acceptable?

CASE HISTORY 11

You are the commissioning officer for an NHS purchaser and must choose between two funding proposals for the next financial year. One proposal is to fund a brand new outreach initiative for young people. The initiative will endeavour to actively seek out those who self-harm and offer them cognitive behavioural therapy to manage their anxiety and low moods and also a risk minimisation approach to self-harm. This will benefit 200 young people per year. The second proposal is to buy two new mobile home dialysis machines for some renal failure patients. This will benefit 15 patients a year.

Which proposal do you favour? What ethical principles lie behind your decision?

CASE HISTORY 12

Amanda has been self-harming since she was 13 and is now 20. Her self-harm is partly in response to tensions in the family. There has been a family row and her stepfather wants her to leave home. She has taken an overdose and in casualty, after receiving treatment for the overdose, sees the duty psychiatrist and says she want to leave and kill herself. She is detained for assessment under Section 2 of the Mental Health Act. On the ward she is denied any materials with which she might self-harm (penknife) and she seems to respond with an escalation of her self-harm with attempts to ligature herself with underwear. She says you are 'taking away my rights to do what I want with my body'.

What ethical principles are involved in this scenario?

LEARNING POINTS: ETHICS AND THE LAW

➤ Without treatment mental illness can persist for many months or even years.

➤ Some mental disorders rob their sufferers of insight and consequently they may fail to take treatment or care for themselves and rarely they may present a danger to others.

➤ There needs to be mental health legislation to enable the provision of appropriate treatment and to prevent as much suffering from mental illness as possible.

➤ Badly drafted or wrongly intentioned mental health legislation has in the past robbed the individual of their ability to reproduce and sometimes robbed them of their lives, so that legislation should be as reasonable, humane and open to scrutiny as possible. Care governed under legislation needs to be carefully monitored to prevent abuses of power and to protect the rights of the individual.

➤ Ethical principles that should guide doctors include: autonomy; beneficence; non-maleficence, and justice.

➤ Sexual activity (and boundary violations) with a current or former patient is/are unethical.

SELF-ASSESSMENT
MCQs

1 Principles of ethical practice in medicine include:
   A ensuring prompt payment for professional services
   B beneficence
   C upholding the autonomy of the individual
   D being a parent figure
   E justice

2 The English Mental Health Act (1983 and 2007):
   A allows surgical operations to be given against the patient's will
   B contains an emergency section for assessment
   C provides for patients to be detained for up to six months without appeal
   D allows for compulsory psychosurgery against the patient's will
   E may compel patients to accept treatment for a mental disorder

MCQ answers
1 A=F, B=T, C=T, D=F, E=T.
2 A=F, B=T, C=F, D=F, E=T.

EXPLORATIONS
LINKS WITH MEDICAL HISTORY
Psychiatry appears to be a discipline with an appallingly bad catalogue of abuses of power, deception and folly.

➤ Is psychiatry different from other subspecialities of medicine in this regard?

➤ Can you find any examples of ethical problems in the history of or current day practice in surgery, medicine or obstetrics and gynaecology?

➤ What are the key factors that allow such abuses or mistakes to occur?

➤ What principles can you identify that might prevent such mistakes occurring in the future?

LINKS WITH FORENSIC PSYCHIATRY

Forensic psychiatry concerns itself with the actions of the mentally disordered or retarded that bring them into conflict with the law.

> ➤ What psychiatric services are available to such people?
> ➤ What happens in criminal law to people who commit serious crimes but are thought to have serious mental illness?
> ➤ What are the prevalence rates for severe mental illnesses in UK prisons?

FURTHER READING AND REFERENCES

Alessi NE, Alessi VA. New media and an ethics analysis model for child and adolescent psychiatry. *Child & Adolescent Psychiatric Clinics of North America.* 2008; **17**(1): 67–92.

Berrios G. *The History of Mental Symptoms: descriptive psychopathology since the nineteenth century.* Cambridge: Cambridge University Press; 1996.

Bloch S, Chodoff P, Green S. *Psychiatric Ethics.* Oxford: Oxford University Press; 1999.

Burleigh M. Psychiatry, German society, and the Nazi 'euthanasia' programme. *Social History of Medicine.* 1994; **7**(2): 213–18.

Freedman R, Ross R, Michels R, Appelbaum P, Siever L, Binder R, Carpenter W, Friedman SH, Resnick P, Rosenbaum J. Psychiatrists, mental illness, and violence. *American Journal of Psychiatry.* 2007; **164**(9): 1315–17.

Green B, Miller PD, Routh CP. Teaching ethics in psychiatry: a one-day workshop for clinical students. *Journal of Medical Ethics.* 1995; **21**(4): 234–8.

Janofsky JS. Lies and coercion: why psychiatrists should not participate in police and intelligence interrogations. *Journal of the American Academy of Psychiatry & the Law.* 2006; **34**(4): 472–8.

Liegeois A, Eneman M. Ethics of deliberation, consent and coercion in psychiatry. *Journal of Medical Ethics.* 2008; **34**(2): 73–6.

Lopez-Munoz F, Alamo C, Dudley M, Rubio G, Garcia-Garcia P, Molina JD, Okasha A. Psychiatry and political-institutional abuse from the historical perspective: the ethical lessons of the Nuremberg Trial on their 60th anniversary. *Progress in Neuro-Psychopharmacology & Biological Psychiatry.* 2007; **31**(4): 791–806.

Sarkar SP. Boundary violation and sexual exploitation in psychiatry and psychotherapy: a review. *Advances in Psychiatric Treatment.* 2004; **10**: 312–20.

Shorter E. *A History of Psychiatry: from the era of the asylum to the age of Prozac.* London: Wiley; 1998.

Simon RI. The natural history of therapist sexual misconduct: identification and prevention. *Psychiatric Annals.* 1995; **25**: 90–4.

RESOURCES

Ethics for student doctors
www.priory.com/ethics.htm

BioethicsWeb
www.intute.ac.uk/healthandlifesciences/bioethicsweb/

Medical ethics: Student BMJ
http://student.bmj.com/topics/non-clinical/medical_ethics.php

Medical ethics
http://en.wikipedia.org/wiki/Medical_ethics

Medical ethics: four principles plus scope
www.bmj.com/cgi/content/full/309/6948/184

Index

References to figures, tables and boxes are in **bold**.